The Carb, Lover's DIET COOKBOOK

Dedication

Ellen

For my mom, who taught me how to cook, and
for my dad, who loved carbs – especially the
chocolate kind! – and enjoyed them every single day.

Frances

For my mother, who taught me the importance of
hearty bread and a well-balanced meal. And for
my wonderful husband, Jon, and sweet kids, Willa
and Leo – thanks for all your love and support.

©2010 Time Home Entertainment Inc.
135 West 50th Street, New York, NY 10020

This edition published 2012 by Hamlyn
a division of Octopus Publishing Group Ltd,
Endeavour House, 189 Shaftesbury Avenue,
London, WC2H 8JY
www.octopusbooks.co.uk

An Hachette UK Company
www.hachette.co.uk

ISBN 13: 978-0-6006-2520-9

A CIP catalogue record for this book is available
from the British Library.

Printed and bound in China

10 9 8 7 6 5 4 3 2 1

HEALTH MAGAZINE
Editor in Chief: Ellen Kunes
Creative Director: Ben Margherita
Design Director: José Fernandez

OCTOPUS PUBLISHING GROUP

Publishing Director: Stephanie Jackson
Editor: Jo Wilson
Design: Yasia Williams-Leedham, Jaz Bahra
UK editors: Nicole Foster, Kate Stanton
Production Manager: Peter Hunt

The Carb, Lover's DIET COOKBOOK

Eat what you love & get slim for life – with 150 new recipes

By **Ellen Kunes,** Editor in Chief,
& **Frances Largeman-Roth,**
Registered Dietician, of **Health** magazine

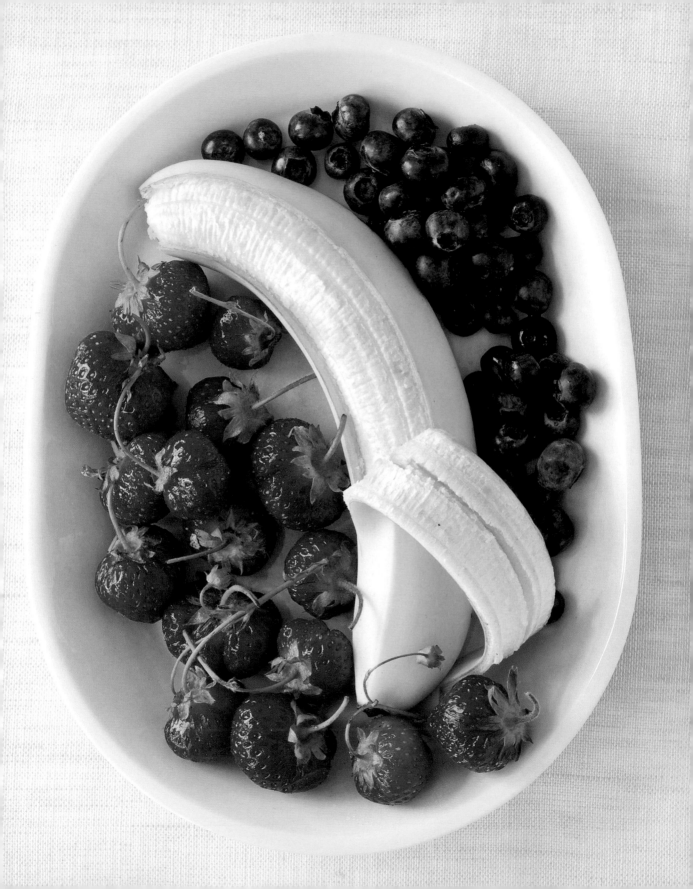

Contents

Acknowledgements

The CarbLovers Diet Cookbook is the culmination of years of researching how we all can achieve our weight-loss goals while still enjoying our favourite foods. But it's also my personal favourite in the *CarbLovers* series, which includes *The CarbLovers Diet Pocket Guide* and the original *CarbLovers Diet* book. I know *Health* and Health.com's audience of nearly 19 million will love the easy, delicious recipes, smart advice and stunning photography as much as I do. Lots of credit goes to my dedicated and talented team, especially my co-author and *Health*'s food and nutrition director, Frances Largeman-Roth, RD, as well as Marc Einsele, Amy O'Connor, Trish McGinty-Boyles, Sarah DiGiulio and Michael Gollust, who worked on *The CarbLovers Diet Cookbook* while putting out a great magazine and website. Thanks also to Sonthe Burge, RD— a tireless resource and advocate for *CarbLovers* dieters – and copy editor Christopher Jagger.

We also want to thank everyone at Time Home Entertainment Inc. and Oxmoor House, especially Richard Fraiman, Jim Childs, Vanessa Tiongson and Helen Wan.

We'd also like to thank Adeena Sussman, Caroline Wright, Sarah Abrams and Kate Slate for their culinary creativity and nutrition wisdom. Special appreciation goes to Andrew McCaul, Stephana Bottom, Jo Miller and Alistair Turnbull for the absolutely gorgeous photography in this book, which will inspire all to make these great dishes. And a big shout-out to our celebrity chefs – Guy Fieri, Wolfgang Puck, Cat Cora, Carla Hall, Michael Chiarello, Donatella Arpaia, Emily Luchetti, Candice Kumai, Cristina Ferrare, Joe Bastianich, Gail Simmons, Allysa Torey, Matt Lewis and Renato Poliafito – for their incredible generosity and amazing carb-filled recipes!

Finally, our deepest gratitude goes to those who enjoyed *The CarbLovers Diet* and asked for more recipes and menus. This book is for all of you!

Ellen Kunes,
Editor-in-Chief, *Health* magazine

PART 1
Cooking the *CarbLovers* Way

Cooking with CarbLovers!

"A diet rich in carbs is the best way to get and stay slim." Believe it or not, that was a controversial statement when it first appeared in *The CarbLovers Diet* just over a year ago. Many were sceptical of the promise of a weight-loss plan based on delicious pasta, pizza and baked potatoes. (To be honest, even we couldn't predict how well it would work!)

We did, however, have faith in the scientific evidence that eating the right carbs would help dieters – even those who failed on other plans – stay slim for life, without ever feeling deprived. And we were excited about encouraging people to eat more foods that contain Resistant Starch, the star ingredient of *The CarbLovers Diet*.

Nearly 200 studies have shown Resistant Starch, found naturally in whole grains, potatoes, beans, and some fruits, to be an extraordinary weight-loss tool. It's 100 per cent safe, and it acts as a powerful appetite suppressant and metabolism booster.

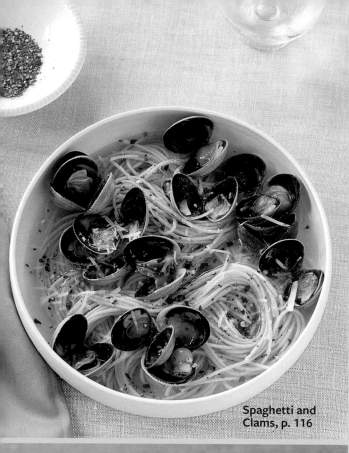

Spaghetti and
Clams, p. 116

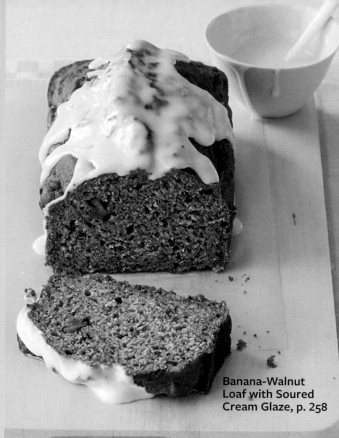

Banana-Walnut
Loaf with Soured
Cream Glaze, p. 258

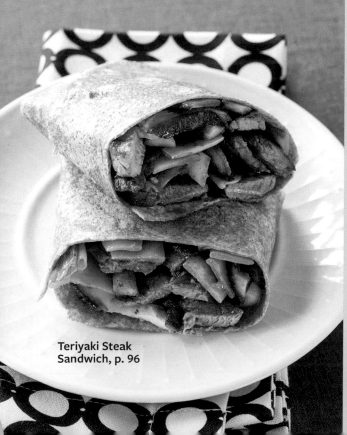

Teriyaki Steak
Sandwich, p. 96

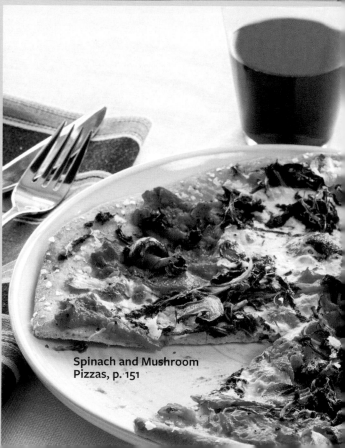

Spinach and Mushroom
Pizzas, p. 151

Today it seems like everyone is talking about Resistant Starch, but not because of a bunch of studies. That carbs make you slim, not heavy, is practically common knowledge, thanks to the incredible success of *The CarbLovers Diet*. The first book spent an amazing nine weeks on *The New York Times* best-seller list, spun off a wildly successful app and *The CarbLovers Diet Pocket Guide*, and generated national media attention. *CarbLovers Diet* fans now include celebrities, renowned chefs and top doctors and researchers. *CarbLovers* even has its own dedicated communities on Facebook and Twitter.

CarbLovers dieters loved the delicious recipes, meal plans anyone can stick to, and easy substitutes and grab-and-go food items. But you told us you wanted more –much more. A breakthrough diet plan that's even simpler to follow. More information about finding and cooking foods with Resistant Starch, the super carb that fills you up and melts fat. More advice for adapting *CarbLovers* to your lifestyle. More drink suggestions – including cocktails. More ideas for following the *CarbLovers Diet* when away from home, during the holidays, with your family, and when you're on the go. More cooking tips. And, most of all, you wanted a whole lot more recipes!

The CarbLovers Diet Cookbook delivers. The Recipe Collection features 150 new, quick and easy, totally yummy recipes – including updated versions of your favourite *CarbLovers* comfort foods. You won't believe what we've cooked up!

In *The CarbLovers Diet Cookbook*, you'll enjoy hearty buckwheat crepes (page 62) or moist, rich banana bread (page 59) for breakfast; decadent Cobb salad (page 200) or silky butternut squash soup (page 80) for lunch; and a succulent spice-rubbed pork fillet (page 165) or prawn tacos (page 162) for dinner. You can even make holiday cookies (page 281) or throw a cocktail party (page 297) with our special-occasion menus, which make entertaining a snap.

As a bonus, we're thrilled to offer you custom recipes from some carb-loving expert chefs, including Guy Fieri, Wolfgang Puck and Cat Cora.

The CarbLovers Diet Cookbook has been created by the same food and nutrition experts who developed the original *CarbLovers*, with a new, proven diet plan and recipes so delicious you'll want to serve them to company. So go ahead: Enjoy our amazing new carb-filled meals!

Ellen **Kunes,**
Editor in Chief, *Health* magazine

How Carbs Make You Thin...For Life

I'm guessing you're digging into this book for one of two (really good) reasons: 1) You lost weight on *The CarbLovers Diet* and want more delicious, easy, carb-rich recipes; or 2) You just love great food – especially dishes bursting with delicious carbs. Learning that your favourite pasta, pizza and potato dishes will actually help you lose weight has made you hungry for more details.

The best news: The research behind *The CarbLovers Diet Cookbook* shows strong evidence that a diet rich in carbs is the healthiest and most effective way to get and stay slim for life. But here's something to keep in mind: These carbs aren't the refined kind, packed with tons of additives and preservatives that come in crinkly packages from a vending machine. *The CarbLovers Diet* isn't about junk food (though you are allowed daily indulgences, including chocolate). The carb-rich foods that make you slender are packed with fibre, antioxidants and Resistant Starch, the star ingredient that has helped so many feel full and lose weight on *The CarbLovers Diet*.

The CarbLovers Diet's Secret Weapon

What exactly is Resistant Starch? Carbohydrate-rich foods contain two types of starch. One is high-glycaemic starch; like sugar, it gets absorbed into the bloodstream quickly and gives you a fast hit of energy. Another is called Resistant Starch, so named because it "resists" digestion. Hundreds of studies have shown Resistant Starch to be a natural appetite suppressant, metabolism booster and overall health promoter. It produces fatty acids that trigger weight loss by turning on enzymes that melt fat, especially in the abdominal area; encouraging your liver to switch to a fat-burning state; and boosting satiety hormones that make you get and stay full longer. Resistant Starch is more than safe; you really can't eat too much of it. In fact, most people consume too little – about 5 grams a day. Researchers believe we need at least twice that amount for optimal health and weight loss. That's why the *CarbLovers* menus include 10 to 15 grams daily of this important fat-burning nutrient, served up in delicious recipes like our Cornflake-Crusted Chicken Strips (p. 182) and Triple-Cheese Mac (p. 126).

The Science of Carbs and Health

The CarbLovers Diet Cookbook doesn't hinge solely on the health and weight-loss benefits of Resistant Starch, though. All of our recipes (which start on page 34) have been created to pack the best possible ratio of the nutrients that research shows help to melt fat, boost satiety, and promote good health – and get you a much flatter stomach. Belly bloat is one of the key symptoms of constipation, a common side effect of not eating enough healthy carbs.

The amazing carb-filled recipes in this book, including Chicken Cacciatore with Rigatoni (p. 122) and Grilled Steak Fajitas (p. 168), taste just as delicious as they sound. But they also contain a mix of carbohydrates that make them healthier and much more filling than most protein- or fat-loaded foods. The Resistant Starch and fibre in our recipes act as powerful appetite suppressants. They fill you up because they are digested more slowly than other types of foods and trigger a greater sensation of fullness in both your brain and your stomach. Eating *The CarbLovers Diet* way, according to research, can help you consume 10 per cent fewer calories a day – without ever feeling hungry!

Scientific evidence bears this out. For instance, one groundbreaking study looked at thousands of people to see what factors determine whether they stayed slim or gained weight over time. Conclusion: The slimmest people ate the most good carbs – the kind you'll find in the recipes in this book – and the chubbiest ate the least. The researchers confirmed that your odds of getting and staying slim are best when carbs comprise up to 64 per cent of your total calorie intake, which mirrors what a day of eating the *CarbLovers* way delivers.

Another recent study found that making a simple lifestyle switch – such as eating more carbs at dinner – can result in both weight loss and a reduction in body fat. Researchers in Israel put 78 overweight or obese police officers on a diet. Half were given a low-calorie weight-loss plan, while the other group followed the same diet but ate most of their carbohydrates at dinner. Incredibly, after six months the carbs-at-dinner group lost both more weight and body fat – and they reported feeling less hungry than other dieters. The evening carb eaters also got healthier, with improvements in both their blood sugar and cholesterol levels. Researchers believe that eating your carbs at night may help elevate satiety hormones during the day, preventing feelings of hunger. Bottom line: Carbs satisfy, no matter what time of day you eat them.

The CarbLovers Diet may actually be one of the healthiest diets you can follow, whether you're trying to lose weight or simply maintain your current weight. Scores of studies conducted at top research institutions worldwide show that eating the right carbs is one of the smartest preventive measures you can take to keep your heart healthy, your cholesterol and blood pressure low, and your blood sugar balanced. A recent study by researchers in the United Kingdom published in *The American Journal of Clinical Nutrition* found that including three servings of wholegrain foods in the diets of healthy people helped significantly lower their blood pressure; the researchers concluded that daily consumption of whole grains could thus decrease the incidence of stroke by 25 per cent and coronary artery disease by 15 per cent.

How Carbs Make You Happy

As you cook and eat according to *The CarbLovers Diet Cookbook*, you might start to feel calmer, happier and less stressed. The reason? Carbs boost mood-regulating, stress-reducing chemicals in the brain, while high-protein, fatty foods may deplete them, says Grant Brinkworth, PhD, lead researcher of a study published in the *Archives of Internal Medicine*. He followed 51 dieters on a carb-rich diet and 55 dieters on a low-carb plan. After a year, the carb eaters felt happier calmer, and more focused than the carb-deprived group, who reported feeling stressed out. Stress produces high levels of hormones, such as cortisol, which boost your appetite and can lead to bingeing, says obesity researcher Elissa Epel, PhD, associate professor in the department of psychiatry at the University of California, San Francisco.

In other words, enjoying the delicious recipes in *The CarbLovers Diet Cookbook* will make you look good and feel great! "Dieters feel so empowered once they lose weight on carbs. For the first time, they are able to lose weight by eating in a balanced manner, without cutting out entire food groups," says Sari Greaves, RD, spokesperson for the American Dietetic Association.

What Foods Contain

FOOD	PORTION	RS
Banana, slightly green	1 medium (18–20cm/7–8")	12.5
Banana, ripe	1 medium (18–20cm/7–8")	4.7
Oats, uncooked/toasted	50g (2oz)	4.6
Beans, cannellini, cooked/canned	125g (4oz)	3.8
Lentils, cooked	100g (3½oz)	3.4
Potatoes, cooked and cooled*	1 potato, small	3.2
Plantain, cooked	75g (3oz)	2.7
Chickpeas, cooked/canned	125g (4oz)	2.1
Pasta, wholewheat, cooked	150g (5oz)	2.0
Barley, pearl, cooked	75g (3oz)	1.9
Pasta, white, cooked and cooled	150g (5oz)	1.9
Beans, kidney, cooked/canned	125g (4oz)	1.8
Potatoes, boiled (skin and flesh)*	1 potato, small	1.8
Rice, brown, cooked	75g (3oz)	1.7
Beans, pinto, cooked/canned	125g (4oz)	1.6
Peas, canned/frozen	75g (3oz)	1.6
Beans, black, cooked/canned	125g (4oz)	1.5
Millet, cooked	75g (3oz)	1.5

*The Resistant Starch content of potatoes varies depending on cooking method and temperature served.

Resistant Starch?

FOOD	PORTION	RS
Pasta, white, cooked	150g (5oz)	1.5
Potatoes, baked (skin and flesh)*	1 potato, small	1.4
Bread, pumpernickel	25g (1oz) slice	1.3
Polenta, cooked	8 tablespoons	1.0
Potato crisps	25g (1oz)	1.0
Yam, cooked	100g (3½oz)	1.0
Bread, rye (whole)	25g (1oz) slice	0.9
Cornflakes	25g (1oz)	0.9
Puffed wheat	15g (½oz)	0.9
Tortillas, corn	25g (1oz), 15cm (6″) tortilla	0.8
English muffin	1 whole muffin	0.7
Bread, sourdough	25g (1oz) slice	0.6
Crackers, rye crispbread	2 crispbreads	0.6
Porridge	240ml (8fl oz)	0.5
Bread, Italian	25g (1oz) slice	0.3
Bread, wholemeal	25g (1oz) slice	0.3
Corn chips	25g (1oz)	0.2
Crackers, crispbread (melba)	25g (1oz)	0.2

In the Kitchen With *CarbLovers*

Cooking the *CarbLovers* way is surprisingly easy. It's fun, affordable, and oh-so-satisfying. But don't take our word for it! Dieters who kicked their fast-food and vending-machine habits tell us they feel an incredible sense of accomplishment shopping for the freshest ingredients and cooking at home, then savouring dishes like Chicken Cacciatore with Rigatoni (page 122) and Maple-Glazed Cod with Baby Pak Choi (page 156) on a daily basis. Some even say cooking gives them an edge when it comes to getting and staying slim for life.

Here's why they might be right: The recipes in *The CarbLovers Diet Cookbook* make dieting almost effortless. They take all the guesswork out of counting calories, tallying Resistant Starch and planning meals. Each is designed to have a specific nutrition profile that allows you to enjoy three full meals a day plus a snack and dessert – while still losing weight. And these recipes are foolproof. We tested each recipe again and again, in real kitchens by real people, so we know they really work!

Read on for details on cooking with *CarbLovers* recipes, plus advice on stocking and organizing your kitchen. Follow our easy tips and soon you'll be cooking the *CarbLovers* way with every meal.

CarbLovers Cooking Basics

Beans and Pulses

Many recipes in *The CarbLovers Diet Cookbook* call for beans, and for good reason. Beans are among the healthiest, most slimming and most affordable foods you can find. Loaded with Resistant Starch, beans and pulses (such as lentils) pack both types of fibre – soluble and insoluble (one fills you up and helps lower cholesterol; the other keeps your digestive system humming along). Getting enough fibre also speeds weight loss: A study of 252 women found that every extra gram of fibre consumed resulted in 250g (8oz) of weight loss. (But you don't have to count grams; *The CarbLovers Diet* makes sure you get 25–35 grams of fibre every day.)

Beans are incredibly easy to cook with. Canned beans are fine to use, as they pack the same nutritional benefits as dried (rinse and drain them first, to lower the sodium that comes in the canning liquid). But do try cooking beans from scratch, in large batches. This method tends to yield better-tasting and sodium-free beans. (It's also super-cheap!) Cooked beans freeze well in airtight containers and will keep for 6 months or longer. To use, thaw, then toss into salads, soups, even pasta. Beans also make a great base for spreads and dips, such as our Layered Spicy Black Bean and Cheddar Dip (page 226).

STOVE-TOP BEANS Sort and wash dried beans, discarding any that look shrivelled or broken. Rinse in a colander, then soak in fresh, unsalted water in a large bowl for at least 8 hours or overnight. Bonus! Soaking beans cuts down on the complex sugars that can cause gas.

When beans have soaked for at least 8 hours, drain and pour into a large saucepan or cast-iron casserole. Cover and bring to the boil, then reduce heat and let simmer for 1 to 3 hours or until beans are tender (the larger the beans, the more time they will take to cook). Salting beans before they're cooked makes them tough, so wait to salt until you are ready to serve.

PRESSURE-COOKER BEANS Pressure-cooking beans is a doddle. Never fill the cooker more than ⅔ full, and be sure to add a teaspoon of oil to the water to prevent foaming. Use 200g (7oz) of beans to 1 litre (1¾ pints water, and check the instructions on your appliance for exact cook times. Cooking time for very dry or large beans will be shorter if you presoak your beans overnight.

> **TIP:**
> Small beans and pulses –such as split peas and lentils – cook quickly, so there's no need to soak or put them in a pressure cooker.

STORAGE Store dried beans at room temperature in an airtight container for up to a year. Just keep them away from sunlight, which may cause their colour to fade. Canned beans last up to 5 years. Refrigerate cooked beans for up to a week or freeze for 6 months.

Store Cupboard

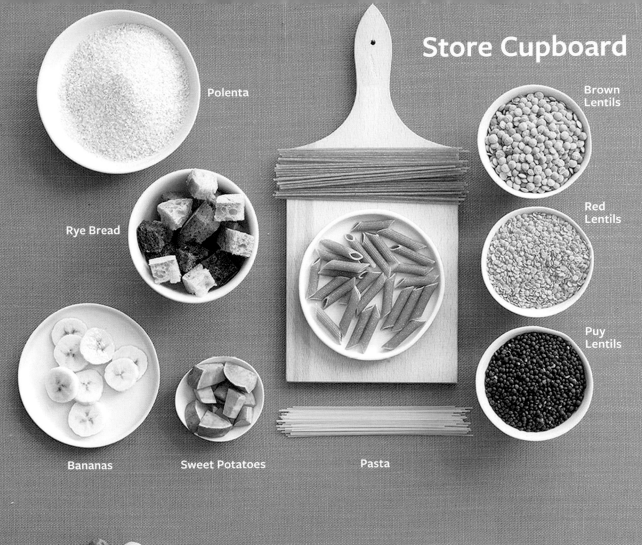

Polenta

Brown Lentils

Rye Bread

Red Lentils

Puy Lentils

Bananas

Sweet Potatoes

Pasta

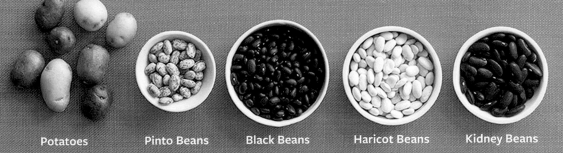

Potatoes

Pinto Beans

Black Beans

Haricot Beans

Kidney Beans

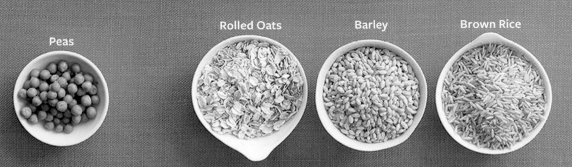

Peas

Rolled Oats

Barley

Brown Rice

Barley

Barley is one of the best grain sources of Resistant Starch and a key source of wholegrains in *The CarbLovers Diet*. Barley has a tight-fitting inedible hull as it grows in the field. It's removed through a process called pearling that scrapes away the hull. Unfortunately, some of the bran gets removed too; try barley labelled "hulled" to be sure that your barley has had the hull removed without removing the bran. Pearl barley, the kind found in most grocery shops and used in our recipes, is also very filling and nutritious. Creamy, chewy, with a subtle flavour that combines well with others, pair barley with any sauce or use as a substitute for rice or pasta.

STOVE-TOP BARLEY Sauté 200g (7oz) dry barley in 1 teaspoon hot oil in a medium saucepan over medium-high heat for 4 minutes or until lightly browned. Stir in 500ml (17fl oz) water. Bring to the boil; cover, reduce heat and simmer 30–40 minutes or until barley is just tender and slightly chewy. Remove from heat; let stand 5 minutes.

STORAGE Cooked barley can be refrigerated for 3–5 days, or you can freeze it in an airtight container for up to 6 months. Store uncooked barley for 6 months or longer in an airtight container at room temperature.

Rice

Although it takes longer to cook than white or yellow rice, brown rice is worth the time because it's a nutritional powerhouse, packing Resistant Starch, fibre, and other nutrients in every nutty bite. That means it will take longer to digest and you'll feel full for a lot longer.

STOVE-TOP RICE In a saucepan, combine 200g (7oz) of uncooked brown rice with 500ml (17fl oz) of water (or in any amounts by volume, using this 1:2 ratio of rice to water). Bring the mixture to the boil, stirring occasionally, then reduce heat. Cover and simmer for about 50 minutes, until cooked.

STORAGE Cooked rice can be kept in the refrigerator for up to 5 days. Uncooked rice can last 6 months or longer stored in an airtight container at room temperature.

Pasta

Who doesn't adore pasta? *The CarbLovers Diet Cookbook* offers loads of mouth-watering pasta dishes, including ones from top chefs, like Michael Chiarello's Fusilli Michelangelo with Roasted Chicken (page 146) and Joe Bastianich's Scoglio (page 148). The pasta recipes we developed for this book include traditional "white" pasta, as well as flavourful and nutritious wholewheat pastas. The wholewheat variety has double to triple the fibre and more protein than regular pasta, so you'll feel fuller faster and eat less now – and later.

STOVE-TOP PASTA Bring a large saucepan filled with water to the boil. Salt the water once it starts boiling and add the pasta. Stir the pasta gently while cooking to prevent clumping, and cook according to packet instructions (though you can test for doneness a minute or two earlier). Reserve 125ml (4 fl oz) of cooking water to add more flavour and body to your sauce. Drain pasta in a colander.

STORAGE While pasta is best when freshly cooked, you can refrigerate it in an airtight container, with or without sauce for 3 days. Fresh (not dried) pasta can be kept in the refrigerator for up to 1 week or frozen for up to a month. Dried pasta lasts longer – up to 2 years – when stored in a dry, cool place.

Oats

Pinhead oatmeal, also called steel-cut oats, is made from wholegrain oats that are cracked, not rolled. These wholegrains are an amazing source of Resistant Starch, especially when cooked and processed as little as possible. They're also rich in soluble fibre, which absorbs water and helps you feel full, so you get – and stay – trim.

The best way to get your Resistant Starch and fibre from oatmeal is to cook pinhead oats on your hob (rolled and instant oats usually don't have the same health and weight-loss benefits as the wholegrain type). Another way to up your oat intake is to replace half your plain flour with shop-bought or homemade oat flour (grind rolled oats in a food processor) for baking biscuits, pancakes and quick breads. You get twice the fibre and fewer calories.

STOVE-TOP PORRIDGE The basic recipe is 1 part oats to 3 parts water. Add both to a saucepan and bring to the boil, then simmer until the liquid is absorbed, about 35 minutes. It's also easy to cook batches of pinhead oats ahead of time. Before bed, combine 100g (3½oz) oats with 750ml (1¼ pints) water, bring the mixture to a boil, then turn off the heat. In the morning, simmer for 5–10 minutes until fully cooked. Keep the extra in the freezer or in the fridge until needed, then warm up.

If all you have time to make is rolled oats, go for it – oats are still one of the healthiest grains you can eat. Combine 1 part oats with 2 parts water or semi-skimmed milk. Bring the mixture to the boil, then reduce heat. You will only need to cook these oats for another couple of minutes – don't leave them cooking for much longer, or they'll get mushy.

MICROWAVE PORRIDGE Combine 50g (2oz) rolled oats or instant porridge oats with 250ml (8fl oz) 1% fat milk or water in a small microwave-safe bowl. Microwave on HIGH for 3–5 minutes.

STORAGE Cooked porridge can be kept in the refrigerator for up to 5 days. Store uncooked oats in an airtight container in a cool, dry place. They can be used for up to 6 months. Some packaged brands of oats last longer – check the packaging before storing.

Potatoes and Sweet Potatoes

{ TIP:
Do not freeze cooked
potatoes, as this can
turn them mushy. }

Potatoes have received a bad rap in the past, but you no longer need an excuse to enjoy your favourite root vegetable. All potatoes are super healthy carbs and a good source of Resistant Starch, especially when cooked and cooled (remember, bringing cooked potatoes to room temperature boosts their Resistant Starch content). They are also a natural source of proteinase inhibitor, a type of protein that may increase levels of satiety hormones and curb hunger. Of course, they're delicious too! That's why baked potatoes, sweet potatoes, mashes of all varieties, yams, oven chips and even potato crisps are allowed on *The CarbLovers Diet*.

Potatoes of every stripe are a dieter's best friend in part because they are incredibly filling. One large baked potato, for instance, will run you fewer than 300 calories. Plus, potatoes are among the richest sources of potassium, the electrolyte that helps to maintain the body's fluid balance (and helps prevent muscle cramps). Sweet potatoes are a great source of beta-carotene; one medium sweet potato packs nearly three times the recommended daily amount. Aside from being rich in potassium, these tasty tubers boast immunity-boosting vitamin C and vitamin B6, key for maintaining a healthy nervous system.

Choose smooth-skinned potatoes and cut out any dark spots with a paring knife or the tip of your peeler (if they've sprouted, throw them out!). If you want to keep the peel on during cooking, check to make sure there is no green tinge to the skin. If there is, simply peel it off.

STORAGE Potatoes keep well for weeks in a cool, dry place, preferably on a worktop or a low-humidity area of your fridge. Remove from plastic before storing.

BAKED POTATOES Preheat the oven to 200°C/400°F/gas mark 6. Pierce the skin with a fork, then cover in foil or simply rub with olive oil. Place on a rimmed baking sheet and cook for about 60 minutes (sweet potatoes will be done sooner, in about 45 minutes). You'll know they're fully cooked when you pierce them with a knife and it slides out easily.

STOVE-TOP POTATOES You can also cook potatoes on the hob. Bring a large saucepan of generously salted water to the boil and place potatoes in one by one (new potatoes can go in whole, but cut or quarter larger potatoes). Simmer for 30 minutes or until potatoes can be pierced with a sharp knife.

MICROWAVE POTATOES Potatoes and sweet potatoes should be baked in the microwave on HIGH for about 10 minutes. Check small and medium potatoes at about the 5-minute mark to make sure they don't get overcooked.

Must-Have Tools for a *CarbLovers* Kitchen

The Essentials

BLENDER A blender is the best and easiest way to whip up the smoothies on page 66, and you don't need a fancy one to get most kitchen jobs done. Blenders are also great for creating homemade salad dressing or puréeing soups.

CAST-IRON FRYING PAN Low-maintenance, hard-working, and super-affordable, every cook needs a cast-iron frying pan for searing, roasting, even baking (nothing is better for making real cornbread in the oven!). Bonus: These pans provide traces of iron, a nutrient many women don't get enough of.

CAST-IRON CASSEROLE These large, heavy-bottomed pots belong in every kitchen. They go from hob to oven and last forever. Use them for everything from batch-cooking beans and porridge to searing meats and making roasts, casseroles, stews and soups.

FOOD PROCESSOR A time-saver when you don't feel like chopping. If you don't want to get a large 4–5 litre (7–8 pint) processor, a mini 1 litre (1¾ pint) version will handle most recipes in this book.

FOOD-STORAGE CONTAINERS The ultimate time- and money-saver! A good selection will keep your leftovers or batch-cooked foods fresh, and allow you to carry *CarbLovers* meals to work or wherever you are headed. Be sure to choose containers that are BPA-free and have secure lids.

KNIVES Like most home cooks, *CarbLovers* cooks will do just fine with these three: a large chef's knife for slicing meat, fish and vegetables; a paring knife for peeling and chopping smaller vegetables like garlic; and a serrated knife for slicing bread and pizza.

MUFFIN TIN Having at least one regular 12-hole tin is a must for baking up several weeks' worth of your favourite *CarbLovers* muffins, page 50.

Also great to have:

HERB CHOPPER Dried herbs are handy, but fresh will rock your world! These mini hand choppers make quick work of parsley, coriander, basil and other fresh herbs that add calorie- and sodium-free flavour to dishes.

STICK BLENDER So much power for so little money! These handy wands, which often cost less than £30, can purée an entire batch of soup or marinara sauce – right in the pan! If you use them to whip up smoothies, make sure to put the ingredients in an oversize glass or plastic container to avoid splashes.

SLOW COOKER There's a good reason more than 80 per cent of American households have one! Slow cookers are great for soups, stews, even casseroles. Just turn the slow cooker on in the morning, set on "low" or "high", and dinner is done when you get home from work. Try serving dinner straight from your cooker, family style!

PIZZA STONE Great for giving our Fresh Mozzarella, Basil and Chicken Sausage Pizza (page 136) a crisp and chewy crust.

The Slim Way to Organize Your Kitchen

Your kitchen can be set up to make your *CarbLovers* cooking easy and even inspiring.

The first place to start? The refrigerator. Ditch the fizzy drinks – regular and diet (carbonation plus artificial sweeteners equals bloat), and replace them with water and iced green tea. Better yet, try the *CarbLovers* Fat-Flushing Cocktail: Take 2 litres (3½ pints) brewed green tea and add the juice of 1 lemon, 1 lime and 1 orange. Mix all ingredients together in a large jug. Store in the fridge for up to 3 days. If you must keep fizzy drinks and fruit juice around for your family, do yourself a favour and store them out of sight. That way, you'll be more likely to grab something diet-friendly.

Invest in fridge- and freezer-friendly stackable containers so the healthy stuff – chopped veggies, herbs, sliced fruit and all your make-ahead beans, barley and brown rice – is easier to grab than fattening fare. These will keep your fridge clutter-free, and encourage you to cook *CarbLovers* meals in large batches that you can use for the whole week. Look for the "make-ahead" icon on some of the recipes. These meals can be made in advance of serving, and many are appropriate for freezing.

Your next stop is the worktop: This is a space that can make or break your diet. Keep your blender close to where you chop fruits or veggies so it's always supereasy to prepare a healthy smoothie or soup. Set out a wooden block or hang a magnetic strip for chopping knives to make it easy to trim excess fat from meat and slice fibre-filled veggies and fruit.

Next to those slicers, use decorative hooks to dangle tools like an apple corer, a citrus zester and a handheld squeezer (to add no-fat flavour to fish, pastas, marinades and salad dressings).

Top your wortop with a big, beautiful basket, and use it to contain kitchen-table clutter, so you won't be tempted to multitask during meals. (Also recommended: a bouquet of fresh flowers, just because you deserve it.) Cooking and eating without distractions will help you focus! Speaking of focus, plug in your iPod and listen to music that de-stresses you. Research suggests that ab fat cells expand in response to the stress hormone cortisol, but cortisol levels decrease faster in people who listen to relaxing music than in those who don't.

> **TIP:**
> Grow your own oregano, thyme and rosemary on your windowsill, and you'll have an easy, no-cal way to jazz up healthy foods like grilled chicken and veggies.

When it comes to the store cupboard, de-cluttering is key! Don't keep unhealthy snacks around to tempt you into mindless munching while you're cooking meals. Instead, keep airtight containers of dry ingredients like pasta and beans on the lowest shelves, so they're convenient for everyday use (check them periodically for freshness).

Build Your *CarbLovers* Kitchen

It's key to have a store cupboard and refrigerator stocked with the right foods. When healthy ingredients are at your fingertips, you won't be tempted to go off your diet. Make sure you have the following within reach at all times:

STORE CUPBOARD

Almonds, walnuts, other nuts and seeds (unsalted)

Almond and peanut butter (natural)

Baked potato crisps

Barley

Brown rice

Bulgar wheat

Canned beans

Canned tomatoes

Coconut, desiccated, unsweetened

Cornflakes

Dates

Dried beans

Dried herbs

Balsamic vinaigrette

Oats
(preferably rolled or pinhead)

Olive oil, both regular and extra virgin

Polenta

Quinoa

Rye crispbread crackers

Tortilla chips, baked

Vinegar

Wholemeal bread

Wholemeal pasta

WORKTOP

Apples

Avocados

Bananas

Garlic

Onions

Pears

Potatoes and sweet potatoes

Tomatoes

REFRIGERATOR

Berries, fresh when in season. Use frozen when not.

Broccoli

Carrots

Celery

Fresh herbs

Lemons

Limes

Low-fat cheese

Olives

Salad greens

Salmon

Semi-skimmed milk

Tortillas

Yogurt, preferably low-fat Greek

FREEZER

Batch-cooked beans and grains

Wholemeal pizza dough

Frozen fruit

Frozen veggies

Frozen *CarbLover*-approved meals (see page 314)

Recipe icons

Gluten-Free These recipes contain no wheat, spelt, kamut, farro, bulgar, semolina, barley, rye or triticale. Some brands of other food products (such as oats, ready-made stocks, canned beans and condiments) may contain gluten, so if you have coeliac disease, always buy products labelled gluten-free.

Kid-Friendly Designed to deter dinnertime meltdowns, our kid-friendly meals are yummy, uncomplicated and healthy for the whole family.

Make-Ahead These meals can be made in advance, and many are appropriate for freezing.

Low-Sodium Defined as less than 500 mg for a meal or less than 250 mg per side or dessert.

Superfast Our collection of Superfast recipes take just 25 minutes (or less) total.

Vegetarian These recipes do not contain any meat or meat products (such as chicken stock), but they may include dairy and eggs. Look for tips on recipes for how to make some of our meat-based meals vegetarian.

BREAKFAST

PART 2
The *CarbLovers* Recipe Collection

Breakfast

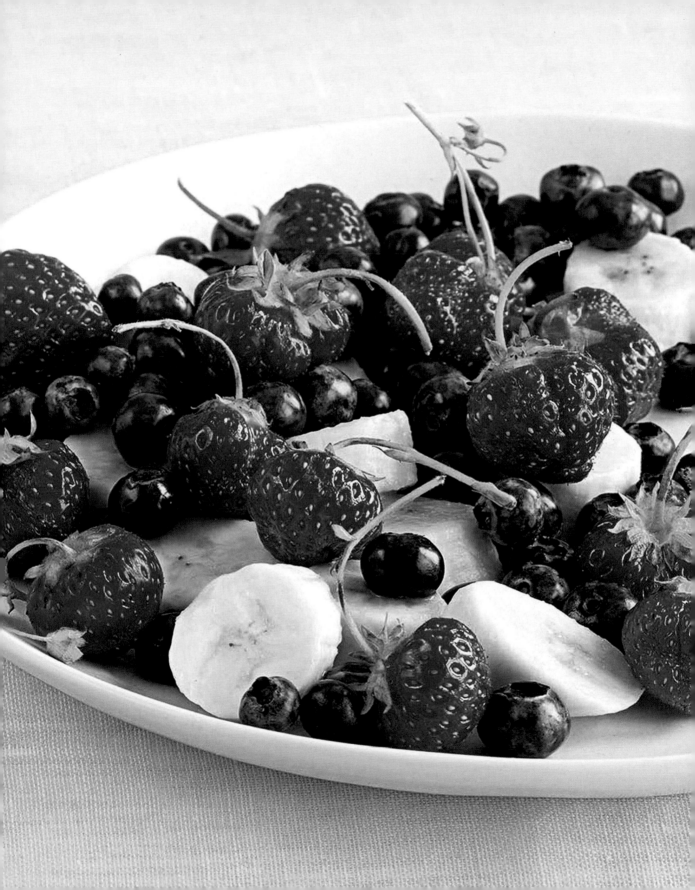

Oat and Honey Pancakes with Strawberry Syrup

Prep: *5 minutes* | **Cook:** *15 minutes* | **Total time:** *20 minutes* | **Makes:** *6 servings*

What could be better for breakfast than a stack of hot pancakes? A stack of pancakes packed with Resistant Starch! And this recipe also features a delicious (and simple) topping of antioxidant-rich strawberries.

Cooking spray
125g (4oz) cup wholemeal flour
50g (2oz) plain flour
25g (1oz) toasted wheat germ
200g (7oz) old-fashioned rolled oats
1 tablespoon baking powder
½ teaspoon salt
½ teaspoon ground cinnamon
2 tablespoons honey
2 tablespoons sugar
500ml (17 fl oz) 1% fat milk
2 large eggs
2 tablespoons vegetable oil
750g (1½lb) strawberries, hulled and quartered
1 tablespoon fresh lemon juice

1. Place flours, wheat germ, oats, baking powder, salt and cinnamon in a food processor; process until combined. Whisk together honey, 1 tablespoon of the sugar, milk, eggs and vegetable oil in a large bowl; stir in flour mixture until well combined. Let stand 5 minutes.

2. Meanwhile, combine strawberries, lemon juice and remaining tablespoon sugar in a large bowl. Crush with clean hands; set aside.

3. Heat a nonstick griddle or frying pan over medium heat. Coat pan with cooking spray. Pour about 4 tablespoons batter per pancake onto pan. Cook for 2 minutes or until tops are covered with bubbles and edges are cooked. Using a spatula, carefully turn pancakes over; cook 1 minute more or until bottoms are lightly browned. Transfer pancakes to a plate; keep warm. Repeat with remaining batter. Serve with strawberry topping (you will have some left over).

Serving size: About 3 pancakes, 4 tablespoons strawberry topping Calories: 395; Fat 10.6g (sat 2g, mono 2.9g, poly 4.7g); Cholesterol 66mg; Protein 14g; Carbohydrate 65g; Sugars 20g; Fibre 8g; RS 7.6g; Sodium 499mg

TIP:
Fresh strawberries are always best, but you can also use frozen, defrosted berries – they're just as nutritious.

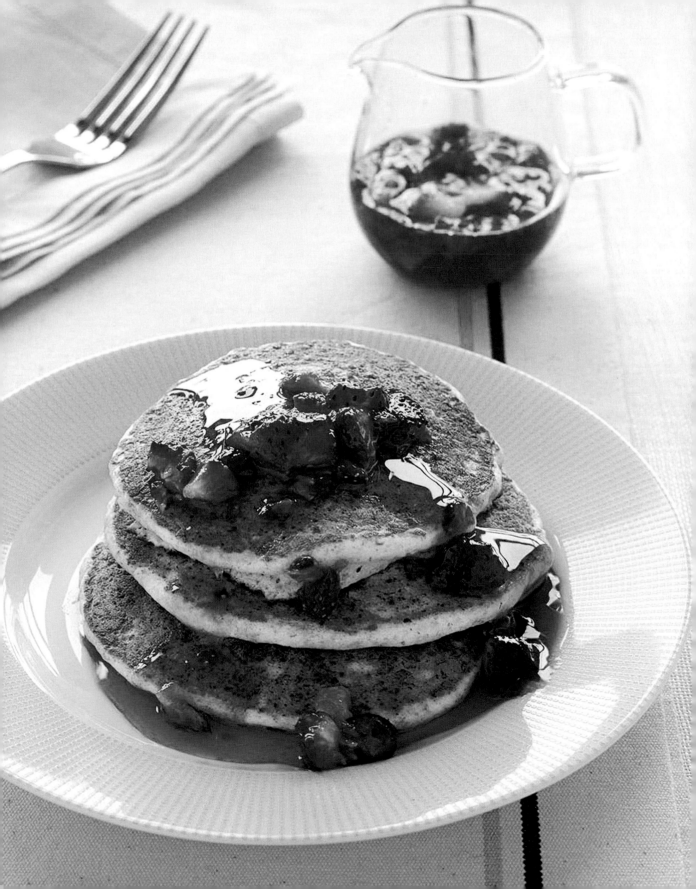

RS
0.6g

Eggs Benedict Florentine

Prep: *10 minutes* | **Cook:** *10 minutes* | **Total time:** *20 minutes* | **Makes:** *4 servings*

Eggs Benedict on a diet? Yes you can! We make ours with a light hollandaise that still tastes incredibly rich. This is the perfect dish for a special Sunday brunch.

1 teaspoon white vinegar
1 teaspoon olive oil
150g (5oz) baby spinach
¼ teaspoon sea salt
⅛ teaspoon freshly ground black pepper
¼ teaspoon freshly grated nutmeg
4 slices sourdough bread, about 25g
  (1oz) each, toasted
5 large eggs
3 tablespoons light mayonnaise
1 tablespoon lemon juice
1 tablespoon melted butter

1. Bring a high-sided sauté pan filled with 5cm (2 inches) of water to a simmer; add vinegar.

2. Heat oil in a large frying pan over medium-high heat. Add spinach; season with salt and pepper. Cook, stirring, until spinach is wilted, about 3 minutes; stir in nutmeg. Arrange toasted bread on 4 plates; divide spinach among toast.

3. Break 1 egg into a ramekin and slide into simmering water. Gently poach 3 minutes; remove with a slotted spoon. Repeat with remaining eggs. Place 1 egg on each toasted slice; reserve last egg.

4. Combine yolk from remaining poached egg (discard white), mayonnaise, lemon juice and 2 teaspoons water in a blender; blend until smooth. Add butter; blend to combine. Spoon hollandaise over eggs and serve immediately.

Serving size: 1 slice bread, 8 tablespoons cooked spinach, 1 tablespoon hollandaise, 1 egg Calories 256; Fat 14.3g (sat 4.7g, mono 4.9g, poly 3.6g); Cholesterol 251mg; Protein 11g; Carbohydrate 21g; Sugars 2g; Fibre 2g; RS 0.6g; Sodium 471mg

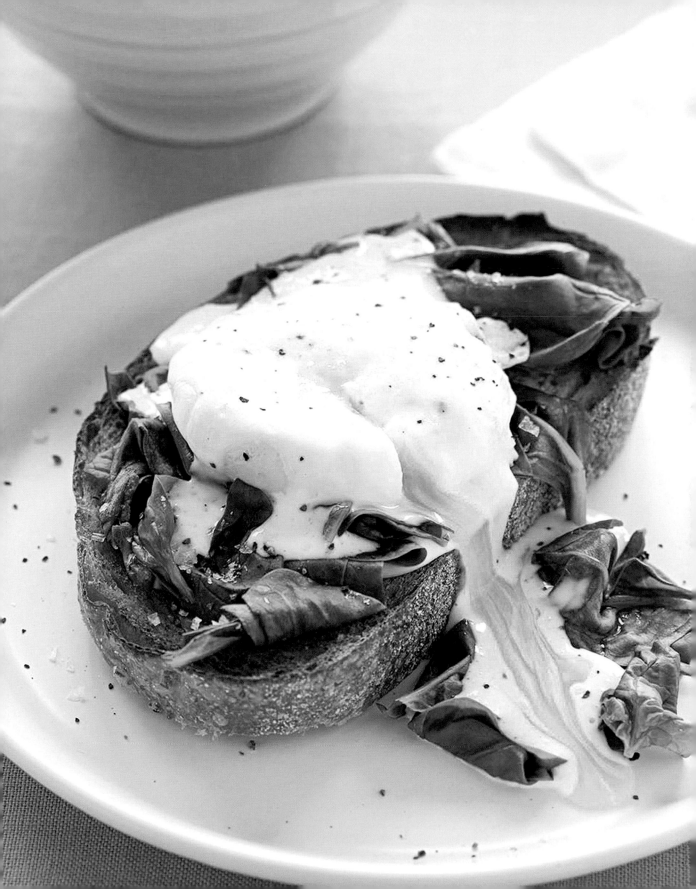

Oatmeal with Salted Caramel Topping

Prep: *5 minutes* | **Cook:** *15 minutes* | **Total time:** *20 minutes* | **Makes:** *4 servings*

Decadent and healthy? They co-exist in this delicious breakfast. It's perfect for company, or just a quick midweek morning meal.

100g (3½oz) uncooked instant porridge oats
750ml (1¼ pints) low-fat milk (1%)
4 tablespoons light brown sugar
½ teaspoon salt
4 tablespoons whipped cream
8 tablespoons fresh berries

1. Preheat oven to 200°C/400°F/gas mark 6.

2. Combine oats and milk in a medium saucepan. Bring to the boil over high heat. Reduce heat and simmer until oats are cooked but not mushy, 7–8 minutes.

3. Remove from heat and distribute oatmeal between four 175ml (6fl oz) ramekins. Arrange ramekins on a rimmed baking sheet.

4. Combine sugar and salt and sprinkle evenly on top of ramekins. Place ramekins (on baking sheet) in oven for 3–4 minutes, until sugar is melted.

5. Remove from oven and heat the grill. Place ramekins under grill until sugar is browned and bubbly, watching carefully to keep them from burning, 2–3 minutes.

6. Remove from grill and top each oatmeal brûlée with 1 tablespoon whipped cream and 2 tablespoons berries. Serve warm.

Serving size: 1 ramekin Calories 242; Fat 5.9g (sat 3.1g, mono 1.7g, poly 0.7g); Cholesterol 19mg; Protein 9g; Carbohydrate 39g; Sugars 25g; Fibre 2g; RS 2.3g; Sodium 229mg

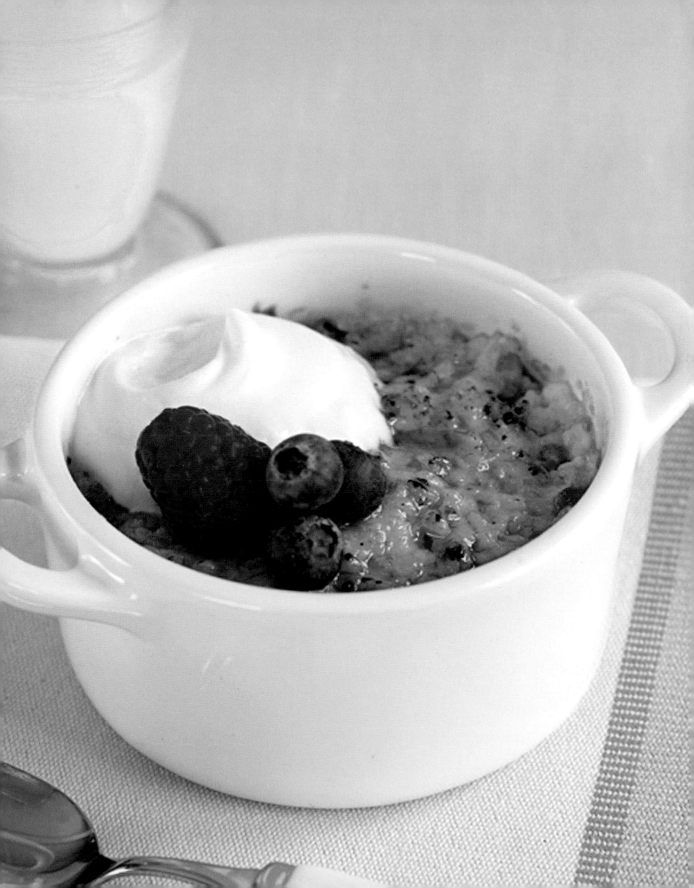

Fresh Citrus with Chopped Crystallized Ginger and Basil

Prep: 10 minutes | *Total time:* 10 minutes | *Makes:* 4 servings

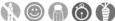

Sunny, bright and packed with vitamin C, this simple fruit salad is a welcome dish at any brunch.

2 large grapefruits, segmented

2 large oranges, segmented

3 tablespoons (25g/1oz) crystallized ginger, thinly sliced

1 tablespoon fresh basil ribbons

1. Gently combine grapefruit and orange segments in a medium bowl.

2. Divide fruit between 4 bowls. Sprinkle evenly with ginger and basil. Serve.

Serving size: About 250ml (8fl oz) Calories 111; Fat 0.3g (sat 0g, mono 0g, poly 0.1g); Cholesterol 0mg; Protein 2g; Carbohydrate 28g; Sugars 20g; Fibre 3g; RS 0g; Sodium 3mg

---

ASK CARBLOVERS

Q: How much fruit can I eat on *CarbLovers*?

A: Our daily plans include 5–6 servings of fruit and vegetables. Fruit is rich in antioxidants and high in fibre, which will help you stay full. It's not unlimited on the diet, but you can eat three servings each day. A medium-sized piece of fruit or 8 tablespoons of sliced fruit equals a serving.

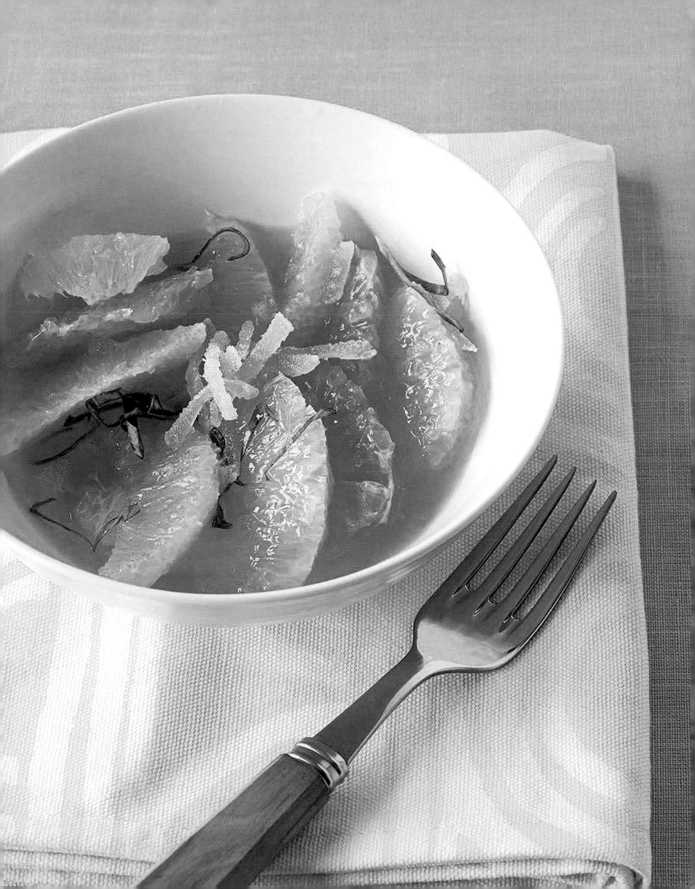

RS
2.7g

Huevos Rancheros

Prep: *10 minutes* | ***Cook:*** *15 minutes* | ***Total time:*** *25 minutes* | ***Makes:*** *4 servings*

Love this Mexican classic? While our version is hearty and filling (and fibre- and protein-packed), we've lightened it up by toasting – not frying – the tortillas and using cooking spray instead of oil for the eggs.

2 teaspoons vegetable oil
1 small onion, finely diced
2 garlic cloves, finely chopped
¼ teaspoon cumin
¼ teaspoon chipotle chili powder
⅛ teaspoon salt
400g (14oz) can reduced-salt black
  beans, rinsed and drained
125ml (4fl oz) reduced-salt chicken stock
1 tablespoon chopped coriander, plus
  more for garnish
Cooking spray
8 eggs
8 corn tortillas, warmed in pan
250ml (8fl oz) tomatillo salsa
200g (7oz) tomatoes, chopped
1 medium avocado, sliced

1. Heat oil in a small saucepan over medium-high heat. Add onion and cook, stirring, until softened, 6–7 minutes. Add garlic, cumin, chipotle chili powder, and salt; cook 1 more minute. Add beans and stock and bring to a boil. Reduce heat and cook until most of liquid is absorbed, 3–4 minutes. Remove from heat, add coriander, and reserve.

2. Heat a large nonstick frying pan coated with cooking spray over medium-high heat. Crack 2 eggs in pan; cook as desired, either sunny-side up or over easy. Repeat with remaining eggs.

3. For each serving: Arrange 2 warmed tortillas on a large plate and slide 1 egg onto each tortilla. To each plate, add 5 tablespoons bean mixture, 4 tablespoons salsa, ¼ cup tomato, and ¼ of the avocado. Garnish with additional coriander and serve.

Serving size: 2 tortillas, 2 eggs, 5 tablespoons bean mixture and toppings Calories 467; Fat 20g (sat 4.3g, mono 8.2g, poly 4.7g); Cholesterol 372mg; Protein 22g; Carbohydrate 50g; Sugars 7g; Fibre 11g; RS 2.7g; Sodium 710mg

TIP:
This is a big breakfast, so if you're on the Kickstart, or just want to go lighter, split it with a friend.

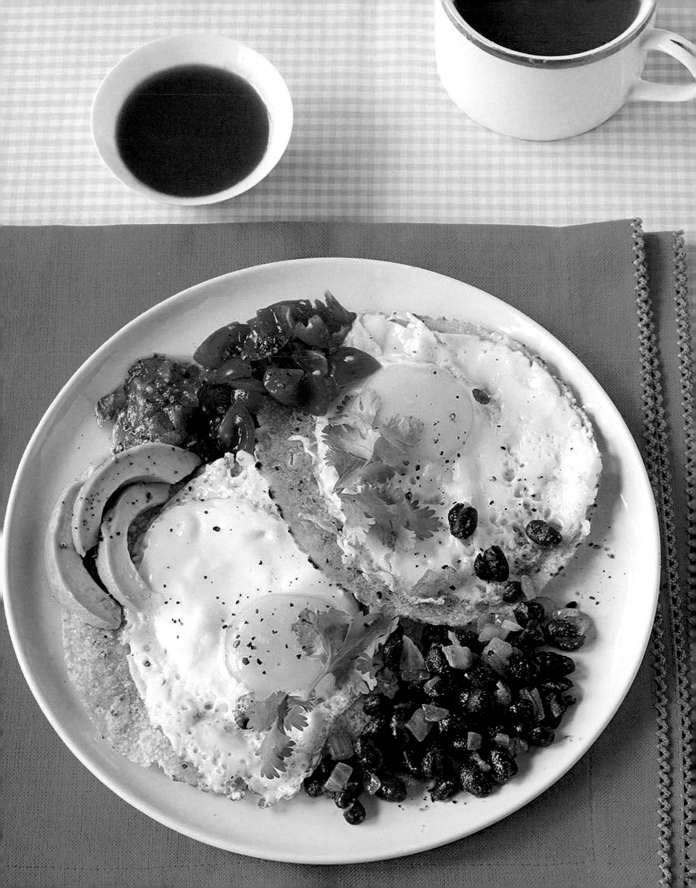

Granola with Pecans, Pumpkin Seeds and Dried Mango

Prep: *5 minutes* | **Cook:** *25 minutes* | **Total time:** *30 minutes* | **Makes:** *6 servings*

Crunchy nuts and chewy mango give a flavor-packed start to your day. This granola also makes a great snack; just cut the portion size to ¼ cup.

300g (10oz) old-fashioned rolled oats
40g (1½oz) puffed millet cereal
50g (2oz) lightly toasted pecans, chopped
2 tablespoons pumpkin seeds
1 tablespoon rapeseed oil
5 tablespoons pure maple syrup
3 tablespoons apple juice
1 teaspoon pure vanilla extract
¼ teaspoon salt
3 tablespoons chopped dried mango

1. Preheat oven to 180°C/350°F/gas mark 4.

2. Line a large rimmed baking sheet with baking paper and reserve.

3. Combine oats, cereal, pecans and pumpkin seeds in a large bowl.

4. Whisk together oil, syrup, juice, vanilla and salt in a small bowl; toss with dry ingredients.

5. Spread on the prepared baking sheet and bake until golden brown, stirring occasionally, 20–25 minutes.

6. Remove from oven, let cool completely and toss with mango.

Serving size: 8 tablespoons granola Calories 330; Fat 11g (sat 1.3g, mono 5.3g, poly 3.7g); Cholesterol 0mg; Protein 8g; Carbohydrate 52g; Sugars 14g; Fibre 5g; RS 4.6g; Sodium 54mg

TIP:
This delicious granola can be stored in an airtight container for up to a week.

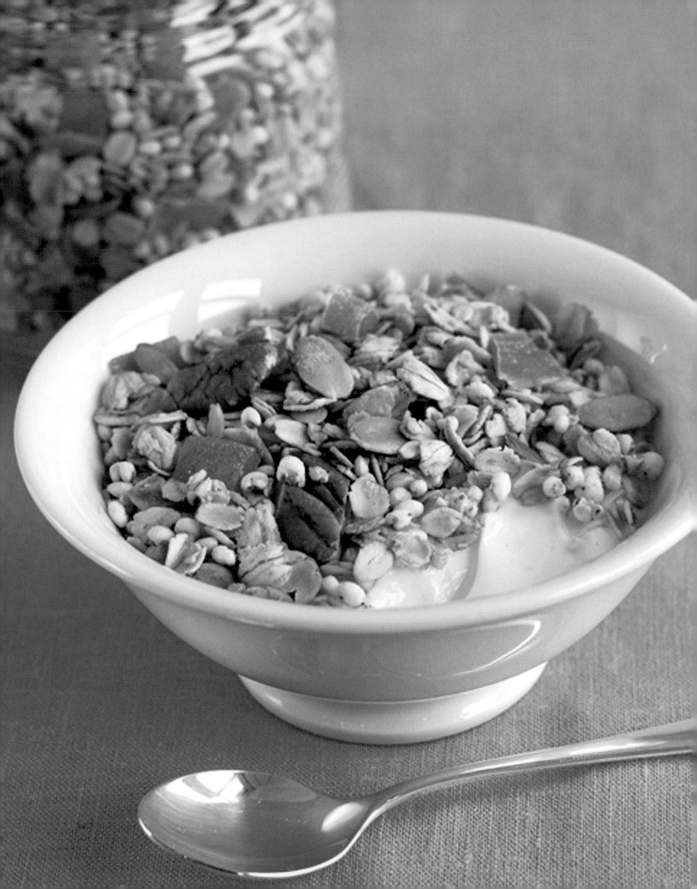

RS
0.2g

Asparagus, Mushroom and Tomato Frittata

Prep: 10 minutes | *Cook:* 30 minutes | *Total time:* 40 minutes | *Makes:* 6 servings

If you want a big, hearty breakfast that also looks gorgeous on the table, a frittata is the way to go. Plus, it cooks up really quickly.

6 eggs
6 egg whites
25g(1oz) Parmesan cheese, finely grated
½ teaspoon freshly ground black pepper
8 tablespoons sliced basil leaves
2 tablespoons olive oil
1 small onion, diced
6 x 75g (3oz) rashers turkey bacon, diced
150g (5oz) mushrooms, sliced
125g (4oz) cooked, sliced potato
250g (8oz) asparagus, trimmed and
 cut into 3.5cm (1½ inch) pieces
250g (8oz) small cherry or grape tomatoes

1. Preheat oven to 200°C/400°F/gas mark 6. Whisk together eggs, egg whites, cheese, pepper and basil; reserve in refrigerator until ready to use.

2. Heat 1 tablespoon oil in a 25cm (10 inch) cast-iron frying pan or oven-proof pan over medium-high heat. Add onion and cook, stirring, until soft and slightly golden, 7–9 minutes.

3. Add turkey bacon and cook, stirring, until crisped, 4–5 minutes. Add mushrooms and cook until softened, 3–4 minutes. Add potato, asparagus and tomatoes; cook 2 more minutes until asparagus just begins to soften.

4. Add remaining oil to pan and stir to incorporate with bacon and vegetables. Add egg mixture and tilt pan to evenly distribute eggs. Cook until eggs just begin to set, 3–4 minutes. Transfer to oven and bake until top is lightly browned and eggs are fully set, 11–12 minutes.

5. Remove from oven and let cool slightly. Cut into 6 equal-sized wedges. (Note: Can be served warm or at room temperature.)

Serving size: 1 wedge Calories 220; Fat 13.7g (sat 3.8g, mono 6.6g, poly 2.2g); Cholesterol 202mg; Protein 16g; Carbohydrate 9g; Sugars 3g; Fibre 2g; RS 0.2g; Sodium 384 mg

TIP:
This is a great make-ahead dish. Prepare the day before, cover with foil, refrigerate, then reheat in a 200°C/400°F/gas mark 6 oven for 11–12 minutes.

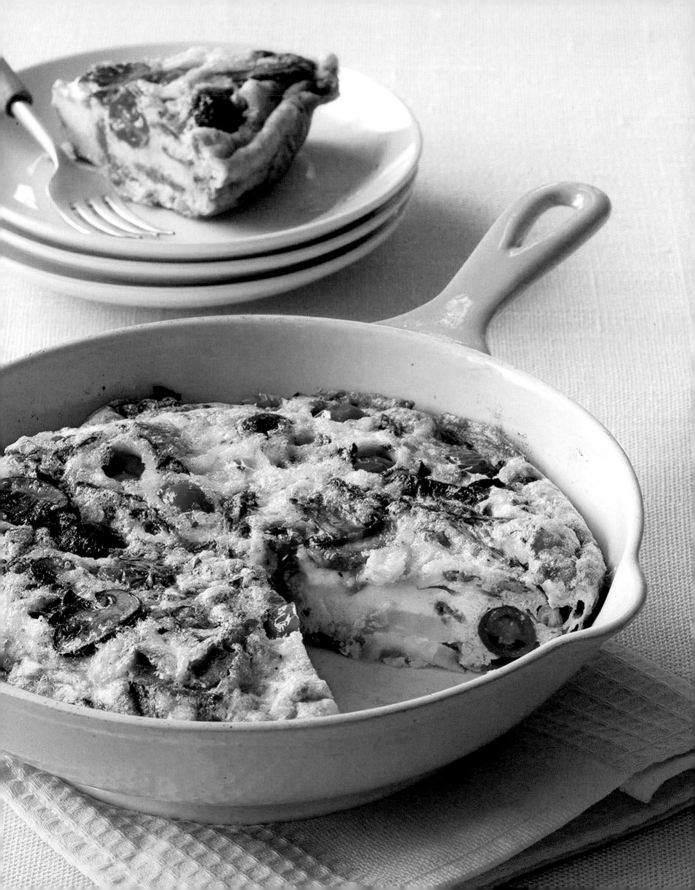

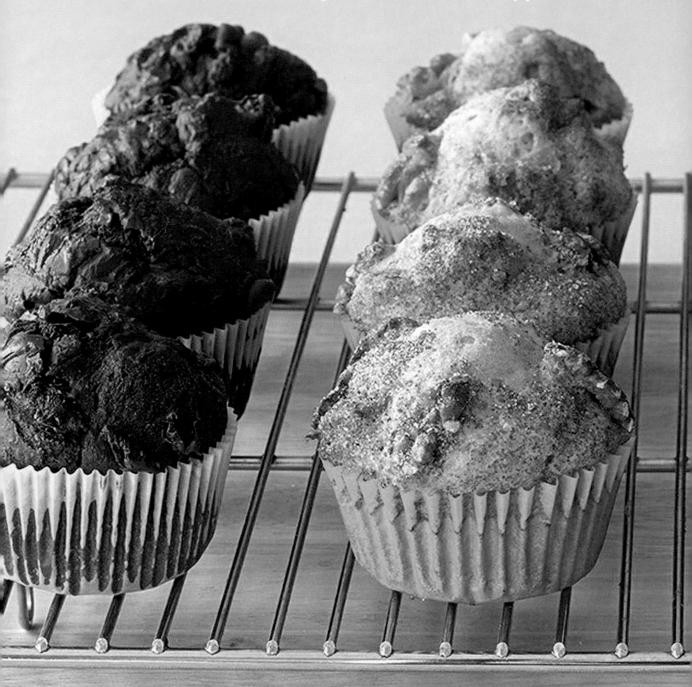

Double Chocolate Cherry   **Cinnamon-Apple Walnut**

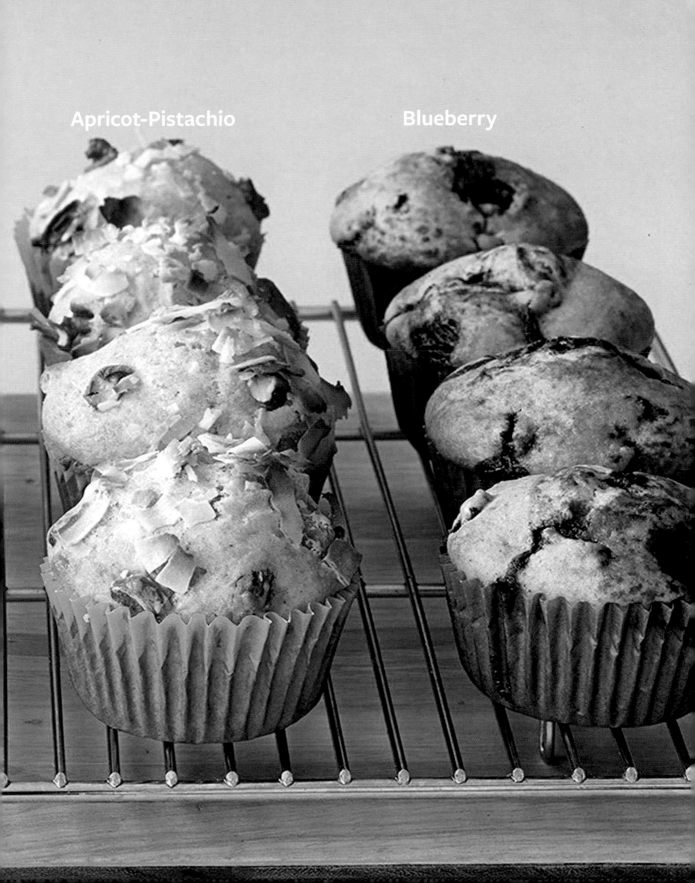

Apricot-Pistachio

Blueberry

CarbLovers Muffin Collection!

Prep: *5 minutes* | **Cook:** *16–20 minutes* | **Total Time:** *25 minutes + 5 to cool* | **Makes:** *12 muffins*

Everyone needs a go-to muffin recipe for special mornings. Start with one great basic recipe and add extras for four delicious variations. Try them all!

Base

100g (3½oz) plain flour
65g (2½oz) wholemeal flour
125g (4oz) sugar
1¼ teaspoons baking powder
¼ teaspoon ground nutmeg
½ teaspoon salt
1 large egg, lightly beaten
175ml (6fl oz) soya milk
2 tablespoons vegetable oil
1 teaspoon pure vanilla extract

MIX-INS: STIR IN THESE INGREDIENTS WHEN YOU GET TO STEP 3 (RIGHT).

Double Chocolate Cherry

*Reduce plain flour in base to
  65g (2½oz)
75g (3oz) plain chocolate chips
75g (3oz) dried cherries
4 tablespoons cocoa powder
  (add to flour mixture)

Serving size: 1 muffin Calories 165; Fat 5.4g (sat 1.6g, mono 1.4g, poly 1.8g); Cholesterol 16mg; Protein 3g; Carbohydrate 27g; Sugars 16g; Fibre 2g; RS 0g; Sodium 173mg

Cinnamon-Apple Walnut

75g (3oz) dried apples, chopped
75g (3oz) chopped walnuts
1 tablespoon sugar + ½ teaspoon cinnamon for topping

Serving size: 1 muffin Calories 159; Fat 6.3g (sat 0.6g, mono 1.2g, poly 4g); Cholesterol 16mg; Protein 3g; Carbohydrate 24g; Sugars 12g; Fibre 2g; RS 0g; Sodium 175mg

Apricot-Pistachio

75g (3oz) dried apricots, chopped
75g (3oz) chopped pistachios
2 tablespoons desiccated unsweetened coconut for topping

Serving size: 1 muffin Calories 162; Fat 6g (sat 1.1g, mono 2g, poly 2.4g); Cholesterol 16mg; Protein 4g; Carbohydrate 24g; Sugars 13g; Fibre 2g; RS 0g; Sodium 172mg

Blueberry

125g (4oz) fresh blueberries

Serving size: 1 muffin Calories 121; Fat 3.2g (sat 0.4g, mono 0.7g, poly 1.8g); Cholesterol 16mg; Protein 3g; Carbohydrate 21g; Sugars 10g; Fibre 1g; RS 0g; Sodium 172mg

1. Preheat oven to 200°C/400°F/gas mark 6. Line a 12-hole muffin tin with paper liners.

2. Combine flours and next 4 ingredients (through to salt) in a large bowl; stir with a whisk. Make a well in centre of mixture.

3. Add egg, milk, oil and vanilla to flour mixture, stirring until just combined. Stir in mix-in ingredients. Divide batter evenly between holes of prepared muffin tin. Add topping as indicated.

4. Bake 16–20 minutes or until a wooden cocktail stick inserted in the centre of a muffin comes out clean. Cool in tin on a wire rack for 5 minutes; remove muffins from tin and cool completely on rack.

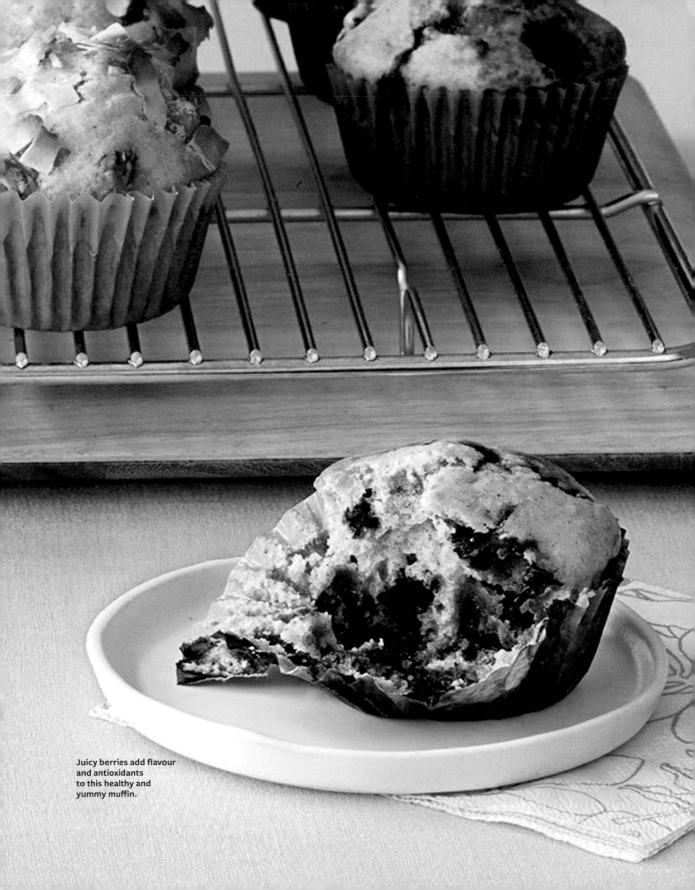

Juicy berries add flavour
and antioxidants
to this healthy and
yummy muffin.

Grilled Banana on Toast

Prep: *5 minutes* | **Cook:** *5 minutes* | **Total time:** *10 minutes* | **Makes:** *1 serving*

No time for breakfast? Try this superfast and yummy open-faced sandwich, which is packed with Resistant Starch from both the bananas and the rye bread.

1 tablespoon brown sugar
½ large banana, removed
from peel and halved lengthways
1 (40g/1½oz) slice rye bread,
  toasted
2 tablespoons reduced-fat
  peanut butter

1. Preheat grill with rack 10cm (4 inches) from heat source. Place sugar on a plate; dip cut sides of banana in sugar. Arrange banana cut side up on a baking sheet or in a heat-proof baking dish; grill 3–5 minutes, rotating sheet often, until banana is browned.

2. Spread toast with peanut butter; top with banana.

Serving size: 1 slice toast Calories 413; Fat 13.6g (sat 2.3g, mono 6.6g, poly 3.9g); Cholesterol 0mg; Protein 12g; Carbohydrate 62g; Sugars 25g; Fibre 6g; RS 4g; Sodium 400mg

ASK CARBLOVERS

Q: I'm not a fan of bananas. What can I do?

A: Bananas are an incredible source of Resistant Starch, but if you don't love 'em, no worries. In this recipe, you could easily substitute an apple or a pear for the banana. Just make sure you're getting enough RS each day from other sources.

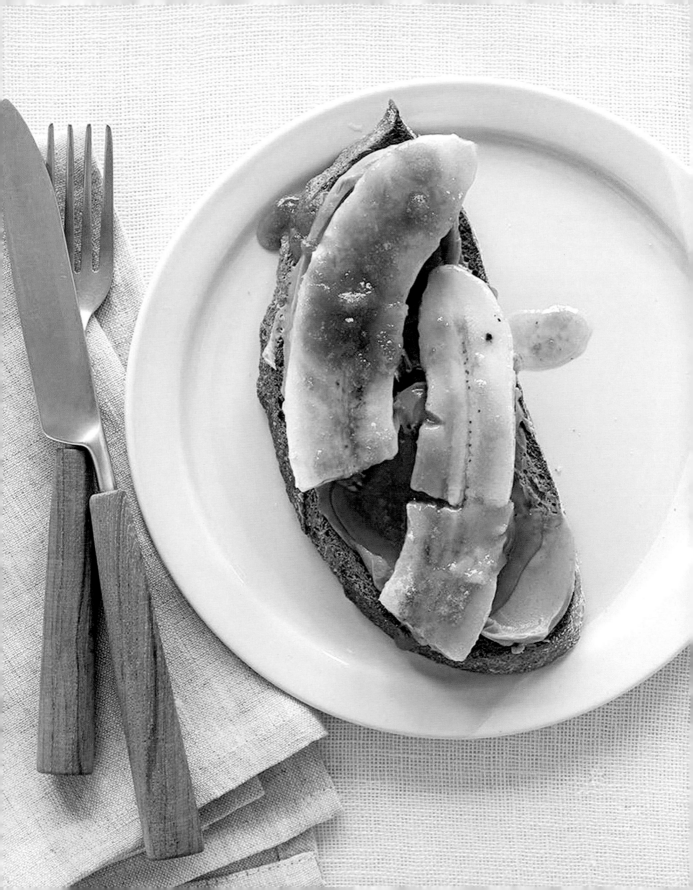

RS
0.3g

Toad in the Hole

Prep: *5 minutes* | ***Cook:*** *15 minutes* | ***Total time:*** *20 minutes* | ***Makes:*** *4 servings*

The name is a total hoot, but trust us, this classic breakfast is the ultimate comfort meal.

Cooking spray
8 large cherry tomatoes, halved
4 slices wholegrain bread
4 teaspoons melted butter
4 eggs

1. Coat a large nonstick pan with cooking spray. Heat pan to medium-high heat; add tomatoes. Cook until just soft and hot, 3–5 minutes. Remove from pan and keep warm.

2. Using a 5cm (2 inch) round cutter, carefully cut circles from each slice of bread. Brush bread and cutouts with butter and place facedown in pan. Toast until golden, 2–3 minutes. Flip bread slices and crack an egg into the centre (the "hole") of each piece. Cook until eggs are partially done, 2–3 minutes. Using a spatula, carefully flip egg-filled toasts and cutouts. Continue cooking until whites are cooked through, 1–2 more minutes. Sprinkle with salt and pepper, if liked.

3. Remove from pan and place each toast on a plate, along with a cutout. Serve with tomatoes.

Serving size: 1 slice bread and egg, plus cutout and 2 tomatoes Calories 184; Fat 10.1g (sat 4.2g, mono 3g, poly 1.6g); Cholesterol 196mg; Protein 10g; Carbohydrate 13g; Sugars 3g; Fibre 2g; RS 0.3g; Sodium 182mg

ASK CARBLOVERS

Q: Can I eat breakfast for dinner – and vice versa – on *CarbLovers*?

A: Sure! Some people feel more in control when they eat the same thing every day – even if it's a shake for dinner or pasta for breakfast! If that sounds like you, then go for it. It will almost certainly make it easier for you to stick to the plan.

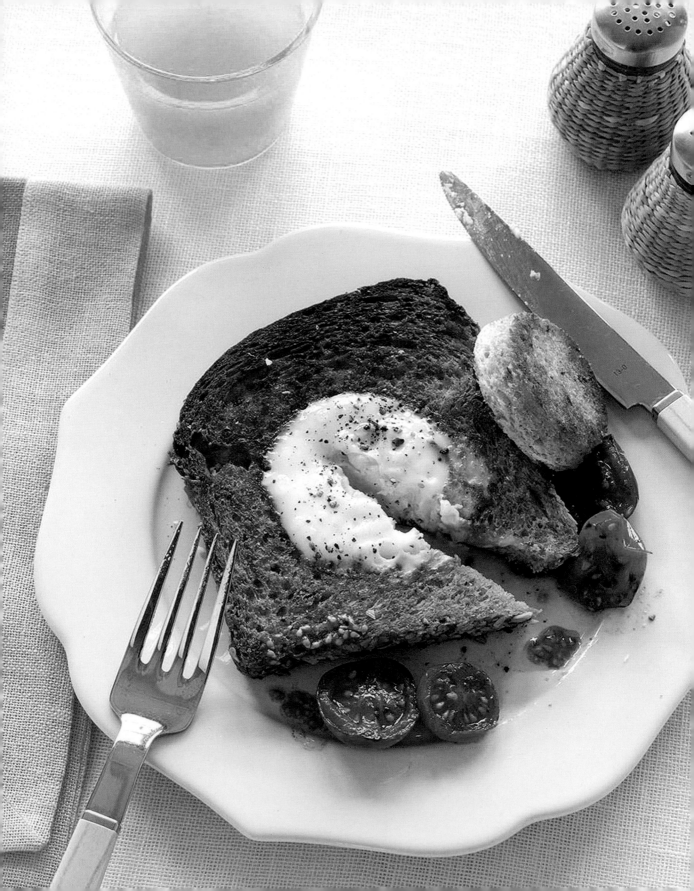

Tartine with Blackberry Thyme Salad

Prep: *3 minutes* | **Total time:** *3 minutes* | **Makes:** *4 servings*

Celebrate berry season with this delicious no-cook breakfast sandwich. You can substitute blueberries if you can't find blackberries.

500g (1lb) fresh blackberries
1 tablespoon fresh thyme leaves
2 teaspoons sugar
1 tablespoon fresh lemon juice
Pinch of sea salt
1 sourdough baguette (about 250g/8oz), split lengthways and cut into 4 pieces
2 tablespoons softened butter
700g (1½lb) natural low-fat yogurt

1. With clean hands or a spatula, crush blackberries, thyme, sugar, lemon juice and salt together in a medium bowl. Spread each baguette piece with ½ tablespoon butter and top with ¼ of the blackberry salad. Serve with ¼ of the yogurt.

Serving size: 1 tartine and 175g (6oz) natural low-fat yogurt Calories 393; Fat 10.2g (sat 5.6g, mono 2.5g, poly 1.1g); Cholesterol 25mg; Protein 18g; Carbohydrate 60g; Sugars 22g; Fibre 9g; RS 1.2g; Sodium 418mg

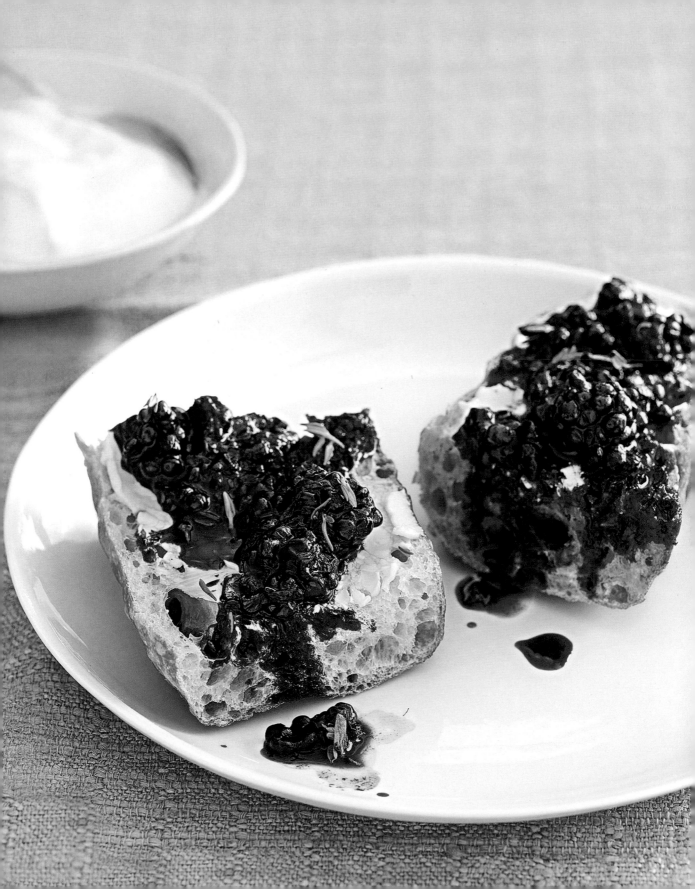

Wholemeal Waffles with Caramelized Pineapple

Prep: *10 minutes* | ***Cook:*** *20 minutes* | ***Total time:*** *30 minutes* | ***Makes:*** *8 servings*

Want a special CarbLovers *weekend brunch? Try these delicious waffles.*

FOR TOPPING:

2 tablespoons melted butter
3 tablespoons dark brown sugar
½ teaspoon pure vanilla extract
250g (8oz) pineapple chunks, fresh
  or frozen, thawed

FOR WAFFLES:

100g (3½oz) plain flour
100g (3½oz) wholemeal flour
2 tablespoons wheat germ
1½ teaspoons baking powder
½ teaspoon bicarbonate of soda
¼ teaspoon salt
475ml (16fl oz) buttermilk, plus more for
  loosening batter if necessary
2 tablespoons melted butter
1 tablespoon pure maple syrup
2 egg whites
1 teaspoon pure vanilla extract
Cooking spray

MAKE TOPPING:

1. Combine butter, brown sugar and vanilla in a saucepan and bring to the boil. Reduce heat, add pineapple to coat, and cook until pineapple is golden brown, 3–4 minutes.

MAKE WAFFLES:

1. Preheat a waffle iron.

2. Place flours, wheat germ, baking powder, bicarbonate of soda and salt in a bowl; whisk to combine. Place buttermilk, butter, maple syrup, egg whites and vanilla in a separate bowl; whisk to combine. Combine dry and wet ingredients; whisk until just incorporated (batter will be thick).

3. Coat waffle iron with cooking spray; pour ¼ of the batter into waffle iron. Cook until golden brown, about 3–4 minutes. Transfer to a plate and keep warm. Repeat with remaining batter.

4. Stack two waffle quarters (or squares) on top of each other. Drizzle with 4 tablespoons pineapple topping and serve.

Serving size: 2 waffle quarters with 4 tablespoons pineapple topping Calories 216; Fat 7.3g (sat 4.1g, mono 2g, poly 0.6g); Cholesterol 18mg; Protein 6g; Carbohydrate 32g; Sugars 13g; Fibre 2g; RS 0g; Sodium 336mg

> **TIP:**
> You can substitute other fruit for the pineapple. Bananas, blueberries and apples are all amazing with these waffles.

RS
0.9g

Banana-Pecan Breakfast Bread

Prep: *10 minutes* | **Cook:** *60 minutes* | **Total Time:** *70 minutes + time to cool* | **Makes:** *16 servings*

Fresh, warm banana bread is a special way to start your day. And it makes great use of your too-ripe bananas!

125g (4oz) plain flour
65g (2½oz) wholemeal flour
50g (2oz) wheat germ
125g (4oz) sugar
½ teaspoon salt
½ teaspoon baking powder
¼ teaspoon bicarbonate of soda
350ml (12fl oz) mashed ripe bananas
  (from 3–4 medium bananas)
75ml (3fl oz) vegetable oil
2 large eggs, lightly beaten
50g (2oz) pecans, coarsely chopped
Cooking spray

1. Preheat oven to 180°C/350°F/gas mark 4.

2. Combine flours, wheat germ, sugar, salt, baking powder and bicarbonate of soda in a large bowl; make a well in centre of mixture. Combine bananas, oil and eggs in a separate bowl; add to flour mixture. Stir until just moist, then stir in pecans.

3. Coat a 20 by 10cm (8 by 4 inch) loaf tin with cooking spray; spoon in mixture. Bake for 1 hour or until a wooden cocktail stick inserted in the centre comes out clean. Cool bread in tin 10 minutes on a wire rack. Remove bread from tin; cool completely on rack.

Serving size: 1 slice Calories 168; Fat 7.5g (sat 0.8g, mono 2.4g, poly 3.8g); Cholesterol 23mg; Protein 3g; Carbohydrate 23g; Sugars 9g; Fibre 2g; RS 0.9g; Sodium 119mg

{ **TIP:**
Make two loaves at a time: Cool the second one, wrap in clingfilm, then freeze. Bring to room temperature before serving. }

Spinach and Egg Breakfast Wrap with Avocado and Pepper Jack Cheese

Prep: *10 minutes* | **Cook:** *5 minutes* | ***Total time:*** *15 minutes* | **Makes:** *4 servings*

We love breakfast sandwiches, so we created this fast take on a burrito, layering it with spicy cheese and creamy avocado. Serve with salsa for an extra kick.

Cooking spray
150g (5oz) baby spinach, chopped
4 eggs
4 egg whites
½ teaspoon salt
¼ teaspoon freshly ground black
  pepper
4 wholemeal tortillas
125g (4oz) pepper jack cheese,
  grated
1 avocado, sliced
Hot sauce or salsa (optional)

1. Heat a nonstick frying pan coated with cooking spray over medium-high heat.

2. Add spinach and cook, stirring, until wilted, 2 minutes.

3. Whisk together eggs and egg whites in a small bowl. Add eggs to pan and cook, stirring, until cooked through, 3–4 minutes. Season with salt and pepper.

4. Place ¼ of egg mixture in the centre of each tortilla; sprinkle with ¼ of the cheese.

5. Top each tortilla with 4 slices avocado and fold, burrito-style. Slice in half and serve.

Serving size: 1 wrap Calories 366; Fat 21.8g (sat 7.7g, mono 6.9g, poly 1.8g); Cholesterol 242mg; Protein 22g; Carbohydrate 30g; Sugars 1g; Fibre 7g; RS 0.6g; Sodium 666mg

TIP:
If you prefer, you can substitute cheddar for pepper jack.

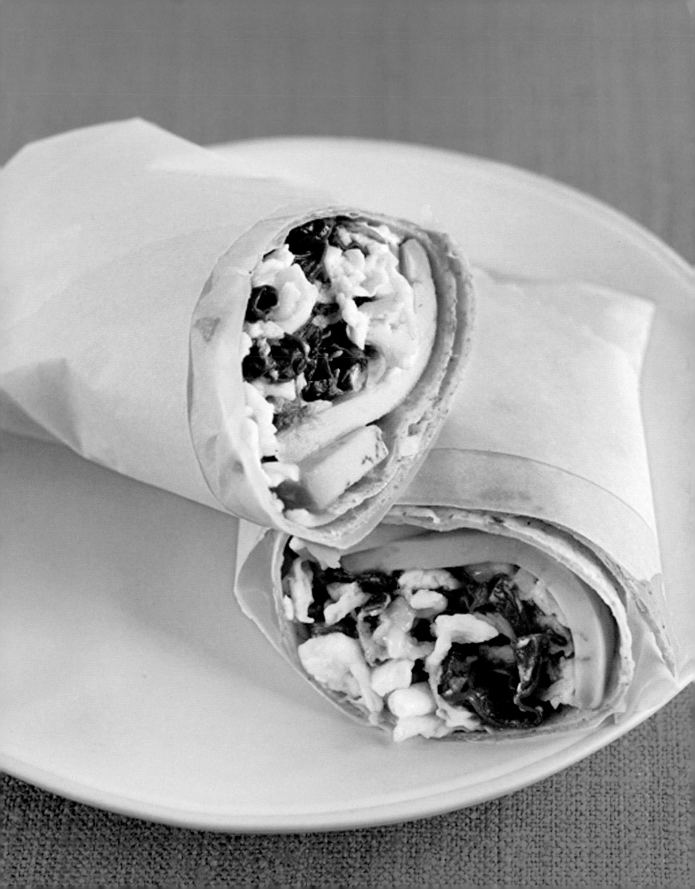

Buckwheat Crepes with Orange-Ricotta Filling

Prep: 10 minutes | **Cook:** 10 minutes | **Total time:** 20 minutes | **Makes:** 6 servings

Crepes might sound cooking-school complicated, but they're just as easy to make as pancakes.

500g (1lb) semi-skimmed ricotta
2 teaspoons finely grated
  orange zest
2 tablespoons fresh-squeezed
  orange juice
2 tablespoons icing sugar, plus
  more for dusting
65g (2½oz) buckwheat flour
65g (2½oz) plain flour
2 large eggs
3 tablespoons vegetable oil
250ml (8fl oz) skimmed milk
½ teaspoon salt
Cooking spray
2 oranges, cut into segments

1. Make filling: Stir together ricotta, orange zest, orange juice and sugar in a medium bowl. Cover and refrigerate mixture until ready to serve.

2. Make batter: Whisk together flours, eggs, oil, milk, 2 tablespoons water and salt in a large bowl until well combined. Let stand 5 minutes.

3. Heat a 25cm (10 inch) nonstick frying pan over medium-high heat; coat pan with cooking spray. Pour about 5 tablespoons batter per crepe onto pan. Cook 30–45 seconds or until crepe is golden on the bottom. Carefully turn crepe over with a spatula; cook 30 seconds or until bottom is lightly browned. Transfer crepes to a plate; keep warm. Repeat with remaining batter.

4. To assemble, spoon about 5 tablespoons filling down the centre of each crepe; roll up to form a cylinder. Place each rolled crepe on a plate, top with a few orange segments, dust with icing sugar and serve.

Serving size: 1 crepe and 5 tablespoons filling, 3–5 orange segments Calories 322; Fat 15.7g (sat 5.2g, mono 4.4g, poly 5.2g); Cholesterol 88mg; Protein 16g; Carbohydrate 31g; Sugars 9g; Fibre 2g; RS 0g; Sodium 340mg

TIP:
With a sharp knife, segment your orange by slicing off the top and bottom, trimming away the peel and white pith, and releasing the pretty segments from the membrane.

Oatmeal-Cranberry Muffins

Prep: *5 minutes* | **Cook:** *30 minutes* | **Total time:** *35 minutes* | **Makes:** *12 muffins*

Make a batch of these on Sunday, and you'll have a healthy grab-and-go breakfast all week. Spread a tablespoon of almond or peanut butter on top for extra protein.

Cooking spray
150g (5oz) old-fashioned rolled oats
100g (3½oz) plain flour
100g (3½oz) wholemeal flour
100g (3½oz) sugar
2½ teaspoons baking powder
1 teaspoon ground cinnamon
½ teaspoon ground nutmeg
½ teaspoon salt
125ml (4fl oz) oil
125ml (4fl oz) apple sauce
2 eggs
65g (2½oz) dried, sweetened cranberries

1. Preheat oven to 180°C/350°F/gas mark 4.

2. Coat a 12-hole muffin tin with cooking spray and set aside.

3. Combine oats, flours, sugar, baking powder, spices and salt in a bowl.

4. Whisk 250ml (8fl oz) water, oil, apple sauce, and eggs in a separate bowl until incorporated.

5. Combine wet and dry ingredients; add cranberries.

6. Distribute batter evenly between muffin holes. Bake until a cocktail stick inserted in the centre of a muffin comes out clean and tops are browned, 30–35 minutes.

Serving size: 1 muffin Calories 227; Fat 11.2g (sat 1.4g, mono 4.6g, poly 4.5g); Cholesterol 35mg; Protein 4g; Carbohydrate 29g; Sugars 10g; Fibre 3g; RS 1.2g; Sodium 194mg

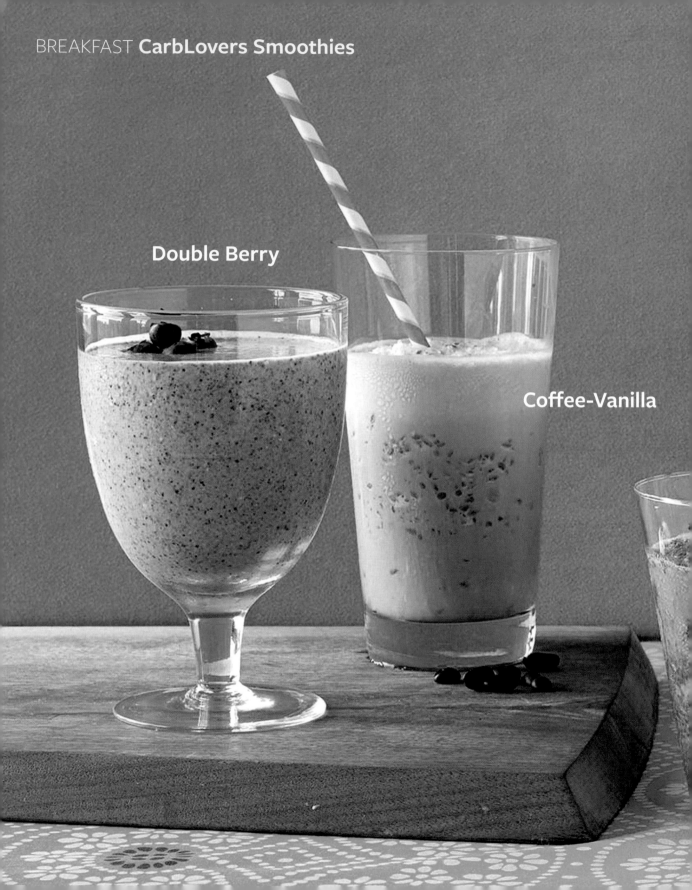

BREAKFAST **CarbLovers Smoothies**

Double Berry

Coffee-Vanilla

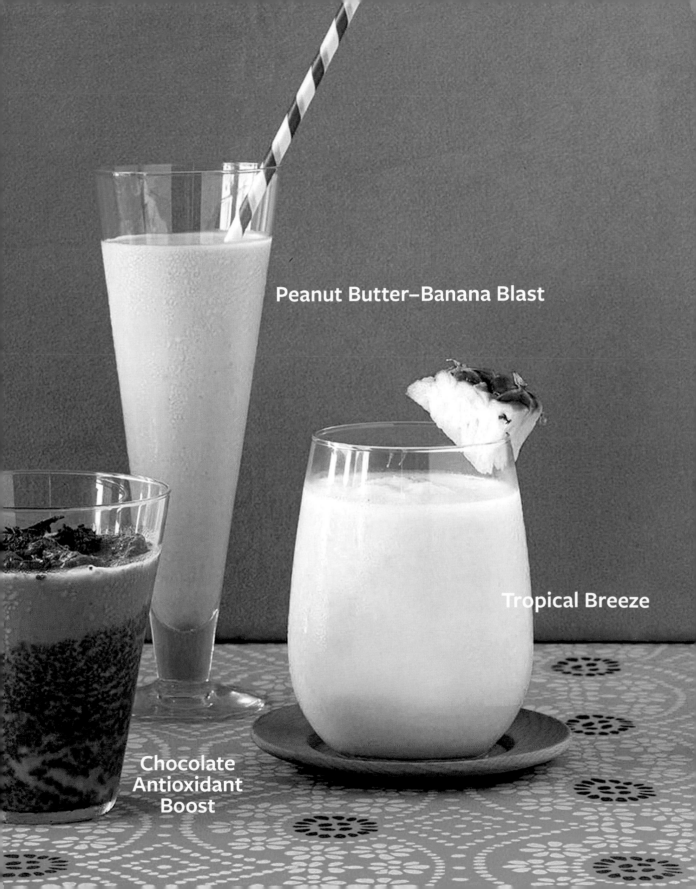

Peanut Butter–Banana Blast

Tropical Breeze

Chocolate Antioxidant Boost

CarbLovers Smoothies 5 Exciting Ways

Prep: 5 minutes | **Total time:** 5 minutes | **Makes:** 1 serving

Wake up to something wonderful! These five energizing smoothie combos will get you fuelled up for whatever your day has in store.

Base

250ml (8fl oz) natural low-fat yogurt
1 teaspoon honey
1 teaspoon pure vanilla extract

Combine base ingredients and add-in ingredients in a blender; blend until smooth. Serve immediately.

MIX-INS:

Double Berry

4 tablespoons prepared quick-cooking oats, cooled
1 additional tablespoon honey
8 tablespoons frozen blueberries
8 tablespoons frozen strawberries
4 tablespoons skimmed milk

Serving size: About 16 ounces Calories 371; Fat 5.2g (sat 2.7g, mono 1.3g, poly 0.4g); Cholesterol 16mg; Protein 18g; Carbohydrate 66g; Sugars 53g; Fibre 5g; RS 0.1g; Sodium 201mg

Coffee-Vanilla

(This one's for caffeine-loving adults only!)

3 tablespoons vanilla whey protein powder
1 tablespoon ground flaxseed
¾ teaspoon coffee granules
125ml (4fl oz) ice

Serving size: About 475ml (16fl oz) Calories 299; Fat 8.1g (sat 3.4g, mono 1.7g, poly 2.4g); Cholesterol 36mg; Protein 25g; Carbohydrate 30g; Sugars 26g; Fibre 2g; RS 0g; Sodium 199mg

Chocolate Antioxidant Boost

2 teaspoons cocoa powder
5 teaspoons additional honey
1 frozen unsweetened acai smoothie pack
75ml (3fl oz) ice

Serving size: About 475ml (16fl oz) Calories 382; Fat 10.1g (sat 4g, mono 4.5g, poly 1g); Cholesterol 15mg; Protein 15g; Carbohydrate 58g; Sugars 54g; Fibre 2g; RS 0g; Sodium 184mg

Peanut Butter–Banana Blast

250g (8oz) sliced frozen bananas
2 tablespoons peanut butter
4 tablespoons ice

Serving size: About 475ml (16fl oz) Calories 509; Fat 20.4g (sat 6g, mono 8.8g, poly 4.8g); Cholesterol 15mg; Protein 23g; Carbohydrate 64g; Sugars 45g; Fibre 6g; RS 6g; Sodium 321mg

Tropical Breeze

100g (3½oz) ineapple chunks
100g (3½oz) mango chunks
4 tablespoons ice

Serving size: About 475ml (16fl oz) Calories 278; Fat 4.2g (sat 2.5g, mono 1.2g, poly 0.2g); Cholesterol 15mg; Protein 14g; Carbohydrate 47g; Sugars 43g; Fibre 2g; RS 0g; Sodium 174mg

RS 0–6g

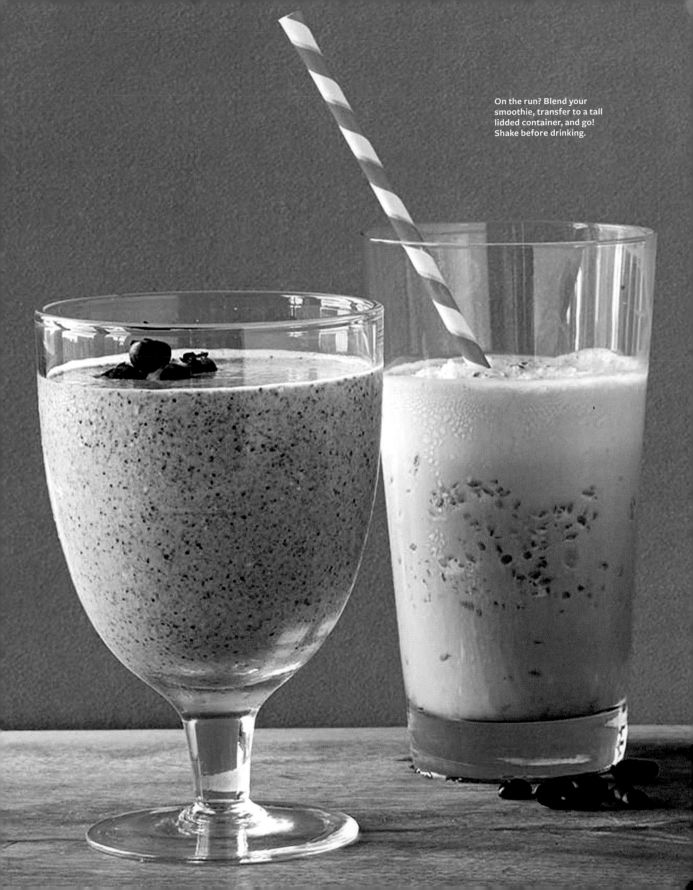

On the run? Blend your smoothie, transfer to a tall lidded container, and go! Shake before drinking.

RS
1.2g

Berry-Kale Smoothie

Prep: *5 minutes* | **Total time:** *5 minutes* | **Makes:** *2 servings*

If you're looking for a quick, high-fiber breakfast, get out your blender and whip up this tasty shake. And please don't be afraid of the kale – you'll never know it's in there!

175g (6oz) fresh or frozen raspberries
50g (2oz) kale, shredded
250ml (8fl oz) ice
175ml (6fl oz) fat-free natural yogurt
½ banana
2 tablespoons honey
1 tablespoon natural almond butter
1 tablespoon wheat germ

Combine all ingredients in a blender; blend until smooth. Serve immediately.

Serving size: 250ml (8fl oz) Calories 248; Fat 5.6g (sat 0.5g, mono 2.7g, poly 1.8g); Cholesterol 2mg; Protein 9g; Carbohydrate 47g; Sugars 30g; Fibre 8g; RS 1.2g; Sodium 77mg

TIP:
This smoothie is also great for a lovely, light lunch, but for a complete meal, we suggest adding a wholemeal English muffin with 1 tablespoon hummus.

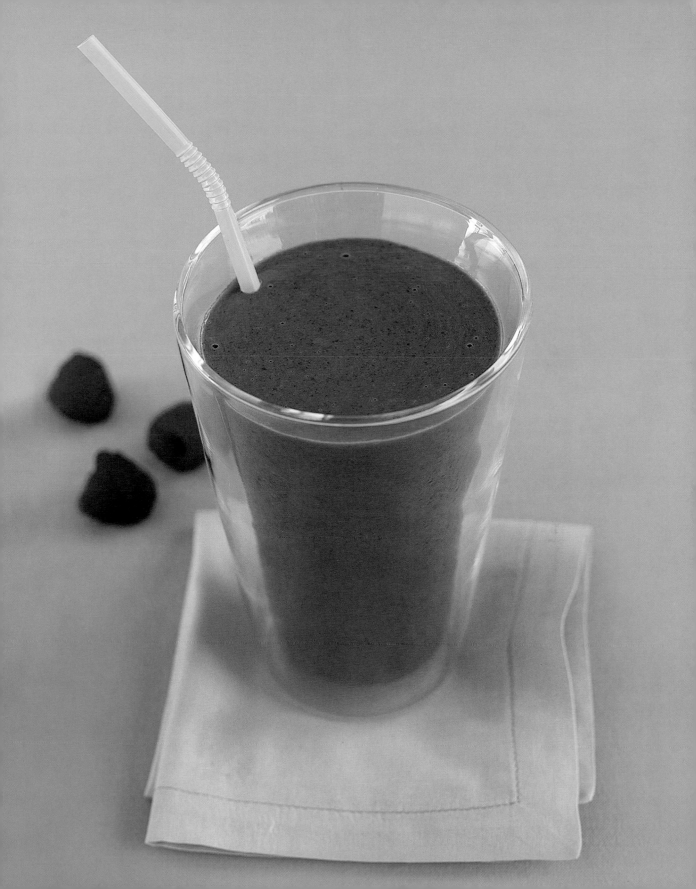

Soups & Sandwiches

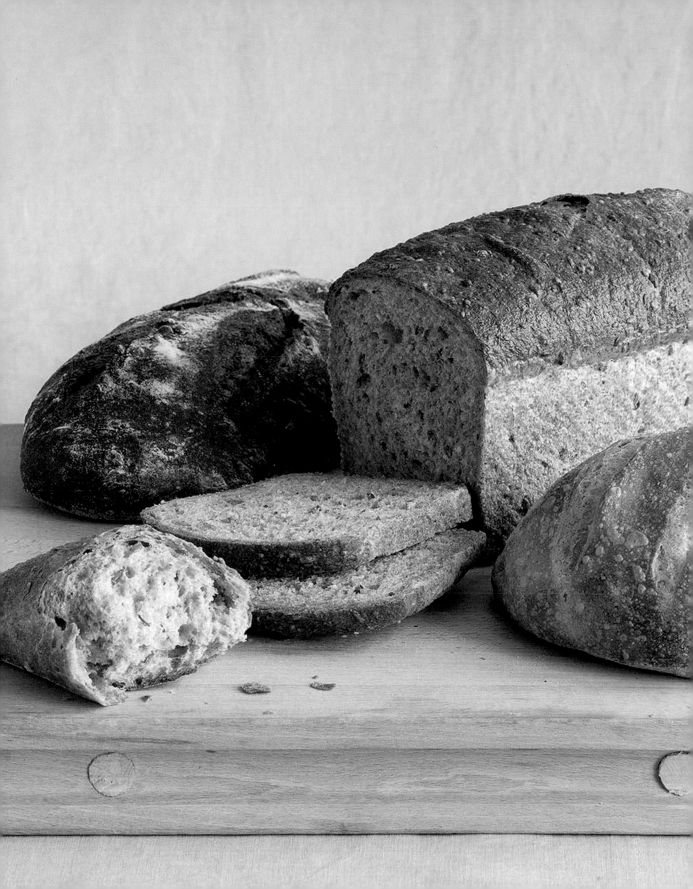

Three-Bean Soup with Bacon

Prep: *10 minutes* | **Cook:** *25 minutes* | **Total time:** *35 minutes* | **Makes:** *4 servings*

This superfast soup is the ultimate slimming, Resistant Starch-rich lunch. Enjoy it with a granary roll.

1 tablespoon olive oil
1 large onion, diced
2 garlic cloves, chopped
1 large courgette, cut into small dice
1 litre (1¾ pints) low-sodium chicken stock
250g (8oz) canned reduced-salt cannellini
  beans, rinsed and drained
250g (8oz) canned kidney beans, rinsed
  and drained
250g (8oz) canned black beans, rinsed
  and drained
¼ teaspoon salt
¼ teaspoon pepper
2 rashers (50g/2oz) smoked back bacon,
  diced
Cooking spray

1. Heat oil in a saucepan over medium-high heat.

2. Add onion and cook until soft, 6 minutes.

3. Add garlic and cook 1 minute.

4. Add courgette and cook, stirring, 4 minutes.

5. Add stock, beans, salt and pepper, and bring to the boil. Reduce heat, and simmer over very low heat until slightly thickened, 15 minutes.

6. While soup is simmering, cook bacon in a large nonstick frying pan coated with cooking spray over medium-high heat until crisp, 3–5 minutes.

7. Divide soup between 4 bowls, and top each bowl with 1 tablespoon crisped bacon.

Serving size: 475ml (16fl oz) soup plus 1 tablespoon crisped back bacon Calories 271; Fat 6.6g (sat 1.3g, mono 3.5g, poly 0.9g); Cholesterol 5mg; Protein 18g; Carbohydrate 38g; Sugars 6g; Fibre 11g; RS 3.5g; Sodium 504mg

TIP:
If you can't find fresh courgettes in winter, try substituting 250g (8oz) chopped kale.

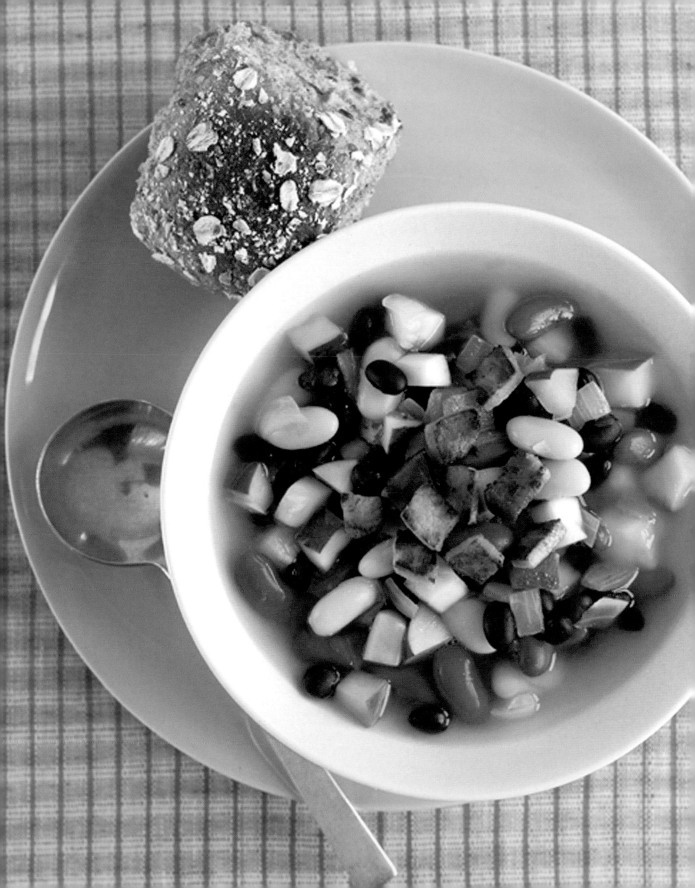

Hearty Chicken Posole Stew

Prep: *10 minutes* | **Cook:** *30 minutes* | **Total time:** *40 minutes* | **Makes:** *4 servings*

If you've never tried posole, you'll love adding this stew to your CarbLovers *menu! It's traditionally served in Mexico at Christmastime, but we think it's delicious any time of year.*

1 tablespoon olive oil
1 small onion, chopped
2 cloves garlic, finely chopped
500g (1lb) boneless, skinless chicken
  breast, cubed
¾ teaspoon cumin
½ teaspoon dried oregano
1 litre (1¾ pints) low-sodium chicken
  stock
475g (15oz) can fire-roasted tomatoes
475g (15oz) can hominy, rinsed
  and drained
1 tablespoon diced green chillies
½ teaspoon salt
¼ teaspoon pepper
Fresh coriander for garnish
Tortilla chips (optional)

1. Heat oil in a medium saucepan over medium heat.

2. Add onion and cook until soft, about 7 minutes.

3. Add garlic and cook, stirring, 2 minutes.

4. Add chicken, cumin and oregano, and cook, stirring, until just cooked through, 5 minutes.

5. Add stock, tomatoes, hominy, green chillies, salt and pepper, and bring to the boil. Reduce heat, skimming foam from top of soup, and simmer,
10 minutes, until liquid has thickened slightly.

6. Divide soup between 4 bowls. Garnish with coriander, and serve immediately with tortilla chips alongside, if liked.

Serving size: 475ml (16fl oz) stew Calories 303; Fat 8.5g (sat 1.8g, mono 4.3g, poly 1.7g); Cholesterol 63mg; Protein 30g; Carbohydrate 26g; Sugars 6g; Fibre 4g; RS 1.3g; Sodium 743mg

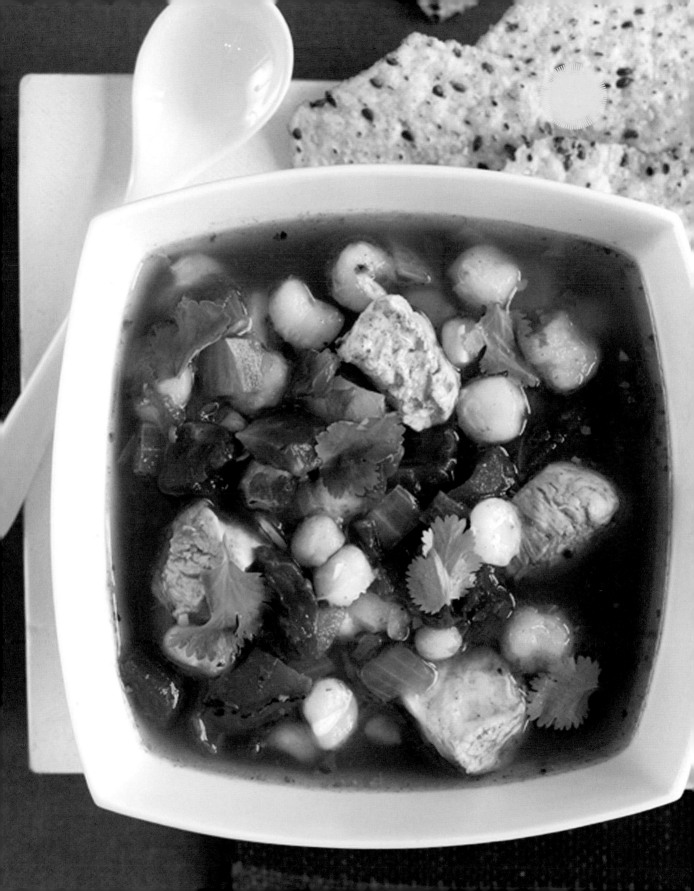

Chunky Tomato-Basil Soup with Pasta

Prep: 5 minutes | **Cook:** 20 minutes | **Total time:** 25 minutes | **Makes:** 4 servings

Take the chill out of a wintry day with this warming, tasty soup. Pair it with half of our Grilled Cheese and Tomato on Rye (page 106) for a satisfying lunch or dinner.

1 tablespoon olive oil, plus more for
   serving if liked
1 small onion, chopped
2 tablespoons tomato purée
1 teaspoon sugar
⅛ teaspoon salt
400ml (14fl oz) low-sodium
   chicken stock
875g (1¾lb) canned chopped tomatoes
   in juice
1 garlic clove, peeled
2 large basil sprigs, leaves coarsely
   torn and stems reserved
50g (2oz) dry, small wholewheat
   pasta (such as rotini, shells
   or broken-up spaghetti)

1. Heat oil in a medium saucepan over medium heat. Add onion; cook, stirring occasionally, until tender, 5–7 minutes. Stir in tomato purée, sugar and salt; cook 2 minutes. Stir in chicken stock, tomatoes and their juice, garlic and basil stems; bring to the boil over high heat.

2. Add pasta; reduce heat to medium and simmer until pasta is tender and flavours are blended, about 10–12 minutes. Remove garlic clove and basil stems; discard. Serve pasta topped with basil leaves and a drizzle of olive oil.

Serving size: 250ml (8fl oz) Calories 156; Fat 4.1g (sat 0.7g, mono 2.5g, poly 0.5g); Cholesterol 2mg; Protein 6g; Carbohydrate 25g; Sugars 10g; Fibre 4g; RS 0.6g; Sodium 211mg

Creamy Clam and Corn Chowder

Prep: *20 minutes* | **Cook:** *45 minutes* | **Total time:** *65 minutes* | **Makes:** *4 servings*

Yes, you can enjoy creamy soup again. This rich-tasting, New England-style chowder is packed with Resistant Starch and delicious flavour.

2 teaspoons vegetable oil

50g (2oz) bacon, diced

1 medium onion, diced

2 celery stalks, diced

4 tablespoons dry white wine

750ml (1¼ pints) 1% fat milk

3 tablespoons flour

125ml (4fl oz) clam juice

1 bay leaf

1 large potato (375g/12oz), peeled
and diced

1 teaspoon Tabasco or other hot
pepper sauce

¼ teaspoon pepper

175g (6oz) fresh or frozen sweetcorn
kernels, thawed

150g (5oz) fresh chopped clams or
canned clams, rinsed and drained

2 tablespoons chopped fresh parsley

1. Heat oil in a medium saucepan over medium-high heat. Add bacon and cook, stirring, until crisped, 4–5 minutes. Add onion and celery and cook, stirring, until onion is softened and celery is cooked, about 6 minutes. Add wine and cook until most of the liquid is dissolved, 3 minutes.

2. Combine milk and flour in a large bowl and whisk until smooth. Add to the saucepan along with clam juice, 125ml (4fl oz) water and bay leaf. Bring to the boil, reduce heat and simmer, whisking, until thickened, 11 minutes. Add potato and cook until tender, about 12 minutes. Add Tabasco, pepper, sweetcorn and clams, and simmer until clams and corn are cooked through, 4–5 minutes.

3. Divide between 4 bowls and garnish with parsley.

Serving size: 350ml (12fl oz) chowder Calories 314; Fat 6.1g (sat 1.8g, mono 1.6g, poly 2g); Cholesterol 34mg; Protein 21g; Carbohydrate 42g; Sugars 13g; Fibre 3g; RS 1.1g; Sodium 739mg

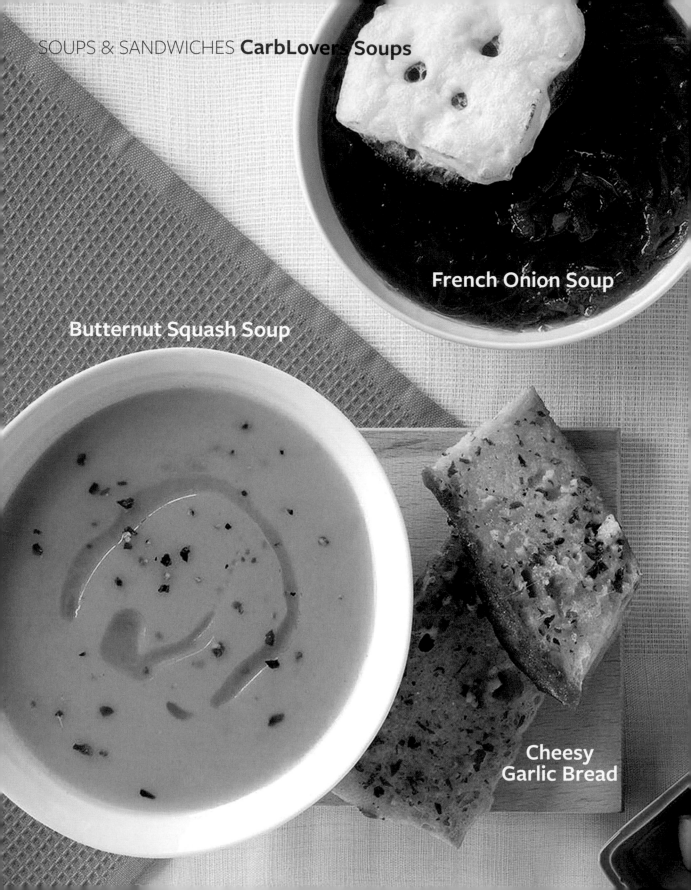

French Onion Soup

Butternut Squash Soup

Cheesy
Garlic Bread

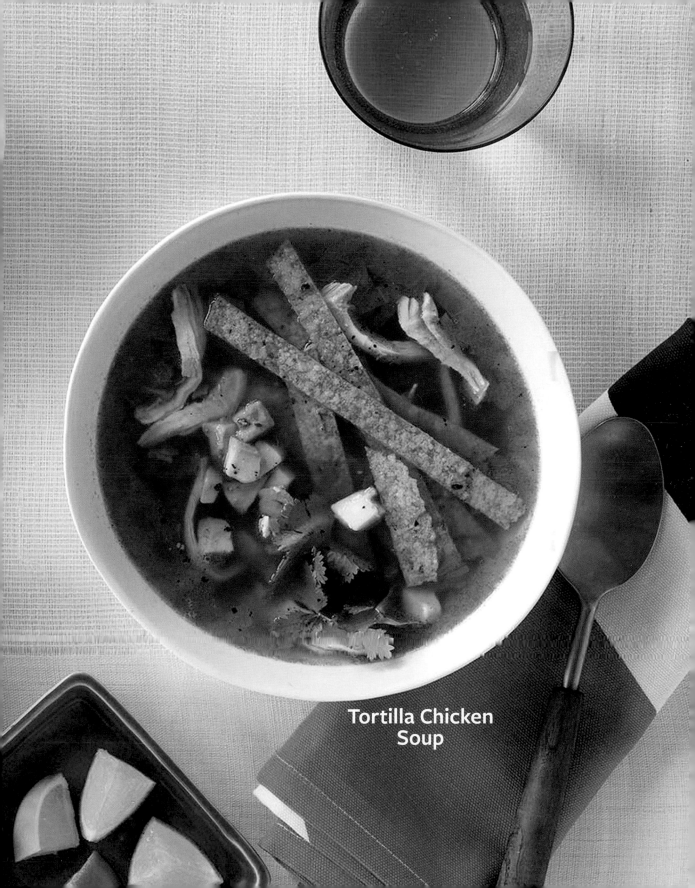

**Tortilla Chicken
Soup**

Butternut Squash Soup

Prep: *10 minutes* | **Cook:** *25 minutes* | **Total time:** *35 minutes* | **Makes:** *4 servings*

Creamy, comforting and packed with beta-carotene, this soup makes a deliciously light lunch or a perfect start to a warming meal.

2 tablespoons olive oil, plus more
for serving
1 medium onion, chopped
2 garlic cloves, chopped
½ teaspoon ground coriander
¼ teaspoon dried chilli flakes, plus
  more for serving
1 tablespoon chopped fresh ginger
1 small butternut squash (750g/1½lb),
  peeled, cut into 1-inch cubes
1 litre (1¾ pints) low-sodium chicken
  stock
2 teaspoons fresh lemon juice

1. Heat oil in a large saucepan over medium heat. Add onion and garlic; cook, stirring occasionally, until tender, 6–8 minutes. Add coriander, chilli flakes and ginger; cook, stirring, 1 minute. Stir in squash, stock and lemon juice; bring to the boil Reduce heat to a simmer and cook 10 minutes or until squash is tender.

2. Working in batches, transfer soup to a blender and blend until smooth (or blend in the pan with a stick blender). To serve, drizzle soup with a small amount of olive oil and sprinkle with dried chilli flakes, if liked.

Serving size: About 250ml (8fl oz) Calories 148; Fat 7g (sat 1g, mono 4.9g, poly 0.8g); Cholesterol 0mg; Protein 4g; Carbohydrate 20g; Sugars 4g; Fibre 5g; RS 0g; Sodium 78mg

TIP:
Pour leftover stock into an ice cube tray, then seal the cubes in a freezer bag for later. Add them when you need a pop of flavour.

French Onion Soup

Prep: *5 minutes* | **Cook:** *50 minutes* | **Total time:** *55 minutes* | **Makes:** *4 servings*

This classic bistro soup is usually packed with sodium and fat, but we lightened up both without compromising flavour.

2 tablespoons vegetable oil

25g (1oz) butter

1.25kg (2½lb) medium onions (about 5),
  halved and thinly sliced

4 tablespoons Marsala wine (or sherry)

4 sprigs fresh thyme

900ml (1½ pints) low-sodium
  beef stock

1 teaspoon red wine vinegar

2 rectangular slices rye bread
(about 75g/3oz each), halved

2 thick slices low-fat Emmental cheese
(about 50g/2oz each), halved

1. Heat oil and butter in a cast-iron casserole or other large saucepan over medium heat. Add onions; cover and cook, stirring occasionally, until onions wilt and begin to brown on bottom of pan, about 20 minutes. Uncover and cook, stirring and adding Marsala 1 tablespoon at a time every 5 minutes, for 15 minutes. Stir in thyme, 750ml (1¼ pints) water, stock and vinegar; bring to the boil. Reduce heat to a simmer and cook 10 minutes or until flavours are blended.

2. Meanwhile, preheat grill with rack in highest position. Arrange bread slices on a large rimmed baking sheet; top with cheese. Grill 2–3 minutes or until cheese is browned. Serve soup with cheese toasts.

Serving size: About 400ml (14fl oz) Calories 429; Fat 16.9g (sat 5.8g, mono 4.6g, poly 5.3g); Cholesterol 25mg; Protein 19g; Carbohydrate 48g; Sugars 15g; Fibre 7g; RS 1.4g; Sodium 429mg

Tortilla Chicken Soup

Prep: *15 minutes* | **Cook:** *25 minutes* | **Total time:** *40 minutes* | **Makes:** *4 servings*

This soup is a spicy Mexican twist on the traditional winter warmer. We love the added crunch of the tortillas on top, plus the creamy avocado.

1 tablespoon olive oi

1 small onion, chopped

2 teaspoons garlic, finely chopped

2 teaspoons seeded finely chopped
  jalapeño chillies

1 teaspoon cumin

½ teaspoon salt

½ teaspoon pepper

1 litre (1¾ pints) low-sodium chicken
  stock

450g (14½oz) can low-sodium
  diced tomatoes

375g (12oz) can no-salt-added
  sweetcorn, drained

1½ teaspoons mild hot sauce

2 (15cm/6 inch) corn tortillas

250g (8oz) cooked chicken, skinned
  and shredded

1 small avocado, diced

4 tablespoons coriander leaves

8 lime wedges

1. Preheat oven to 190°C/375°F/gas mark 5.

2. Heat 2 teaspoons oil in a medium saucepan over medium-high heat. Add onion and cook, stirring occasionally, until softened, 6 minutes. Add garlic, jalapeños, cumin, salt, and pepper, and cook 2 minutes. Add stock, tomatoes and their juice, sweetcorn and hot sauce, and bring to the boil.

3. Reduce heat and simmer for 15 minutes. While soup is simmering, brush both sides of tortillas with remaining teaspoon oil. Using a pizza cutter or knife, cut tortillas into 5mm (¼ inch) strips. Transfer to a baking sheet and bake until crisp and slightly browned, 7–8 minutes. Remove from oven and cool. When soup is done, divide between 4 bowls. Top with ¼ of the chicken, diced avocado and tortilla strips and a few coriander leaves. Serve with lime wedges.

Serving size: 350ml (12fl oz) soup Calories 306; Fat 11.9g (sat 1.8g, mono 6.9g, poly 1.7g); Cholesterol 50mg; Protein 23g; Carbohydrate 31g; Sugars 8g; Fibre 7g; RS 0.5g; Sodium 649mg

Cheesy Garlic Bread

Prep: *10 minutes* | **Cook:** *15 minutes* | **Total time:** *25 minutes* | **Makes:** *8 servings*

Who doesn't love garlic bread? Our crunchy version is excellent dunked in any of our soups or with saucy dishes like spaghetti and meatballs.

50g (2oz) grated Parmesan cheese
2 tablespoons olive oil
1 tablespoon softened butter
1 tablespoon reduced-fat
   mayonnaise
1 tablespoon finely chopped garlic
¼ teaspoon salt
¼ teaspoon pepper
4 tablespoons chopped parsley
30cm (12 inch) French stick, split

1. Preheat oven to 200°C/400°F/gas mark 6.

2. Combine Parmesan, oil, butter, mayonnaise, garlic, salt and pepper, and spread evenly on both bread halves. Wrap bread loosely in foil and place on a baking sheet. Bake until golden brown and crust is crisp, 13–15 minutes. Remove bread halves from oven and cut each (using a serrated bread knife) into 4 pieces.

Serving size: 7cm (3 inch) piece bread Calories 144; Fat 7.2g (sat 2.3g, mono 3.4g, poly 0.8g); Cholesterol 9mg; Protein 4g; Carbohydrate 15g; Sugars 1g; Fibre 1g; RS 0.3g; Sodium 364mg

RS
1.9g

Mexican Mole Chilli

Prep: *15 minutes* | **Cook:** *45 minutes* | **Total time:** *1 hour* | **Makes:** *6 servings*

This hearty bowl has some kick from two different types of chilli powder, plus dried chilli flakes. And it's fibre-packed! Make a batch for a post-match get-together.

1 tablespoon olive oil
1 large onion, chopped
1 tablespoon finely chopped garlic
500g (1lb) lean minced beef or bison
3 tablespoons cocoa powder
1 tablespoon chilli powder
1 teaspoon cumin
1 teaspoon chipotle chilli powder
¾ teaspoon salt
½ teaspoon pepper
½ teaspoon dried chilli flakes
2 green peppers, deseeded
 and chopped
2 x 475g (15oz) cans low-sodium diced
 tomatoes in juice
475g (15oz) can kidney beans
475g (15oz) can black beans
4 tablespoons chopped fresh coriander
2 tablespoons diced red onion
Light soured cream (optional)

1. Heat oil in a large saucepan over medium-high heat. Add onion and cook until softened, 6–7 minutes. Add garlic and cook 1 minute. Add meat and cook, breaking up with a spoon, until just cooked through, 5 minutes. Add cocoa, chilli powder, cumin, chipotle powder, salt, pepper, and chilli flakes, and cook for 1 minute until fragrant. Add peppers, tomatoes and beans, and bring to the boil. Cover, reduce heat, and simmer until liquid is absorbed, 40–45 minutes.

2. Divide between 6 bowls and garnish with coriander, onion and soured cream, if liked.

Serving size: 350ml (12fl oz)   Calories 355; Fat 11.1g (sat 3.6g, mono 5g, poly 0.9g); Cholesterol 49mg; Protein 27g; Carbohydrate 38g; Sugars 7g; Fibre 11g; RS 1.9g; Sodium 624mg

TIP:
Our perfectly sized Mini Corn and Feta Muffins are an ideal partner for this spicy chilli. Find the recipe on page 234.

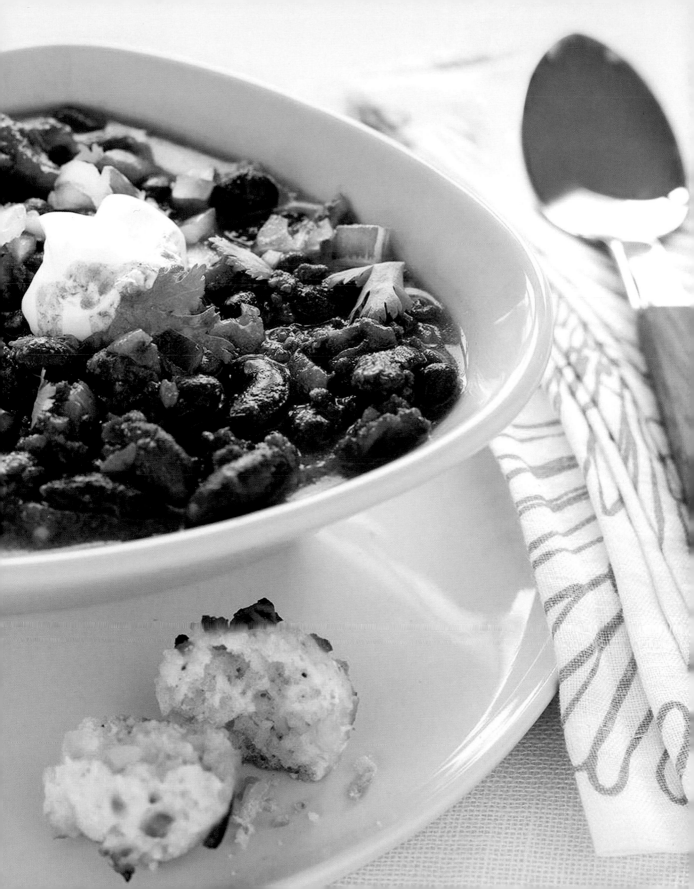

Chicken Noodle Soup with Autumn Vegetables

Prep: 5 minutes | **Cook:** 20 minutes | **Total time:** 25 minutes | **Makes:** 4 servings

Other than a hug from Mum, nothing makes you feel as good as a warm bowl of homemade chicken soup. This healthy variation gets a touch of sweetness from the parsnips and nutmeg.

1 tablespoon olive oil
1 garlic clove, finely chopped
1 small onion, chopped
1 celery stalk, cut into 1cm (½ inch) pieces
1 parsnip, halved and sliced crossways
1 carrot, halved and sliced crossways
1 litre (1¾ pints) reduced-sodium chicken broth
2 boneless, skinless chicken breasts (about 500g/1lb total)
¼ teaspoon sea salt
¼ teaspoon freshly ground black pepper
¼ teaspoon freshly grated nutmeg
4 sprigs fresh thyme
175g (6oz) wholewheat medium egg noodles

1. Heat oil in a large saucepan over medium-low heat. Add garlic, onion, celery, parsnip and carrot; cook, stirring occasionally, until vegetables are crisp-tender, 5–7 minutes. Add stock, chicken, salt, pepper, nutmeg and thyme. Bring to the boil; reduce heat to medium and simmer 10–15 minutes or until chicken is cooked through. Remove chicken; set aside.

2. Return stock mixture to the boil. Add noodles; simmer 5–8 minutes or until tender. Pull chicken apart into thin strips; return to soup and serve.

Serving size: 300ml (½ pint) Calories 343; Fat 8.7g (sat 1.6g, mono 4g, poly 1.4g); Cholesterol 103mg; Protein 31g; Carbohydrate 34g; Sugars 3g; Fibre 3g; RS 1.7g; Sodium 729mg

TIP:
Have a hot bowl of chicken soup ready in minutes by making extra and freezing it. Chill first, then place portions in freezer-safe containers. Thaw, heat and enjoy!

RS
0.6g

Apple, Gouda and Turkey Wrap with Bacon

Prep: *5 minutes* | ***Cook:*** *10 minutes* | ***Total time:*** *15 minutes* | ***Makes:*** *4 servings*

Crispy, sweet apples and salty Gouda cheese are a natural pairing. Add in some turkey and a little bacon, and you've got one delicious wrap

4 rashers bacon
4 (25cm/10 inch) wholemeal wraps
75g (3oz) Gouda, sliced
125g (4oz) thinly sliced roasted
  deli turkey
1 medium crisp apple (such as
  Gala), thinly sliced
50g (2oz) gourmet salad mix

1. Heat a large nonstick frying pan over medium heat; add bacon. Cook, turning often, until bacon is crispy, 6–8 minutes. Drain on kitchen paper, and set aside.

2. Arrange wraps on a clean work surface. Place ¼ of the cheese and turkey slices in the centre of each wrap. Top turkey with ¼ of the apple slices, 1 rasher of the cooled bacon and ¼ of the salad leaves; roll wraps, folding in sides, to enclose filling.

Serving size: 1 wrap Calories 256; Fat 12.5g (sat 4.9g, mono 4.6g, poly 1.5g); Cholesterol 43mg; Protein 23g; Carbohydrate 26g; Sugars 7g; Fibre 13g; RS 0.6g; Sodium 734mg

Chicken Parmesan Hero

Prep: 20 minutes | **Cook:** 30 minutes | **Total time:** 50 minutes | **Makes:** 4 servings

Zesty homemade marinara sauce, gooey cheese, and crispy chicken meld together in this dream of a sandwich. Save time by using shop-bought wholemeal bread crumbs.

4 slices wholemeal bread
¾ teaspoon paprika
½ teaspoon garlic powder
1 tablespoon olive oil
1 small onion, diced
2 garlic cloves, finely chopped
875g (1¾ lb) chopped tomatoes
65g (2½oz) plain flour
½ teaspoon black pepper
3 egg whites, whisked
4 (125–150g/4–5oz) boneless, skinless
  chicken breasts, pounded
  to ½-inch thickness
Olive oil cooking spray
2 wholegrain rolls (12–15cm/5–6 inches),
  split
50g (2oz) baby spinach leaves
75g (3oz) shredded semi-skimmed
  mozzarella cheese, grated

1. Preheat oven to 190°C/375°F/gas mark 5.

2. Process bread in a food processor until crumbs form, about 20 seconds. Toast crumbs on a baking sheet until golden, tossing occasionally, 7–8 minutes. Remove from oven and cool. Transfer to a shallow dish; toss with ½ teaspoon paprika and the garlic powder. Set aside.

3. Heat oil in a medium saucepan over medium-high heat. Add onion and cook until soft and translucent, 6–7 minutes. Add garlic and cook 1 minute. Add tomatoes and their juices and bring to the boil. Reduce heat and simmer until sauce thickens slightly, 10 minutes. Remove from heat; reserve. In a resealable plastic bag, combine flour, remaining paprika and pepper. Shake each piece of chicken in flour mixture, then dip in egg, then in reserved breadcrumbs, shaking off excess.

4. Place chicken in a baking dish and coat each side with cooking spray. Bake until cooked through and browned, about 12–13 minutes.

5. Place rolls on a baking sheet. Spoon about 4 tablespoons marinara sauce onto one side of a roll and top with ¼ of the spinach. Top with an escalope, an additional 4 tablespoons marinara sauce and 3 tablespoons mozzarella. Return to oven until cheese is melted, about 5 minutes.

Serving size: ½ roll, 8 tablespoons marinara sauce, 1 escalope, 15g (½oz) spinach leaves, 3 tablespoons mozzarella Calories 563; Fat 14.9g (sat 4.4g, mono 5.4g, poly 3.2g); Cholesterol 90mg; Protein 48g; Carbohydrate 58g; Sugars 5g; Fibre 11g; RS 0.8g; Sodium 552mg

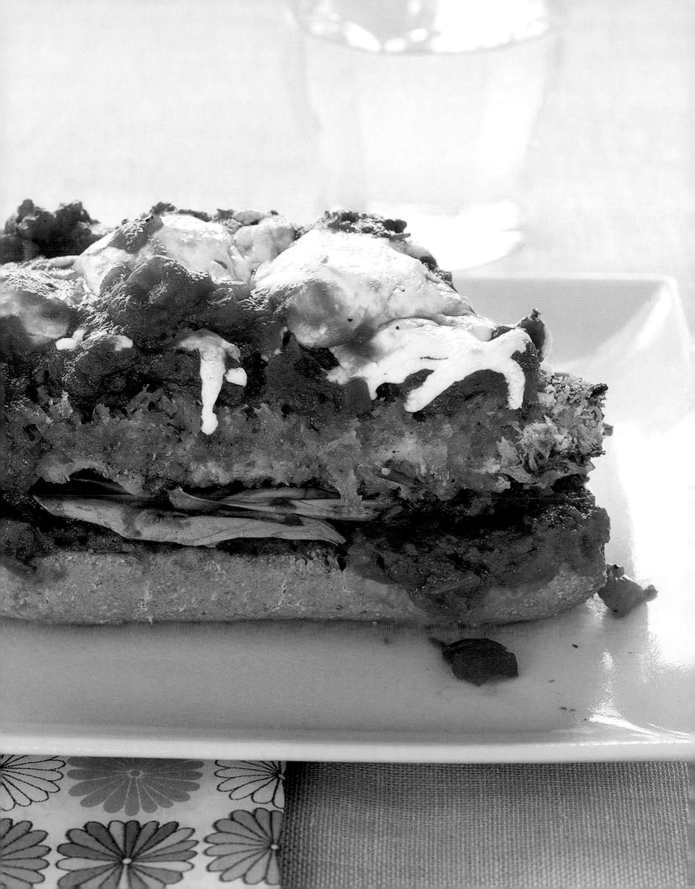

CarbLovers Club Sandwich

Prep: *15 minutes* | **Cook:** *10 minutes* | **Total time:** *25 minutes* | **Makes:** *4 servings*

Bite into the amazing combination of creamy avocado, salty bacon and cool tomato. Perfection on a plate!

175g (6oz) canned reduced-salt
  cannellini beans, rinsed and drained
2 roasted garlic cloves
1 tablespoon olive oil
¼ teaspoon salt
¼ teaspoon pepper
12 thin slices wholemeal bread,
  toasted
8 leaves round lettuce
1 beefsteak tomato, sliced
1 avocado, stoned and sliced
8 rashers turkey bacon, cooked
  according to packet instructions
  and drained on kitchen paper

1. Mash beans, garlic, oil, salt and pepper with a fork and reserve.

2. Arrange 4 bread slices on a work surface. Spread 3 tablespoons white-bean mixture on each slice of bread.

3. Top with 2 lettuce leaves and 2 tomato slices.

4. Layer another slice of bread on each sandwich, and top each with 4 avocado slices and 2 turkey bacon slices. Top with last piece of bread.

5. Halve sandwiches diagonally, and secure with cocktail sticks.

Serving size: 1 sandwich Calories 412; Fat 17.5g (sat 2.4g, mono 10.1g, poly 3.6g); Cholesterol 14mg; Protein 16g; Carbohydrate 47g; Sugars 5g; Fibre 12g; RS 2.2g; Sodium 572mg

TIP:
Make extra bean spread when you're whipping up this sandwich, and use it as a dip for fresh vegetables and tortilla chips.

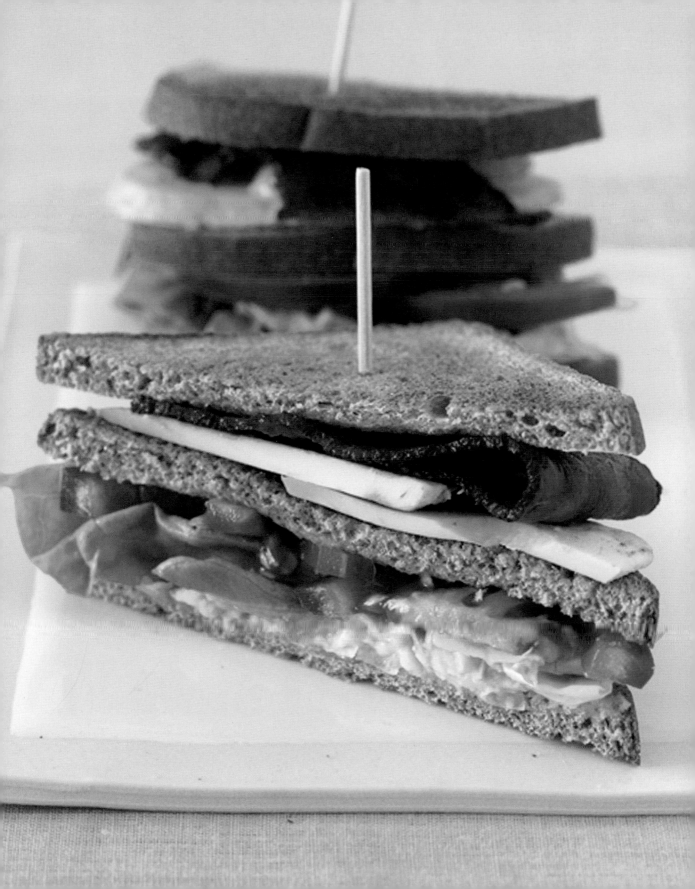

Stacked Deli Sandwiches with Homemade Coleslaw

Prep: *5 minutes* | **Cook:** *15 minutes* | **Total time:** *20 minutes* | **Makes:** *4 servings*

These impressive (and Resistant Starch-loaded!) sandwiches are stacked to the hilt with tasty ingredients. Serve them at your next book club meeting or picnic.

FOR RUSSIAN DRESSING:

3 tablespoons light mayonnaise
3 tablespoons reduced-fat soured cream
1 tablespoon ketchup
1 teaspoon red wine vinegar
1 teaspoon chopped dill pickles

FOR COLESLAW:

300g (10oz) bagged coleslaw mix
250g (8oz) red cabbage, shredded
2 tablespoons cider vinegar
1 tablespoon vegetable oil
2 teaspoons lightly toasted
  caraway seeds
2 teaspoons Dijon mustard

FOR SANDWICHES:

8 (40g/1½oz) slices dark
  pumpernickel bread
175g (6oz) thinly sliced roast beef
175g (6oz) thinly sliced fresh roasted
  turkey breast
4 (15g/½oz) slices reduced-fat
  Emmental cheese
1 large beefsteak tomato, cut into 8
  slices

MAKE RUSSIAN DRESSING:

1. Whisk together mayonnaise, soured cream, ketchup, red wine vinegar and pickles in a small bowl; reserve.

MAKE COLESLAW:

2. Toss coleslaw mix, cabbage, cider vinegar, oil, caraway seeds, and mustard in a large bowl; reserve.

MAKE SANDWICHES:

3. Spread about 1 tablespoon Russian dressing on each slice of bread. Top 4 slices with 40g (1½ oz) roast beef and a tomato slice. Add 40g (1½ oz) turkey, then another tomato slice. Top with cheese. Finish with second slice of bread, dressing side down. Serve with 65g (2½ oz) coleslaw, either on the sandwich or alongside (you'll have some left over).

Serving size: 1 sandwich plus about 65g (2½ oz) coleslaw Calories 497; Fat 15g (sat 4.8g, mono 3.4g, poly 4.5g); Cholesterol 76mg; Protein 36g; Carbohydrate 56g; Sugars 15g; Fibre 6g; RS 6.9g; Sodium 744mg

> **TIP:**
> If you're packing these for a picnic or road trip, leave off the coleslaw and dressing. Add to the sandwiches before serving.

RS 1g

Curried Tuna Salad Sandwiches

Prep: *15 minutes* | ***Total time:*** *15 minutes* | ***Makes:*** *4 servings*

Spice up ordinary tuna with a hint of curry and the unexpected sweetness of sultanas.

4 tablespoons light mayonnaise
1½ teaspoons curry powder
¼ teaspoon salt
½ teaspoon pepper
2 x 150g (5oz) cans water-packed light
   tuna, drained
2 stalks celery, chopped
75g (3oz) water chestnuts, chopped
3 tablespoons finely minced red onion
3 tablespoons sultanas
4 lettuce leaves
8 tomato slices
8 slices wholemeal bread, toasted

1. Whisk together mayonnaise, curry powder, salt and pepper in a medium bowl. Add tuna, celery, water chestnuts, onion and sultanas and mix well.

2. Place a lettuce leaf and 2 tomato slices on a piece of toasted bread. Add about 10 tablespoons tuna mixture and top with another slice of bread. Serve immediately.

Serving size: 1 sandwich Calories 433; Fat 10.8g (sat 1.7g, mono 2.5g, poly 5.7g); Cholesterol 27mg; Protein 27g; Carbohydrate 60g; Sugars 10g; Fibre 8g; RS 1g; Sodium 621mg

Falafel Pitta with Tahini Sauce

Prep: *15 minutes* | **Cook:** *10 minutes* | **Total time:** *25 minutes* | **Makes:** *6 servings*

Even meat eaters will love these veggie burgers! The patties are a spin on falafel, but instead of deep-frying, we give them a light pan-fry. And since the recipe takes less than 30 minutes, it's great for a quick and tasty weeknight meal.

65g (2½oz) uncooked bulgar
250ml (8fl oz) boiling water
475g (15oz) can chickpeas,
  rinsed and drained
1 large egg white
8 tablespoons parsley leaves
4 tablespoons mint leaves
1 garlic clove, roughly chopped
¼ teaspoon cayenne pepper
1 teaspoon ground cumin
¼ teaspoon salt
¼ teaspoon pepper
1 tablespoon olive oil
4 tablespoons tahini
2 tablespoons fresh lemon juice
6 (15cm/6 inch) pittas
300g (10oz) torn lettuce
3 roasted red peppers

1. Combine bulgar and boiling water in a medium bowl. Cover and let stand 10 minutes or until just warm; drain. Transfer to a food processor with chickpeas, egg white, parsley, mint, garlic, cayenne, cumin, salt and pepper. Form mixture into 6 (approximately 7cm/3 inch) patties and place on a large plate. Refrigerate 20 minutes or until firm.

2. Heat oil in a large nonstick frying pan over medium-high heat. Cook falafels until browned and heated through, 3 minutes per side. Transfer to a plate.

3. Whisk together tahini, lemon juice and 4 tablespoons water in a medium bowl until light and fluffy. Serve in pittas with lettuce, roasted red peppers, and falafels.

Serving size: 1 burger, 2 tablespoons tahini mixture
Calories 396; Fat 10g (sat 1.4g, mono 4g, poly 3.6g);
Cholesterol 0mg; Protein 15g; Carbohydrate 64g; Sugars 5g;
Fibre 10g; RS 2.4g; Sodium 602mg

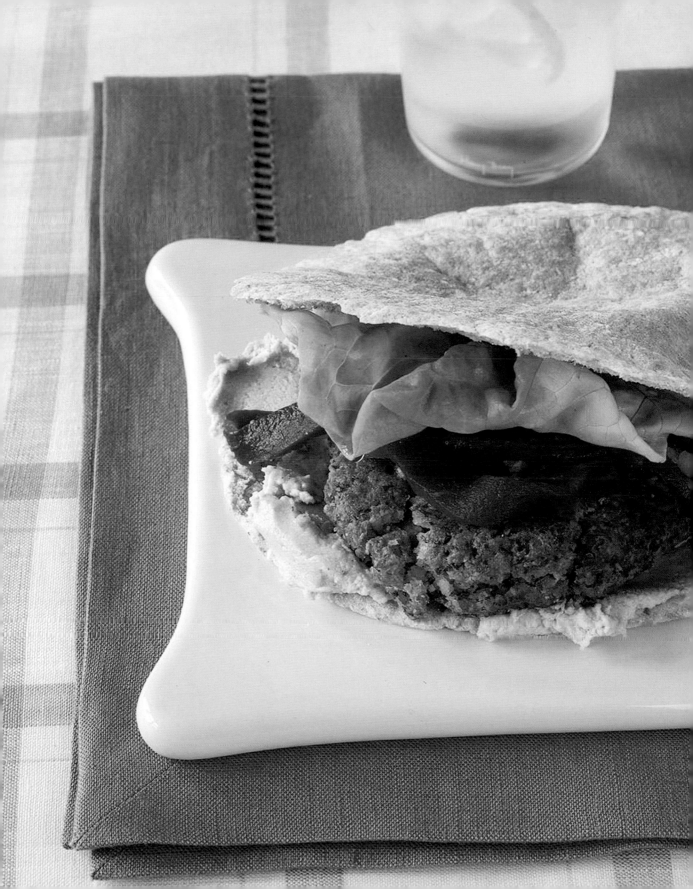

Teriyaki Steak Sandwich

Prep: 20 minutes | **Cook:** 15 minutes | **Total time:** 35 minutes | **Makes:** 4 servings

Looking for a sandwich with a bit more flair? This is it! The delicious teriyaki flavour makes this great for lunch or dinner, and the 26 grams of protein and 15 grams of fibre will keep you satisfied for hours.

FOR TERIYAKI SAUCE:

2 tablespoons low-sodium soy sauce
3 tablespoons light brown sugar
1 tablespoon finely chopped fresh ginger
2 teaspoons finely chopped garlic
1 teaspoon cornflour
1 teaspoon sesame oil
½ teaspoon chilli-garlic sauce (such as Sriracha)

FOR SANDWICH:

4 teaspoons vegetable oil
375g (12oz) lean sirloin steak, very thinly sliced
2 bunches spring onions, trimmed, cut into 5cm (2 inch) lengths, whites and greens separated
175g (6oz) shiitake mushrooms, sliced
125g (4oz) mangetout
4 x 25cm (10 inch) wholemeal wraps

MAKE TERIYAKI SAUCE:

1. Whisk together soy sauce, 4 tablespoons water, sugar, ginger, garlic, cornflour, sesame oil and chilli-garlic sauce in a bowl. Reserve.

MAKE SANDWICH:

2. Heat 2 teaspoons oil in a large frying pan over medium-high heat. Add steak and cook until browned and just cooked through, 2–3 minutes per side. Transfer steak (with its juices) to a bowl. Add remaining 2 teaspoons oil to pan, then add spring onion whites and cook, stirring, until charred, 2 minutes. Add mushrooms and cook until softened, 3–4 minutes. Return beef to pan, add spring onion greens, mangetout and teriyaki sauce and cook until heated through and entire mixture is thickened, 2–3 minutes.

3. Place about 175ml (6fl oz) mixture in middle of wrap and wrap tightly. Slice in half and serve warm.

Serving size: 1 wrap and 175ml (6fl oz) mixture Calories 342; Fat 15.1g (sat 2.8g, mono 5.3g, poly 4.9g); Cholesterol 41mg; Protein 26g; Carbohydrate 39g; Sugars 15g; Fibre 15g; RS 0.6g; Sodium 640mg

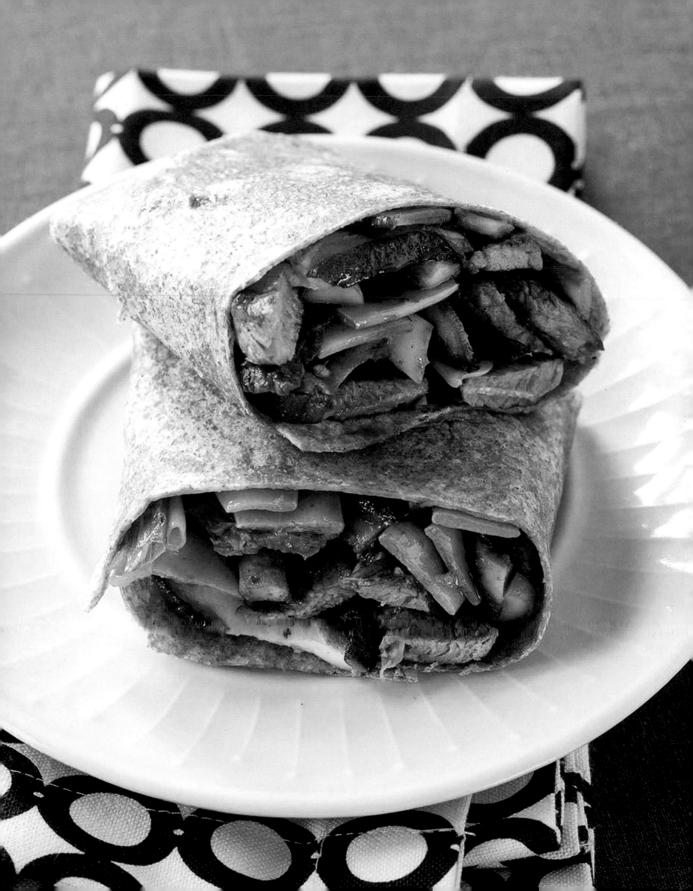

Roast Beef Pumpernickel Sandwich with Roasted Red Pepper, Rocket and Goats' Cheese

Prep: *10 minutes* | **Total time:** *10 minutes* | **Makes:** *4 servings*

Juicy deli sandwiches have probably been on your "no-no" list for years. Ours lets you indulge without the bulge, and has almost 3 grams of Resistant Starch!

75g (3oz) goats' cheese, softened
8 slices pumpernickel bread
4 lettuce leaves
375g (12oz) thinly sliced lean roast beef
4 roasted red peppers from a jar
 (50g/2oz each), rinsed, drained, patted
 dry and halved
4 teaspoons balsamic vinegar

1. Spread the cheese on 4 slices of bread.

2. Arrange 1 lettuce leaf on each cheese-topped bread slice, then layer each with ¼ of the roast beef.

3. Top with red peppers, drizzle with vinegar and cover with remaining bread slices. Serve.

Serving size: 1 sandwich Calories 380; Fat 11.4g (sat 5.1g, mono 3.7g, poly 1.1g); Cholesterol 74mg; Protein 33g; Carbohydrate 38g; Sugars 3g; Fibre 4g; RS 2.9g; Sodium 653mg

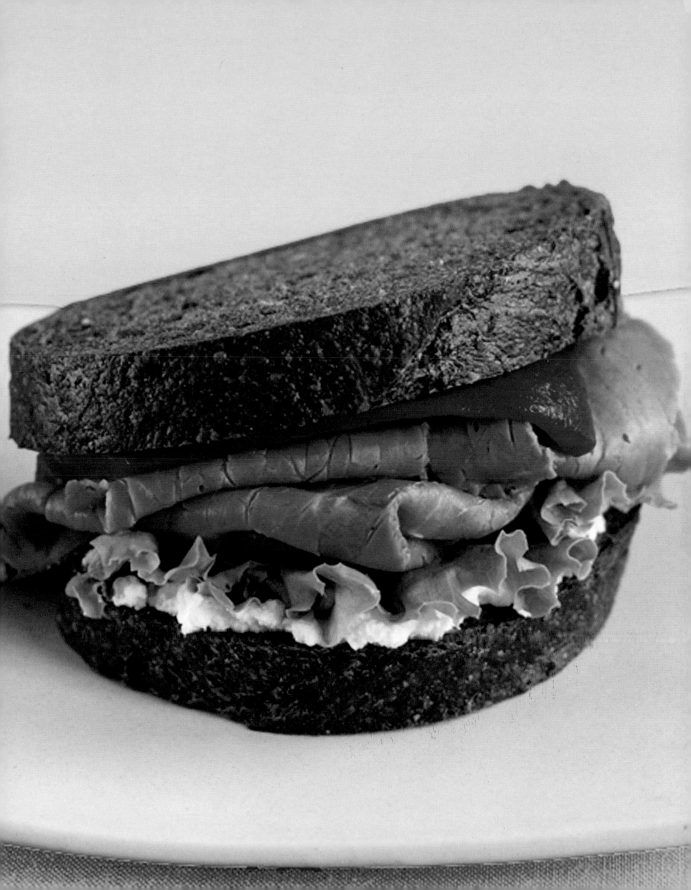

Tuna and White Bean Crostino

Prep: *2 minutes* | **Cook:** *3 minutes* | **Total time:** *5 minutes* | **Makes:** *4 servings*

Got 5 minutes? Then you can whip up this tasty, Resistant Starch-packed crostino.

150g (5oz) can tuna in olive oil,
 drained and flaked
475g (15oz) can cannellini beans,
 drained
1 tablespoon chopped parsley
2 tablespoons fresh lemon juice
¼ teaspoon sea salt
¼ teaspoon freshly ground black
pepper
4 slices wholemeal rustic bread
 (about 50g/2oz each)
50 g(2oz) Fontina cheese, coarsely
 grated

Preheat grill with rack in highest position. Stir together tuna, beans, parsley, lemon juice, salt and pepper in a medium bowl. Arrange bread on a baking sheet; divide tuna salad between bread slices. Top crostino with cheese; grill until golden, 2–3 minutes.

Serving size: 1 crostino Calories 394; Fat 10.7g (sat 3.8g, mono 3g, poly 3g); Cholesterol 23mg; Protein 26g; Carbohydrate 50g; Sugars 3g; Fibre 8g; RS 3.9; Sodium 754mg

> **TIP:**
> Convert this from a lunch to a starter
> by using slices of toasted baguette.
> Mash the beans for a creamier texture.

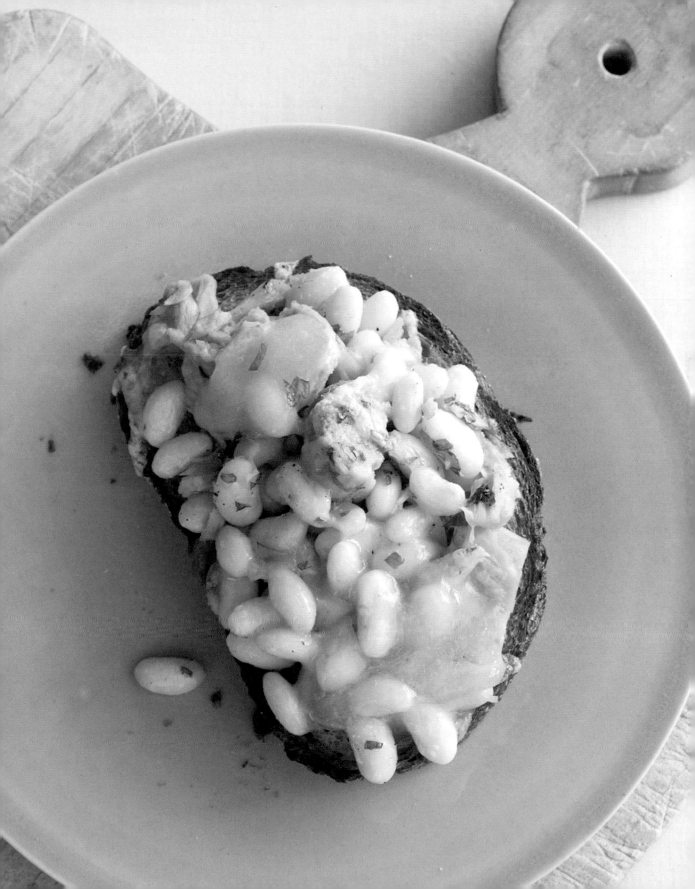

RS
2.7g

Black Bean, Avocado, Brown Rice and Chicken Wrap

Prep: 15 minutes | **Total time:** 15 minutes | **Makes:** 4 servings

Superfast and satisfying, this wrap is one of our favourites. It's also great for a make-your-own-burrito night with the kids. Just put all the ingredients in little bowls, and let them get creative.

½ teaspoon salt
¼ teaspoon freshly ground black pepper
375g (11oz) reduced-salt black beans, rinsed and drained
1 teaspoon chilli powder
½ teaspoon cumin
¼ teaspoon dried chilli flakes
4 (25cm/10 inch) wholemeal wraps
175g (6oz) cooked brown rice
250g (8oz) grilled chicken breast, sliced
1 small carrot, grated
½ avocado, stoned and diced
Hot sauce for serving (optional)
1 plum tomato, deseeded and chopped (½ cup)

1. Place salt, pepper, beans, chilli powder, cumin and chilli flakes in a small bowl and toss to combine.

2. Place one wrap on a clean work surface. Spoon 5 tablespoons rice onto bottom of wrap. Add 5 tablespoons bean mixture, 50g (2oz) chicken and ¼ cup of the carrot, then top with about 1 tablespoon avocado and 2 tablespoons tomato.

3. Seal wrap, slice in half and serve immediately with hot sauce on the side, if desired.

Serving size: 1 wrap Calories 425; Fat 9g (sat 1.3g, mono 3.4g, poly 1.2g); Cholesterol 48mg; Protein 31g; Carbohydrate 60g; Sugars 7g; Fibre 12g; RS 2.7g; Sodium 636mg

ASK CARBLOVERS

Q: I am a vegetarian. How do I modify the *CarbLovers* diet to fit my needs?

A: Since it's mainly built around grains, beans and vegetables, *CarbLovers* is perfect for vegetarians. And you can always make tweaks to recipes like the one above, substituting firm tofu for the chicken, or adding a side of beans to grain dishes.

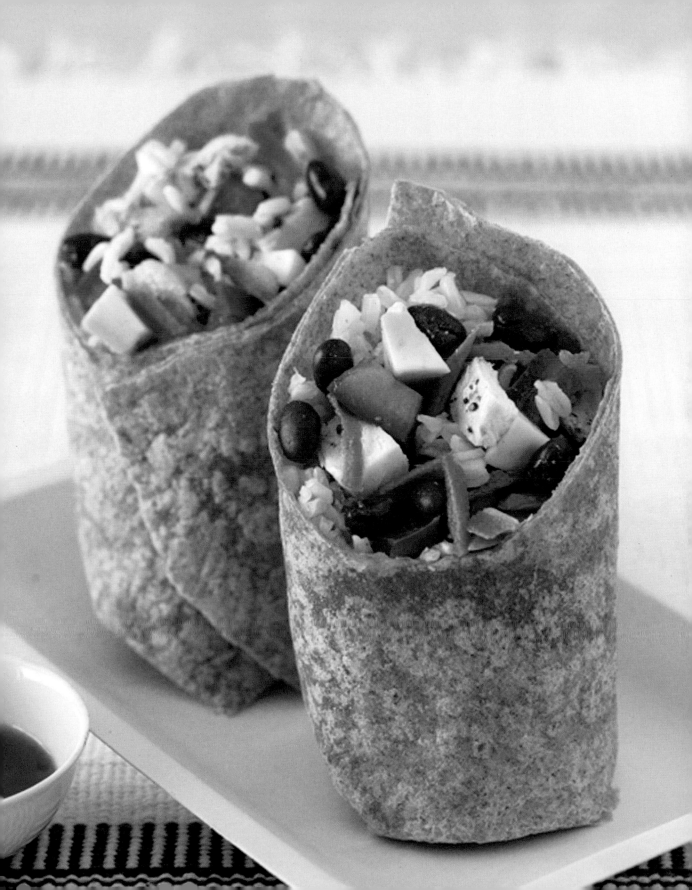

Roasted Corn and Black Bean Burrito

Prep: *10 minutes* | **Cook:** *5 minutes* | **Total time:** *15 minutes* | **Makes:** *4 servings*

Black beans are an amazing source of Resistant Starch and fibre (this recipe has 20 grams!). But not only is this burrito filling and healthy, it's also packed with flavour from the fresh lime juice and coriander.

175g (6oz) sweetcorn kernels, thawed
  and patted dry
475g (15oz) can black beans,
  rinsed and drained
4 tablespoons finely diced red onion
¼ teaspoon chipotle chilli powder
1 tablespoon fresh lime juice
1 teaspoon olive oil
4 tablespoons chopped fresh coriander
¼ teaspoon salt
¼ teaspoon pepper
4 x 25 cm(10 inch) wholemeal tortillas
125g (4oz) hot cooked white rice
75g (3oz) shredded romaine lettuce
50g (2oz) Monterey Jack or Cheddar
  cheese, grated

1. Heat a large cast-iron or other heavy frying pan over high heat until very hot, 3 minutes. Add sweetcorn; cook, stirring occasionally, until charred, about 3 minutes. Remove from heat and toss with next 8 ingredients (through to pepper).

2. Spread 4 tablespoons cooked rice over the bottom half of a tortilla, leaving a 2.5cm (1 inch) border. Top rice with generous 8 tablespoons corn and bean mixture, ¼ of the shredded lettuce and 2 tablespoons cheese; roll up. Repeat with remaining ingredients. Slice each burrito in half, and serve.

Serving size: 1 burrito with 8 tablespoons corn and bean mixture Calories 331; Fat 9.3g (sat 3g, mono 3.7g, poly 1.6g); Cholesterol 13mg; Protein 21g; Carbohydrate 56g; Sugars 3g; Fibre 20g; RS 2.3g; Sodium 705mg

{
TIP:
Boost the Resistant Starch in
this recipe even higher by using
brown rice instead of white.
}

Saucy Turkey Meatball Sub

RS 1.1g

Prep: 25 minutes | **Cook:** 25 minutes | ***Total time:*** *50 minutes* | **Makes:** *4 servings*

We've taken a huge diet no-no and turned it into a "Yes, please!" This sub sandwich will satisfy even your most die-hard meat eaters. Serve with plenty of napkins.

475ml (16fl oz) marinara sauce
500g (1lb) minced turkey
4 tablespoons fresh breadcrumbs
50g (3oz) Pecorino Romano cheese, grated
½ carrot, finely grated
4 tablespoons finely chopped onion
2 garlic cloves, finely chopped
3 tablespoons chopped parsley
2 tablespoons ketchup
¼ teaspoon salt
¼ teaspoon pepper
Cooking spray
4 wholemeal hot dog rolls, split and lightly toasted

1. Place marinara sauce in a medium saucepan and keep warm on low.

2. Combine turkey, breadcrumbs, ½ the cheese, the carrot, onion, garlic, parsley, ketchup, salt and pepper in a bowl and mix with clean hands until well incorporated. Using slightly wet hands, form into 16 equal-sized meatballs. Heat a large nonstick frying pan coated with cooking spray over medium-high heat; brown meatballs on all sides, about 5–6 minutes.

3. Add meatballs to sauce, increase heat to medium, and simmer until meatballs have absorbed some of the sauce and are heated through, 10–15 minutes. Spoon 4 meatballs and some sauce onto a roll and sprinkle with ¼ of the remaining cheese.

Serving size: 1 sub Calories 431; Fat 15g (sat 4.4g, mono 3g, poly 2.5g); Cholesterol 88mg; Protein 34g; Carbohydrate 43g; Sugars 12g; Fibre 5g; RS 1.1g; Sodium 1,131mg

TIP:
If you're on a low-sodium diet, use no-salt-added marinara and skip the cheese and added salt.

Grilled Cheese and Tomato on Rye

Prep: 5 minutes | *Cook:* 6 minutes | *Total time:* 11 minutes | *Makes:* 4 servings

Sometimes the simplest ingredients can be the most satisfying. That's the case with this toasty spin on grilled cheese. Enjoy it with a piece of fresh fruit for a filling lunch.

Cooking spray
2 tablespoons wholegrain mustard
8 slices rye bread
250g (8oz) reduced-fat Cheddar
  cheese, sliced
1 beefsteak tomato, sliced

1. Heat a large nonstick frying pan coated with cooking spray over medium-high heat.

2. Spread ½ tablespoon mustard on each of 4 slices of bread, then top each with 2 slices cheese and 1 slice tomato. Top with remaining bread slices.

3. Place sandwiches in pan; place another pan on top of the sandwiches.

4. Cook until bottoms of sandwiches are browned, 2–3 minutes. Flip and cook, 2–3 minutes, until bread is golden and cheese is melted.

Serving size: 1 sandwich Calories 328; Fat 12.5g (sat 6.6g, mono 3.6g, poly 0.9g); Cholesterol 32mg; Protein 22g; Carbohydrate 31g; Sugars 4g; Fibre 3g; RS 1.8g; Sodium 851mg

ASK CARBLOVERS

Q: I love bread! What kinds can I eat on *CarbLovers*?

A: You can enjoy rye, pumpernickel, sourdough and wholemeal bread on *CarbLovers*. Make sure the first ingredient listed is "whole" rye, wheat, etc., and look for 3 grams of fibre per slice.

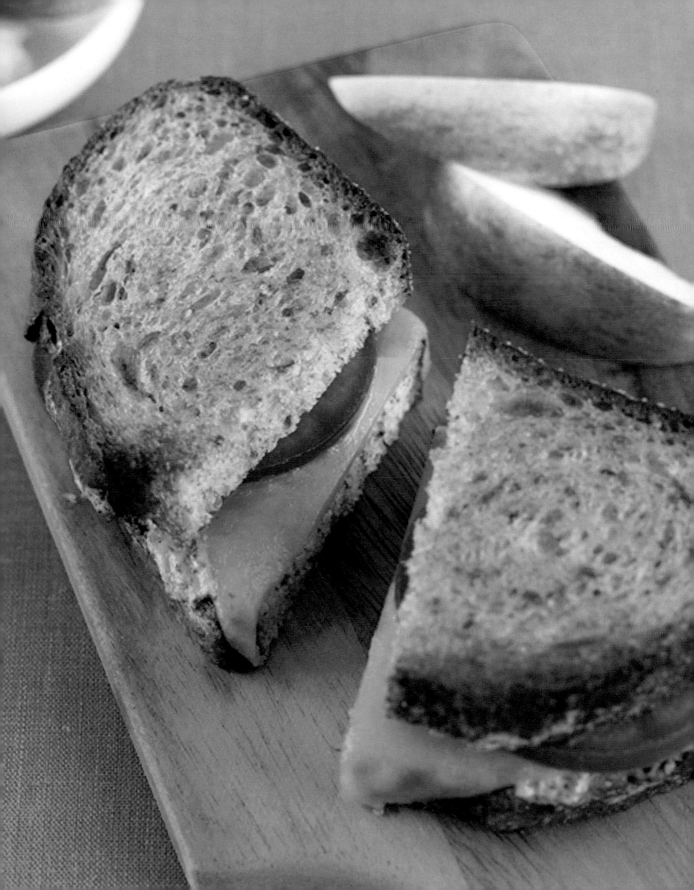

RS
3g

Banana-Nut Elvis Wrap

Prep: 5 minutes | **Total time:** 5 minutes | **Makes:** 4 servings

Elvis Presley was famous for eating a fried version of this sandwich. We skipped the King's melted butter and bacon and went with a wholemeal wrap, but the PB and bananas make for a yummy combo.

8 tablespoons chunky natural-style
  peanut butter
4 x 15cm (6 inch) wholemeal wraps
2 large bananas, sliced
8 teaspoons honey

1. Spread 2 tablespoons peanut butter on bottom third of each wrap, leaving a 5cm (2 inch) border on each side.

2. Top each wrap with ½ banana and about 2 teaspoons honey.

3. Roll up wrap, cut in half and serve immediately.

Serving size: 1 wrap Calories 372; Fat 18.2g (sat 2.7g, mono 7.9g, poly 4.8g); Cholesterol 0mg; Protein 11g; Carbohydrate 46g; Sugars 23g; Fibre 12g; RS 3g; Sodium 247mg

Pan Bagnat

Prep: *15 minutes* | ***Total time:*** *15 minutes* | ***Makes:*** *4 servings*

This sandwich reflects the flavours of a traditional niçoise salad, and also hails from the French city of Nice. We love the briny combination of the olives, mustard and tuna.

3 tablespoons light mayonnaise
2 tablespoons finely chopped pitted
niçoise olives
3 teaspoons Dijon mustard
2 teaspoons red wine vinegar
½ teaspoon black pepper
60cm (24 inch) French baguette, sliced
  into 4 pieces, then halved
4 red-leaf lettuce leaves
2 medium vine-ripened tomatoes,
  each cut into 6 slices
2 hard-boiled eggs, each cut into
  6 slices
1 small red onion, cut into 8 rings
2 medium red-skinned potatoes,
  cooked and cooled, each cut into
  4 slices
2 x 200g (7oz) cans oil-packed tuna,
well drained

1. Whisk together mayonnaise, olives, mustard, vinegar and pepper until smooth; chill until ready to use.

2. Spread about 2¼ teaspoons of the mayo mixture on each side of bread. Layer 1 lettuce leaf, 3 tomato slices, 3 egg slices, 2 onion rings, 2 potato slices and about 75g (3oz) of tuna on bottom half of bread. Top with other bread half, slice in half on the diagonal and serve.

Serving size: 1 sandwich Calories 507; Fat 14.1g (sat 2.9g, mono 4.8g, poly 5.2g); Cholesterol 108mg; Protein 34g; Carbohydrate 61g; Sugars 5g; Fibre 4g; RS 1.8g; Sodium 746mg

Pasta & Pizza

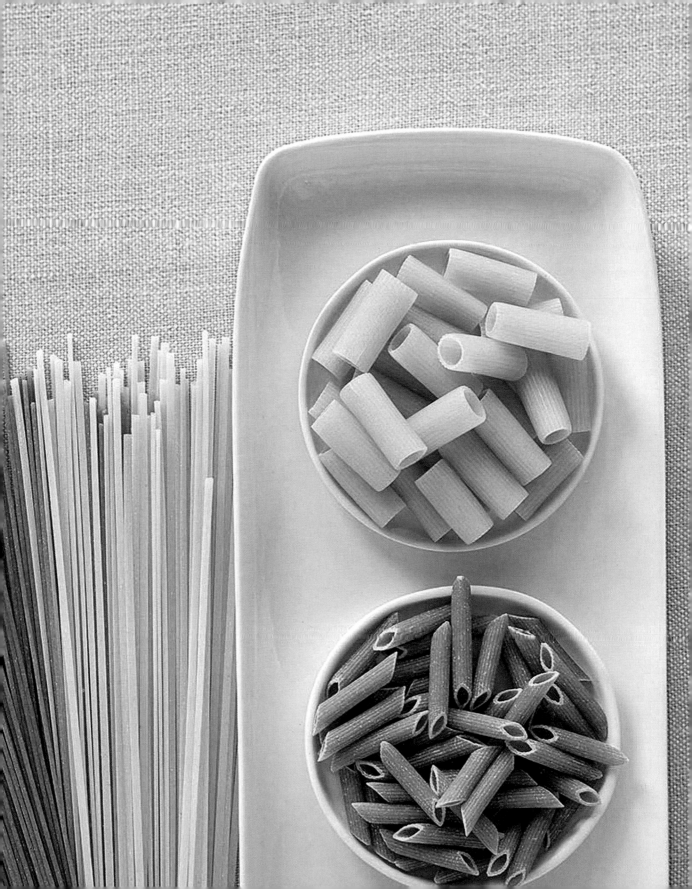

RS 0.6g

Pasta Primavera

Prep: 25 minutes | *Cook:* 30 minutes | *Total time:* 55 minutes | *Makes:* 4 servings

This delightful pasta is as gorgeous on the plate as it is delicious. We love the whimsical bow-tie shape, but feel free to substitute any pasta.

1 tablespoon olive oil
1 small onion, sliced
3 garlic cloves, thinly sliced
250g (8oz) small multicoloured cherry tomatoes
750ml (1¼ pints) 1% fat milk
3 tablespoons flour
½ teaspoon salt
½ teaspoon pepper
250g (8oz) farfalle (bow-tie) pasta
3 small carrots (175g/6oz), peeled and diced
250g (8oz) thin asparagus, trimmed and cut into 5cm (2 inch) pieces
1 small courgette, halved and cut into 5cm (2 inch) matchsticks
4 tablespoons basil leaves
50g (2oz) Parmesan cheese, finely grated

1. Bring a large pan of water to the boil.

2. While water is heating, heat oil in a large nonstick frying pan over medium-high heat.

3. Add onion and cook, stirring, until soft, 6–7 minutes. Add garlic and cook 1 minute. Add tomatoes and cook (do not stir) until slightly bursting, 5 minutes.

4. Whisk together milk and flour and add to vegetables. Bring mixture to the boil; reduce heat and simmer. Stir until thickened, 2–3 minutes. Add salt and pepper, stir to incorporate, remove from heat and cover with foil to keep warm.

5. Cook pasta according to packet instructions. During last 3 minutes of cooking, add carrots to boiling pasta. During last minute of cooking, add asparagus and courgette.

6. Drain pasta and vegetables (do not rinse); add immediately to warmed vegetable-cream sauce.

7. Toss gently and divide between 4 pasta bowls.

8. Divide basil and Parmesan between the bowls.

Serving size: 300g (10oz) pasta and 2 tablespoons cheese Calories 286; Fat 7.2g (sat 2.5g, mono 3.4g, poly 0.8g); Cholesterol 12mg; Protein 14g; Carbohydrate 43g; Sugars 15g; Fibre 5g; RS 0.6g; Sodium 473mg

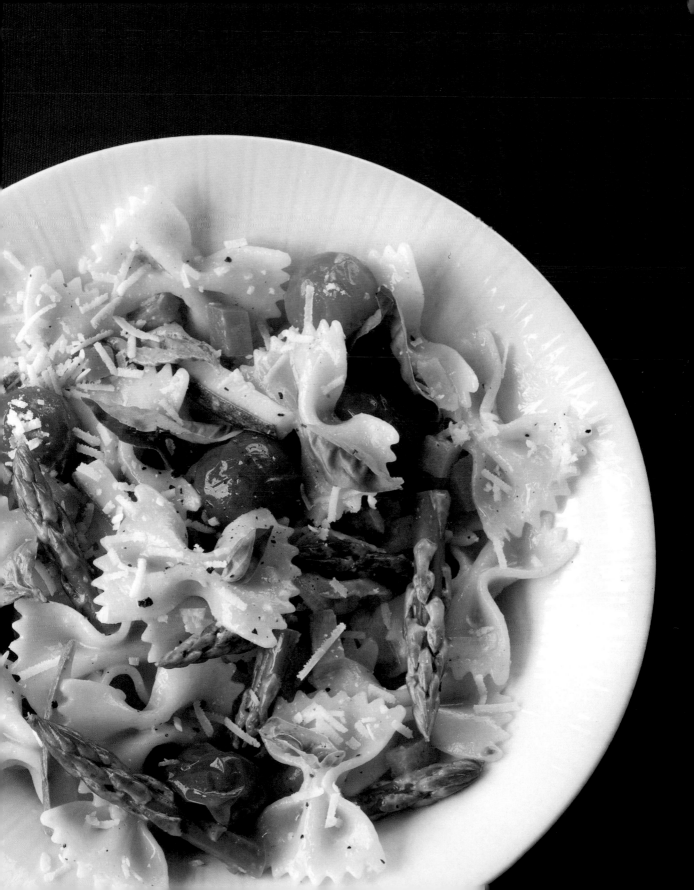

Ultimate Spinach and Turkey Lasagne

Prep: 25 minutes | **Cook:** 1 hour 15 minutes | **Total time:** 1 hour 40 minutes | **Makes:** 9 servings

Cheesy, meaty and unbelievably good, this saucy lasagne is a real crowd-pleaser. Serve it with a crisp green salad.

1 tablespoon olive oil

1 medium onion, chopped

2 garlic cloves, finely chopped

375g (12oz) minced turkey breast

750ml (1¼ pints) low-sodium marinara sauce

375g (12oz) semi-skimmed ricotta cheese

300g (10oz) frozen spinach, completely defrosted and squeezed of all excess liquid

4 tablespoons chopped parsley

2 egg whites

¼ teaspoon salt

¼ teaspoon pepper

12 lasagne sheet, cooked al dente according to packet instructions

50g (2oz) semi-skimmed mozzarella cheese, grated

4 tablespoons grated Parmesan cheese

1. Preheat oven to 190°C/375°F/gas mark 5.

2. Heat oil in a large high-sided sauté pan and cook onion, stirring occasionally, until softened, 6–7 minutes. Add garlic and cook 1 minute. Add turkey and cook, breaking up with a spoon, until no longer pink and cooked through, 4–5 minutes. Add marinara, bring to the boil, reduce heat and simmer 2–3 minutes. Remove pan from heat and cool slightly.

3. Combine ricotta, spinach, parsley, egg whites, salt and pepper in a large bowl.

4. Coat the bottom of a 35 x 28cm (14 x 11 inch) lasagne dish with 8 tablespoons sauce. Arrange three lasagne sheets on the bottom of the dish. Spread 12 tablespoons sauce evenly over the pasta. Spoon 10 tablespoons ricotta-spinach mixture evenly on top of sauce. Repeat layers two more times.

5. Cover top with three lasagne sheets and remaining sauce. Sprinkle with mozzarella and Parmesan. Cover loosely with foil and bake for 45 minutes. Remove foil and bake 10–15 minutes, until cheese is bubbly. Cut into 9 squares and serve.

Serving size: 1 (10 by 7 cm/4 by 3 inch) piece Calories 346; Fat 11.3g (sat 4.3g, mono 3.7g, poly 1.5g); Cholesterol 44mg; Protein 23g; Carbohydrate 38g; Sugars 5g; Fibre 4g; RS 1g; Sodium 321mg

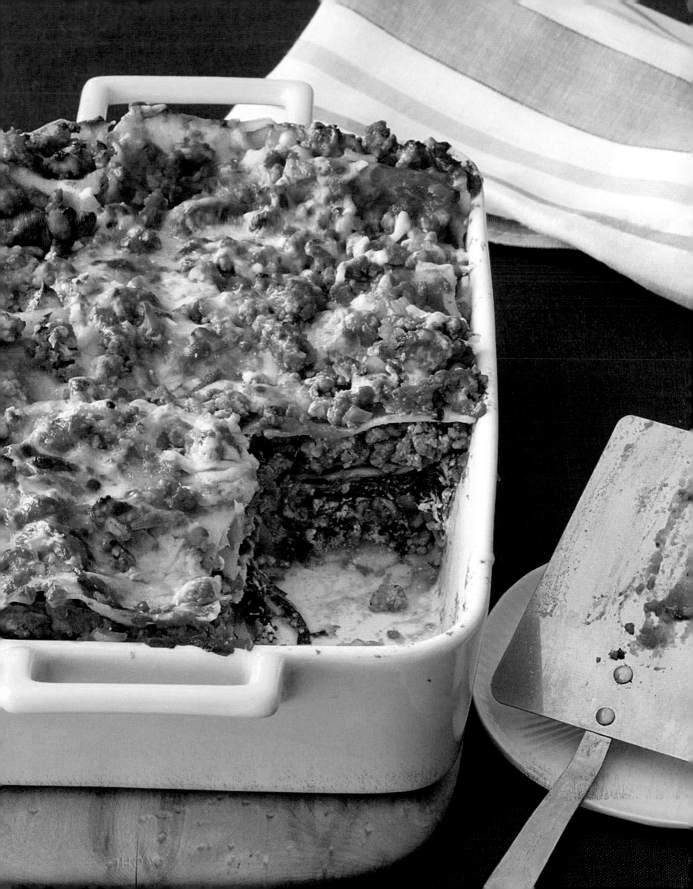

RS
2.2g

Spaghetti and Clams

Prep: *5 minutes* | **Cook:** *20 minutes* | **Total time**: *25 minutes* | **Makes:** *4 servings*

Clams have a wonderful sweet-briny flavour and add a touch of sophistication for very few calories. They're also a good source of iron.

250g (8oz) wholewheat spaghetti
15g (½oz) unsalted butter
1 garlic clove, thinly sliced
1kg (2lb) clams, scrubbed
¼ teaspoon dried chilli flakes
1 tablespoon fresh lemon juice
1 tablespoon grated Parmesan
  cheese

1. Cook spaghetti according to packet instructions. Reserve 125ml (4fl oz) of the cooking water before draining. Drain pasta and set aside.

2. Melt butter in a large frying pan over medium heat. Add garlic and cook 1 minute.

3. Add clams, chilli flakes, lemon juice and the reserved cooking water; stir gently to combine. Cover and simmer until clams open and release their juices, about 6 minutes. Use tongs to transfer clams to a bowl.

4. Add cooked pasta and Parmesan to the pan with sauce. Cook, tossing, 3 minutes or until slightly thickened. Divide the pasta and clams between 4 shallow bowls and serve.

Serving size: About 300g (10oz) Calories 276; Fat 4.8g (sat 2.3g, mono 1g, poly 0.7g); Cholesterol 32mg; Protein 18g; Carbohydrate 44g; Sugars 1g; Fibre 4g; RS 2.2g; Sodium 208mg

> **TIP:**
> When buying fresh, live clams, make sure they are closed. Open clams should be discarded.

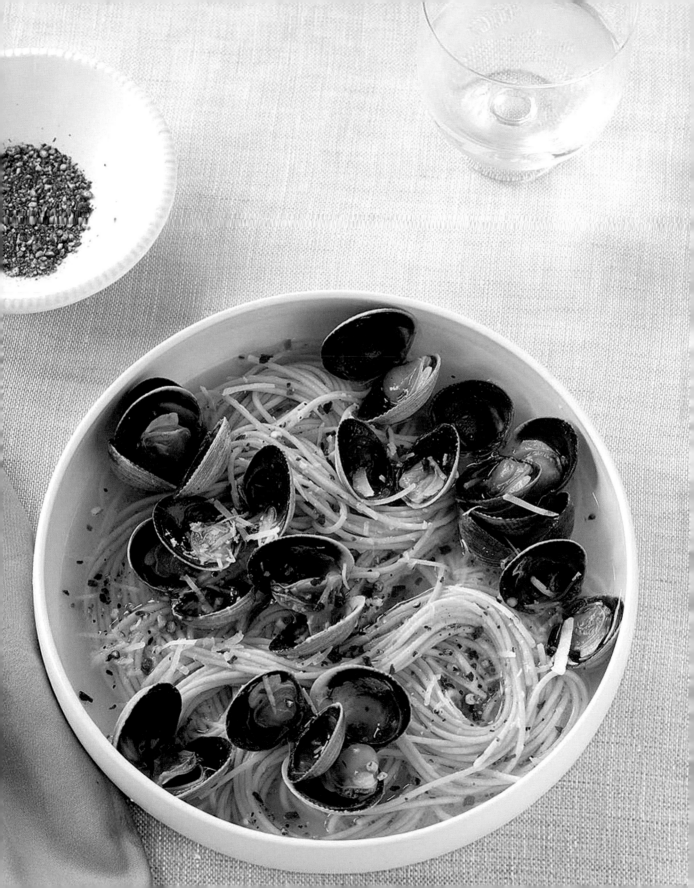

RS
1.8g

Individual Baked Macaroni Cheese

Prep: 10 minutes | **Cook:** *45 minutes* | **Total time:** *1 hour 5 minutes* | **Makes:** *6 servings*

What's better than the ultimate comfort food? Your very own personal dish of it!

600ml (1 pint) 1% fat milk
4 tablespoons flour
⅛ teaspoon ground or freshly
  grated nutmeg
75g (3oz) reduced-fat Cheddar
  cheese, grated
50g (2oz) smoked Gouda cheese,
  grated
50g (2oz) reduced-fat Gruyère or
  Emmental cheese, grated
¼ teaspoon cayenne pepper
¼ teaspoon pepper
875g (1¾lb) cooked short-cut
  macaroni
50g (2oz) breadcrumbs
2 tablespoons freshly grated
  Parmesan cheese
2 teaspoons chopped thyme
2 teaspoons chopped parsley
1 teaspoon olive oil or butter
¼ teaspoon salt
¼ teaspoon pepper

1. Preheat oven to 200°C/400°F/gas mark 6.

2. Whisk together milk and flour in a medium saucepan and bring to the boil over high heat. Reduce heat, add nutmeg, and cook, stirring until thickened, about 10 minutes.

3. Add Cheddar, Gouda, Gruyère, cayenne and pepper; whisk until melted, 1 minute. Add macaroni and stir to combine.

4. Toss breadcrumbs, Parmesan, thyme, parsley, oil, salt and pepper in a small bowl.

5. Place six individual crocks, ramekins or ovenproof bowls on a rimmed baking sheet. Divide the macaroni mixture between the ramekins and sprinkle with breadcrumb topping.

6. Bake until topping is browned and cheese is bubbling, 30–35 minutes. Serve hot.

Serving size: 150g (5oz) macaroni mixture and 15g (½ oz) breadcrumb topping Calories 433; Fat 12.1g (sat 6.7g, mono 1.9g, poly 0.7g); Cholesterol 34mg; Protein 22g; Carbohydrate 58g; Sugars 7g; Fibre 3g; RS 1.8g; Sodium 424mg

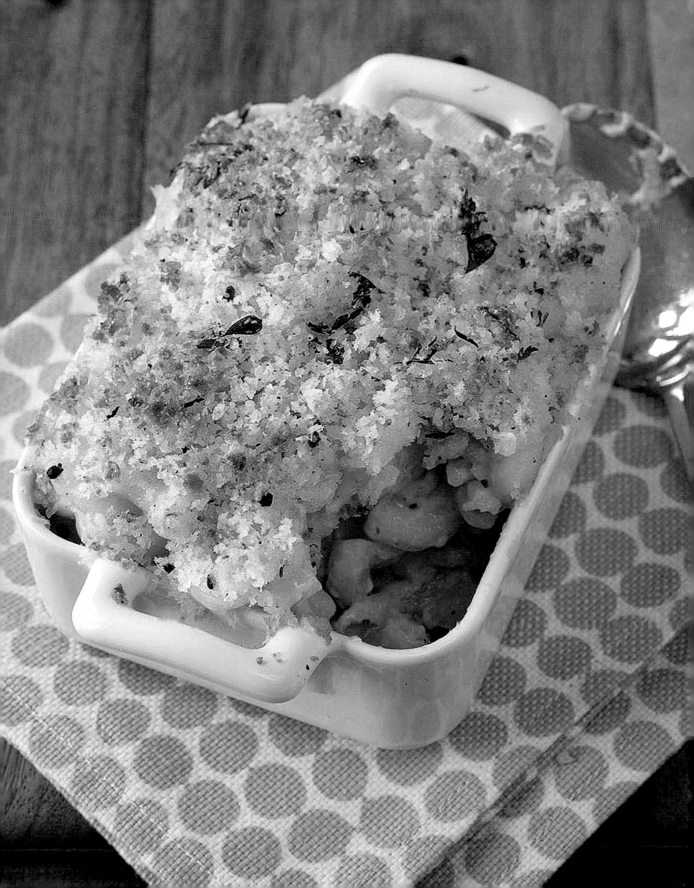

Sausage, Tomato, White Bean and Corkscrew Pasta Toss

Prep: *5 minutes* | **Cook:** *20 minutes* | **Total time:** *25 minutes* | **Makes:** *4 servings*

Looking for a pasta meal that will keep you full for hours? This flavourful dish fits the bill with Italian sausage, beans, tomatoes – and more than 5 grams of Resistant Starch.

1 tablespoon olive oil

175g (6oz) Italian sausages

800g (26oz) can diced tomatoes in juice

475g (15oz) can unsalted cannellini beans, rinsed and drained

2 teaspoons dried oregano or 1 teaspoon fresh

½ teaspoon dried chilli flakes

250g (8oz) wholewheat fusilli (corkscrew) pasta, cooked according to packet instructions

4 tablespoons freshly grated Parmesan cheese

2 tablespoons chopped parsley

1. Heat oil in a frying pan over medium-high heat.

2. Add sausages and cook until browned and cooked through, 6–8 minutes. Transfer to a chopping board and thinly slice.

3. Add tomatoes with juice, beans, oregano and chilli flakes; bring to a low boil.

4. Reduce heat; cook until the liquid reduces slightly, about 3–4 minutes.

5. Stir in pasta; heat through, 2–3 minutes.

6. Divide between 4 bowls. Garnish each bowl with 1 tablespoon Parmesan and ½ tablespoon of the chopped parsley.

Serving size: 325g (11 oz) pasta Calories 435; Fat 10.1g (sat 2.9g, mono 4.6g, poly 1g); Cholesterol 17mg; Protein 24g; Carbohydrate 65g; Sugars 8g; Fibre 12g; RS 5.3g; Sodium 365mg

ASK CARBLOVERS

Q: I'm on a budget. Can *CarbLovers* help?

A: Absolutely! Most of the ingredients on *CarbLovers* are wallet-friendly. To save even more money, try buying grains – pasta, barley, and brown rice – in bulk. Then store them in airtight containers away from heat and light. This will help them last a whole lot longer.

Penne with Grilled Chicken and Vodka Sauce

Prep: 10 minutes | **Cook:** 30 minutes | **Total time:** 40 minutes | **Makes:** 6 servings

This restaurant favourite is usually made with bucket-loads of double cream and butter. We opted to use a little olive oil and single cream, which still gives you a wonderful, creamy texture.

1 tablespoon olive oil
1 small onion, finely diced
2 garlic cloves, finely chopped
800g (26oz) low-sodium can diced tomatoes in juice
250ml (8fl oz) can no-salt-added tomato sauce
125ml (4fl oz) vodka
¼ teaspoon dried chilli flakes
4 tablespoons single cream
¼ teaspoon salt
¼ teaspoon freshly ground pepper
625g (1¼lb) cooked wholewheat penne pasta
125g (4oz) grilled boneless, skinless chicken breasts
2 tablespoons chopped basil

1. Heat oil in a medium saucepan over medium-high heat. Add onion and cook until soft and translucent, 6–7 minutes. Add garlic and cook 1 minute.

2. Add tomatoes with juice, tomato sauce, vodka and chilli flakes, then bring to the boil.

5. Reduce heat and cook, stirring occasionally, until sauce reduces slightly, about 10 minutes.

6. Add cream, and cook until sauce reduces, 5 minutes. Stir in salt and pepper.

8. Divide the pasta between 6 bowls and top with 8 tablespoons vodka sauce.

9. Arrange the grilled chicken on top of the pasta and garnish with chopped basil.

Serving size: 100g (3½oz) pasta, 8 tablespoons sauce and 50g (2oz) chicken Calories 360; Fat 6.3g (sat 1.8g, mono 2.8g, poly 1g); Cholesterol 42mg; Protein 21g; Carbohydrate 52g; Sugars 7g; Fibre 4g; RS 1g; Sodium 206mg

RS 1g

TIP:
If you can't find pre-grilled chicken breasts, cook fresh breasts 5 minutes per side in a griddle pan over high heat.

Chicken Cacciatore with Rigatoni

Prep: *15 minutes* | **Cook:** *45 minutes* | **Total time:** *1 hour* | **Makes:** *4 servings*

The word cacciatore *means hunter in Italian, and this hearty, rich dish is certainly fit for a hunter's appetite. We suggest choosing a glass of red wine to pair with the meal as one of your daily snacks.*

1 tablespoon olive oil
500g (1lb) boneless, skinless chicken thighs
1 medium onion, chopped
4 garlic cloves, sliced
150g (4oz) mushrooms, sliced
1 tablespoon chopped fresh oregano
850g (28oz) can whole tomatoes in juice, chopped
1 tablespoon tomato purée
4 tablespoons dry red wine
¼ teaspoon salt
¼ teaspoon black pepper
625g (1¼lb) cooked rigatoni pasta
4 tablespoons chopped parsley

1. Heat oil in a large nonstick frying pan over medium-high heat. Add chicken to pan and brown until golden, turning once, 3 minutes per side. Remove chicken from pan and reserve.

2. Reduce heat to medium; add onion and cook until soft and translucent, 6–7 minutes. Add garlic and cook 1 minute. Add mushrooms and oregano and cook until mushrooms release their water, 5 minutes.

3. Add tomatoes with juices, tomato purée, wine, salt and pepper; simmer until slightly reduced, 5 minutes. Return chicken to pan; spoon with some of sauce. Reduce heat to medium-low, cover and simmer until chicken is cooked through, 20–25 minutes. Remove from heat; transfer chicken to a plate.

4. Toss pasta with sauce in a large bowl. Divide the pasta and sauce between each of 4 serving bowls. Top with 2 chicken thighs, sprinkle with parsley and serve.

Serving size: 1–2 thighs, 175ml (6fl oz) sauce from pan and 150g (5oz) pasta Calories 462; Fat 9.6g (sat 1.9g, mono 4.1g, poly 2.1g); Cholesterol 94mg; Protein 34g; Carbohydrate 58g; Sugars 8g; Fibre 6g; RS 1.5g; Sodium 567mg

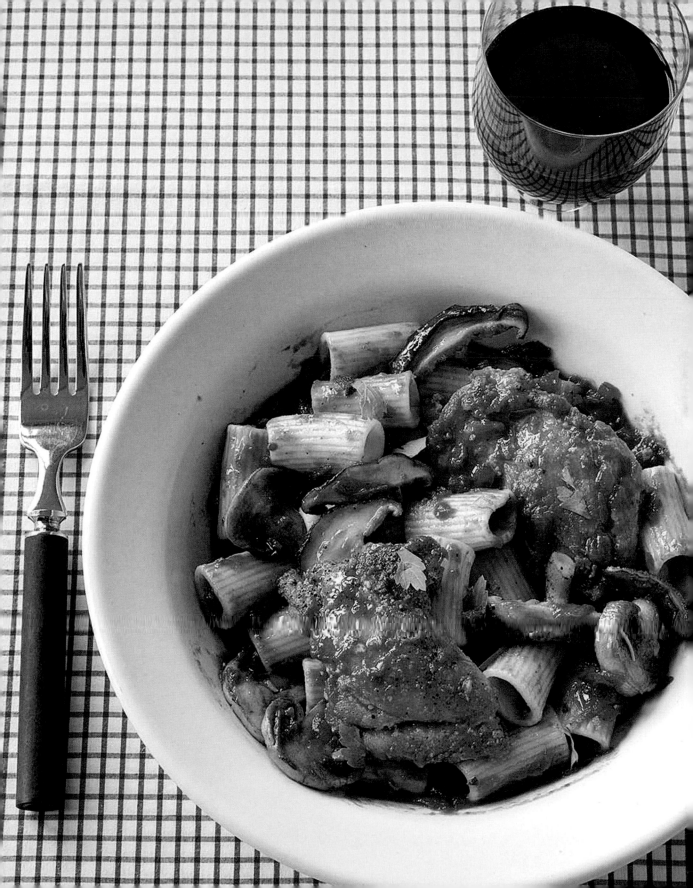

RS
1.6g

Capellini with Bacon and Breadcrumbs

Prep: *10 minutes* | **Cook:** *15 minutes* | **Total time:** *25 minutes* | **Makes:** *4 servings*

Friends coming for dinner? This quick recipe delivers restaurant-quality flavour and appeal in no time.

250g (8oz) wholewheat or
 regular capellini
2 bacon rashers, chopped
1 garlic clove, sliced
¼ teaspoon dried chilli flakes,
 optional
500g (1lb) grape tomatoes, halved
250ml (8fl oz) low-sodium chicken
 stock
1 tablespoon olive oil
4 tablespoons panko breadcrumbs
¼ teaspoon salt
⅛ teaspoon freshly ground black
 pepper
1 tablespoon freshly grated
 Parmesan cheese
4 tablespoons coarsely chopped
 parsley

1. Cook pasta according to packet instructions until al dente. When pasta is done, reserve 125ml (4fl oz) cooking water; drain pasta and return to pot.

2. Meanwhile, heat a large frying pan over medium heat; add bacon. Cook, stirring, until bacon is crispy, about 5 minutes. Add garlic and chilli flakes; stir 1 minute or until fragrant. Add tomatoes; cook, stirring occasionally, until tomatoes begin to soften, about 3 minutes.

3. Add stock to pan. Simmer the mixture until stock is thick and has reduced to about 4 tablespoons, 5–8 minutes.

4. While sauce cooks, heat oil in a small frying pan over medium heat. Add panko and toast, stirring occasionally, until golden, 2–3 minutes.

5. Season with salt and pepper.

6. Remove sauce from heat; stir in 2 teaspoons Parmesan and parsley.

7. Toss sauce with pasta in pan; add cooking water to reach desired consistency, if needed.

8. Divide between 4 serving plates. Top with reserved bread crumbs and remaining Parmesan.

Serving size: About 300g (10oz) Calories 274; Fat 9.5g (sat 2.5g, mono 4.9g, poly 1.2g); Cholesterol 9mg; Protein 10g; Carbohydrate 39g; Sugars 4g; Fibre 6g; RS 1.6g; Sodium 290mg

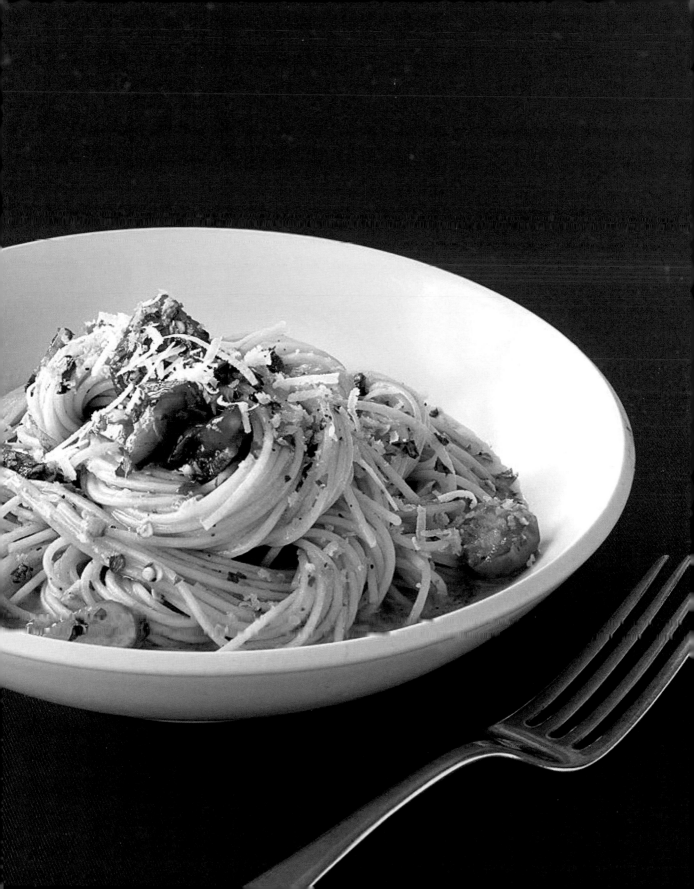

Triple-Cheese Mac

Prep: *10 minutes* | **Cook:** *20 minutes* | **Total time:** *30 minutes* | **Makes:** *6 servings*

Macaroni cheese needn't be a diet disaster. We added high-fibre cauliflower to this version, which virtually blends into the smooth sauce. And the three cheeses provide unbelievable flavour and creaminess – yum!

375g (12oz) can evaporated fat-
  free milk

2 teaspoons Dijon mustard

⅛ teaspoon cayenne pepper

¼ teaspoon ground nutmeg

1 garlic clove, finely grated

300g (10oz) frozen cauliflower
  florets, thawed

1 tablespoon cornflour

400g (13oz) wholewheat pasta shells

50g (2oz) Cheddar cheese,
  coarsely grated

50g (2oz) Gouda cheese,
  coarsely grated

2 tablespoons grated Parmesan
  cheese

2 tablespoons chopped parsley, for
  serving (optional)

1. Combine evaporated milk, mustard, cayenne, nutmeg, garlic and cauliflower in a medium saucepan. Cook over medium heat, stirring occasionally, until cauliflower is tender, 5 minutes.

2. Carefully transfer to a blender; add cornflour and blend until smooth. Return cauliflower mixture to saucepan and heat over low heat.

3. Meanwhile, cook pasta shells according to packet instructions. Reserve 125ml (4fl oz) cooking water; drain.

4. Bring sauce to a simmer until thickened; stir in cheeses. Stir until smooth. Toss sauce with pasta and, if needed, some of the cooking water. Divide between 6 bowls, top with parsley if liked, and serve immediately.

Serving size: 175g (6oz) Calories 358; Fat 7.4g (sat 4.2g, mono 1.9g, poly 0.6g); Cholesterol 24mg; Protein 20g; Carbohydrate 57g; Sugars 9g; Fibre 6g; RS 2.5g; Sodium 283mg

TIP:
This cheesy dish packs ⅓ of your daily calcium needs and 2.5g of Resistant Starch, so you can feel great about digging in!

Creamy Barley Risotto with Peas and Pesto

Prep: *5 minutes* | **Cook:** *25 minutes* | **Total time:** *30 minutes* | **Makes:** *4 servings*

Once you try this dish, you'll be a convert to barley. Its wonderful nutty flavour and slightly chewy texture make it a star in creamy dishes, as well as in cold salads.

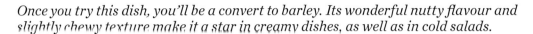

1 tablespoon olive oil
1 shallot, finely chopped
2 garlic cloves, finely chopped
400g (13oz) pearl barley
475ml (16fl oz) reduced-sodium
  chicken stock
½ teaspoon salt
¼ teaspoon freshly ground
  black pepper
150g (5oz) frozen peas, thawed
2 tablespoons finely grated
  Parmesan cheese
3 tablespoons shop-bought pesto,
  for serving

1. Heat oil in a medium frying pan over medium-high heat. Add shallot and garlic; cook 4–5 minutes until onion begins to brown.

2. Reduce heat to medium; stir in barley and stock. Cook, stirring occasionally, until liquid is absorbed, about 10 minutes. Add 475ml (16fl oz) water; cook until vegetables are tender and most of the liquid has been absorbed, 10–15 minutes. Season with salt and pepper.

3. Stir in peas; remove from heat. Let risotto rest 1–2 minutes until peas are thawed but still bright green. Stir in Parmesan just before serving. Serve topped with pesto.

Serving size: 200g (7oz) Calories 423; Fat 10.5g (sat 2.1g, mono 2.8g, poly 0.9g); Cholesterol 6mg; Protein 10g; Carbohydrate 74g; Sugars 3g; Fibre 11g; RS 6.5g; Sodium 637mg

Gnocchi with Walnut-Rocket Pesto

Prep: 5 minutes | **Cook:** 5 minutes | **Total time:** 10 minutes | **Makes:** 4 servings

These little Italian potato dumplings make for a delicious, filling and superfast meal.

275g (9oz) rocket
125g (1½oz) Parmesan cheese,
  freshly grated
4 tablespoons walnuts
½ teaspoon salt
¼ teaspoon freshly ground black
  pepper
2 tablespoons olive oil
425g (14oz) frozen, shop-bought
  potato gnocchi

1. Place 175g (6oz) rocket, 100g (4oz) Parmesan, walnuts, salt and pepper in a food processor; pulse until incorporated, 30 seconds. With motor running, drizzle in oil and 1 tablespoon water; process until smooth, 30 seconds, adding more water by the tablespoon if necessary.

2. Cook gnocchi according to packet instructions; drain. Return gnocchi to pan; add pesto.

3. Divide remaining rocket between 4 bowls; toss with the gnocchi. Sprinkle with remaining Parmesan, and serve immediately.

Serving size: 300g (10oz) gnocchi-rocket mixture
Calories 358; Fat 25.1g (sat 9.9g, mono 9.6g, poly 4.4g); Cholesterol 41mg; Protein 14g; Carbohydrate 21g; Sugars 1g; Fibre 2g; RS 1.6g; Sodium 605mg

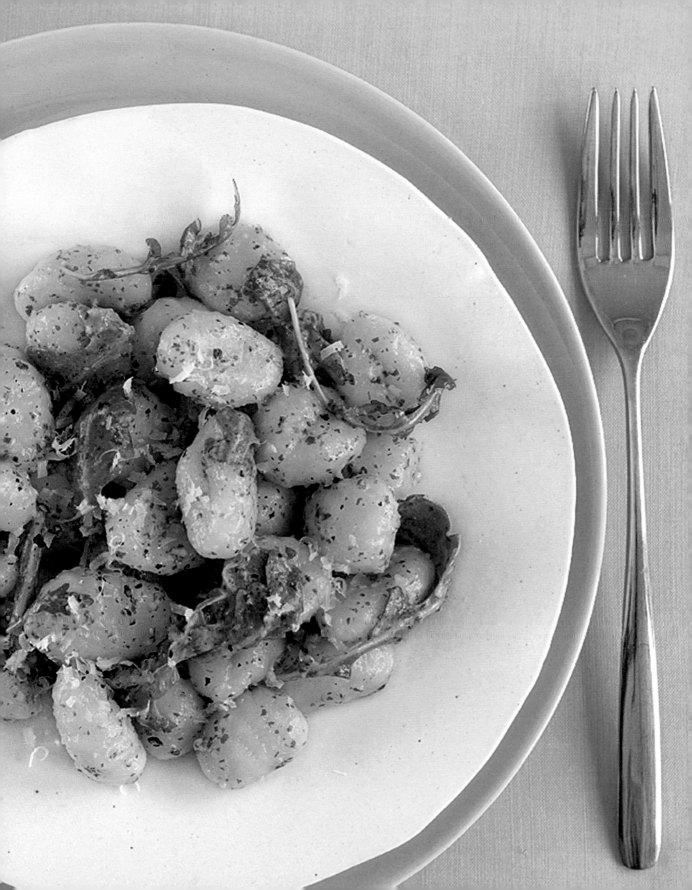

RS
2.5g

Spaghetti and Turkey Meatballs in Tomato Sauce

Prep: *15 minutes* | **Cook:** *30 minutes* | **Total time:** *45 minutes* | **Makes:** *5 servings*

The whole family will love this yummy and ultra-satisfying dish. We took classic spaghetti and meatballs and made it healthier by using lean turkey and adding beans to boost the Resistant Starch. The end result is as delicious as you'd expect!

500g (1lb) lean minced turkey meat

75g (3oz) Parmesan cheese, finely grated

4 tablespoons chopped parsley, plus more for garnish

4 tablespoons fresh wholemeal breadcrumbs (from 1 slice bread)

1 egg, beaten

¾ teaspoon salt

½ teaspoon pepper

1 tablespoon olive oil

1 small onion, finely chopped

2 garlic cloves, finely chopped

750g (1½lb) low-sodium passata

250g (8oz) canned pinto beans, rinsed and drained

250g (8oz) wholewheat spaghetti, cooked according to packet instructions and kept warm

1. Combine turkey, 50g (2oz) Parmesan, parsley, breadcrumbs, egg, ½ teaspoon salt and ¼ teaspoon pepper in a bowl; form into 15 meatballs. Place meatballs on a plate and set aside.

2. Heat oil in a large saucepan over medium-high heat. Add onion; cook until soft, 5 minutes. Add garlic; cook 2 minutes.

3. Add passata, beans and remaining salt and pepper; bring to the boil.

4. Add meatballs; return to a boil. Reduce heat and simmer over low heat until meatballs are cooked through and sauce has thickened, 15 minutes.

5. Divide spaghetti between 5 bowls, then divide meatballs and sauce between bowls. Garnish with additional parsley and remaining Parmesan.

Serving size: 150g (5oz) pasta, 3 meatballs and about 175ml (6fl oz) sauce Calories 439; Fat 12.2g (sat 3.4g, mono 2.7g, poly 1g); Cholesterol 98mg; Protein 33g; Carbohydrate 55g; Sugars 2g; Fibre 9g; RS 2.5g; Sodium 623mg

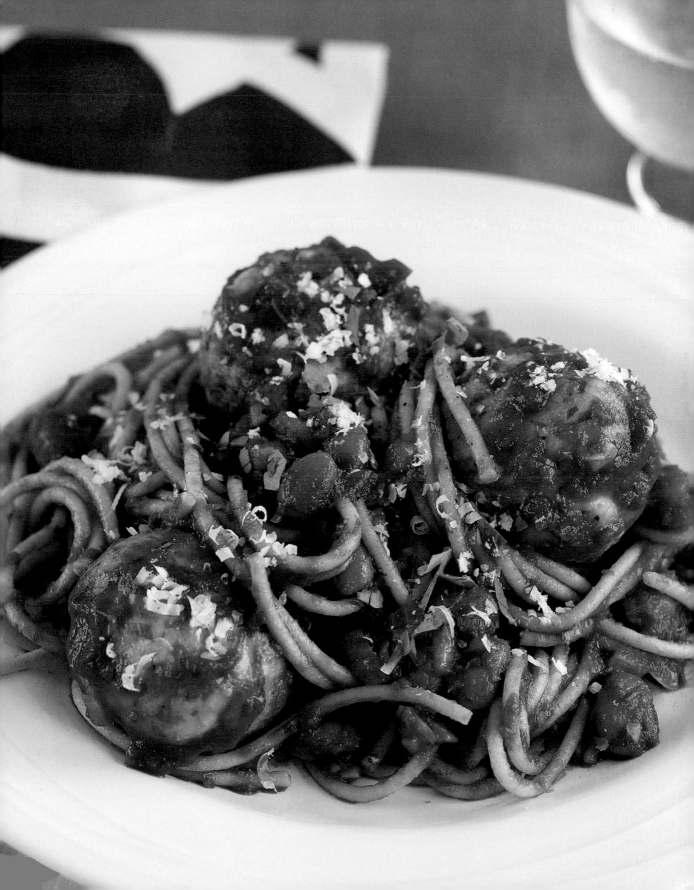

RS
3.5g

Pasta with Peas, Ham and Parmesan Cheese

Prep: *5 minutes* | **Cook:** *15 minutes* | **Total time:** *20 minutes* | **Makes:** *4 servings*

We tossed bow ties, sweet peas and salty ham in a creamy sauce to create a really rich-tasting, but still light dish you will absolutely love.

125ml (4fl oz) light soured cream

300g (10oz) frozen peas, thawed

250g (8oz) uncooked wholewheat
  orecchiette or bow-tie pasta

125g (4oz) lean, boneless ham, thinly
  sliced

100g (3½oz) Parmesan cheese,
  finely grated

2 tablespoons chopped tarragon,
  plus more for garnish

½ teaspoon salt

½ teaspoon pepper

1. Combine soured cream and peas in a small bowl.

2. Cook pasta according to packet instructions. Drain, reserving 125ml (4fl oz) of the cooking water.

3. Return pasta to pan. Fold in soured cream mixture, ham, 75g (3oz) Parmesan, tarragon, salt and pepper. Stir in enough reserved cooking water to create a thin sauce.

4. Divide between 4 bowls; garnish with additional tarragon and remaining Parmesan.

Serving size: 300g (10oz) pasta Calories 434; Fat 12.7g (sat 6.6g, mono 4g, poly 1g); Cholesterol 55mg; Protein 29g; Carbohydrate 54g; Sugars 5g; Fibre 8g; RS 3.5g; Sodium 538mg

ASK CARBLOVERS

Q: **I haven't really eaten pasta in years. How can I make friends with this food again?**

A: Pasta should be enjoyed in modest portions with fresh herbs, vegetables, lean meats, interesting sauces, and even nuts and beans. Experiment!

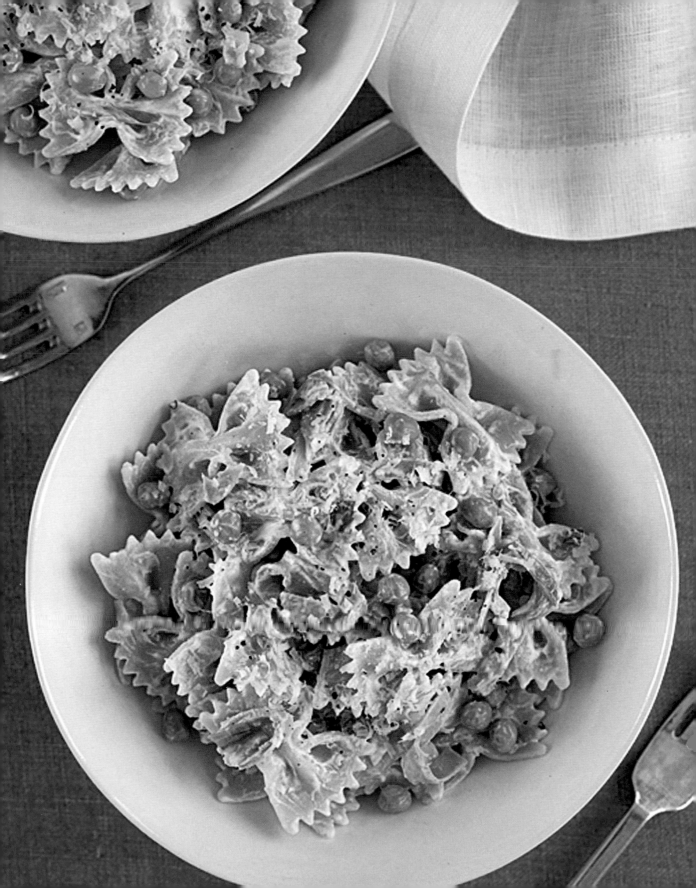

Penne with Sausage and Spinach

Prep: *5 minutes* | ***Cook:*** *20 minutes* | ***Total time:*** *25 minutes* | ***Makes:*** *4 servings*

It's tough to find dishes that are satisfying both to your taste buds and to your health standards, but this one delivers both. You get to indulge in tasty sausage and pasta while getting 8 grams of fibre and more than 3 grams of Resistant Starch.

375g (12oz) wholewheat penne

1 tablespoon olive oil

3 Italian turkey sausages

250ml (8fl oz) reduced-sodium chicken stock

¼ teaspoon dried chilli flakes (optional)

150g (5oz) baby spinach

2 tablespoons grated Pecorino cheese

1 tablespoon fresh lemon juice

1. Cook pasta according to packet instructions.

2. Meanwhile, heat oil in a large frying pan over medium-high heat. Remove sausages from casing; form each sausage into 4 balls.

3. Add meatballs to pan; cook, tossing occasionally, until browned, about 5 minutes. Add stock and, if using, chilli flakes; simmer 8 minutes or until stock is almost fully evaporated.

4. Add the cooked pasta to the pan, then stir in spinach to wilt.

5. Toss pasta and spinach with Pecorino and lemon juice. Transfer to 4 bowls and serve while hot.

Serving size: 375g (12oz) Calories 447; Fat 11g (sat 3g, mono 2.6g, poly 0.9g); Cholesterol 56mg; Protein 26g; Carbohydrate 66g; Sugars 2g; Fibre 8g; RS 3.3g; Sodium 600mg

RS
5.3g

Roasted Aubergine and Ricotta Calzones

Prep: 20 minutes | **Cook:** 35 minutes | **Total time:** 55 minutes | **Makes:** 6 servings

Filled with lots of rich cheese and pepperoni, calzones generally aren't considered diet fare. We slimmed ours down by using semi-skimmed ricotta and swapping sausag for roasted aubergine, which adds a ton of flavour and fibre with low calories.

1 medium (500g/1lb) aubergine,
  cubed
2 tablespoons olive oil
½ teaspoon pepper
750ml (1¼ pints) marinara sauce
250g (8oz) semi-skimmed
  ricotta cheese
2 tablespoons chopped parsley
4 tablespoons chopped basil
¼ cup polenta
500g (1lb) wholewheat pizza dough
  divided into 6 equal-sized pieces
1 egg white, beaten

1. Preheat oven to 240°C/475°F/gas mark 9.

2. Toss aubergine with oil and ¼ teaspoon pepper. Place in a single layer on a foil-lined baking sheet; bake until soft and edges are charred, 15 minutes. Remove aubergine from oven and cool to room temperature.

3. Transfer cooked aubergine to a bowl and toss with 475ml (16fl oz) marinara.

4. Combine ricotta, parsley, basil and remaining pepper in a small bowl until incorporated.

5. Sprinkle 2 tablespoons polenta on a clean, dry work surface. Place one dough ball on surface and roll out to a 23cm (9 inch) circle. Place about 12 tablespoons aubergine filling and about 4 tablespoons ricotta mixture in centre of circle. Moisten edges with water, fold into a half moon, and crimp tightly with fingers to close. Repeat with remaining pieces of dough.

6. Transfer calzones to a baking paper-lined baking sheet and brush with egg white. Bake until golden brown, 16–17 minutes.

7. Serve with additional warmed marinara sauce for dipping.

Serving size: 1 calzone and about 2½ tablespoons sauce
Calories 380; Fat 12.9g (sat 2.7g, mono 4.3g, poly 0.7g); Cholesterol 13mg; Protein 14g; Carbohydrate 53g; Sugars 6g; Fibre 7g; RS 5.3g; Sodium 798mg

Fresh Mozzarella, Basil and Chicken Sausage Pizza

Prep: *5 minutes* | **Cook:** *20 minutes* | **Total time:** *25 minutes* | **Makes:** *6 servings*

Delicious mozzarella: check. Sausage: check. Spicy tomato sauce: check. Resistant Starch: check! Finally, even dieters can have an amazing, pizzeria-style pie at home.

500g (1lb) fresh or frozen wholemeal
  pizza dough, thawed
1 tablespoon olive oil
2 medium tomatoes (about 300g/10z)
¼ teaspoon dried chilli flakes
¼ teaspoon dried oregano
8 tablespoons basil leaves
250g (8oz) fresh mozzarella, pulled
  into 2.5cm (1 inch) chunks
175g (6oz) pre-cooked Italian chicken
  sausage, sliced

1. Position one oven rack in middle of oven and another on the lowest setting. Place a flat baking sheet on the bottom rack. Preheat oven to 240°C/475°F/gas mark 9.

2. Roll dough into a large, thin oval (about 18 inches long). Brush oil over dough.

3. Remove preheated baking sheet from oven. Slide dough onto sheet and return to bottom rack. Bake for 8 minutes, then remove from oven.

4. Meanwhile, with clean hands, crush tomatoes, chilli flakes, oregano and 4 tablespoons basil in a medium bowl.

5. Spread sauce in an even layer over base, leaving a 5mm (¼ inch) border. Top with mozzarella and sausage. Bake on middle rack an additional 10 minutes or until base is golden brown and cheese melts. Sprinkle with remaining basil; cut into 12 slices or wedges and serve.

Serving size: 2 slices pizza Calories 360; Fat 17.9g (sat 7.4g, mono 2.4g, poly 0.7g); Cholesterol 51mg; Protein 17.2g; Carbohydrate 32g; Sugars 1g; Fibre 3g; RS 2.2g; Sodium 322mg

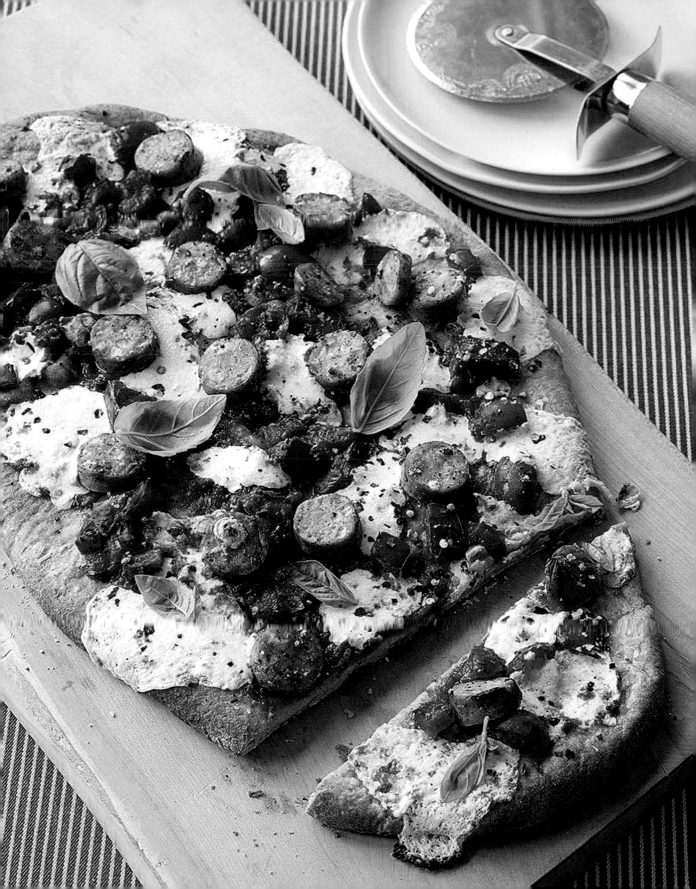

RS
2g

Pizza with Parma Ham, Tomatoes and Parmesan Cheese

Prep: *5 minutes* | **Cook:** *15 minutes* | **Total time:** *20 minutes* | **Makes:** *4 servings*

Dinner in 20 is easy to pull off with this tempting pizza. Serve it with a fresh green salad dressed with olive oil and balsamic vinegar.

30cm (12 inch) pre-baked wholemeal pizza base

175ml (6fl oz) low-sodium marinara sauce

50g (2oz) semi-skimmed mozzarella cheese, grated

4 tablespoons freshly grated Parmesan cheese

2 thin slices (25g/1oz) Parma ham, coarsely chopped

3 small tomatoes, sliced

8 basil leaves

1. Preheat oven to 200°C/400°F/gas mark 6.

2. Place pizza base on a baking sheet.

3. Spread sauce evenly over base, leaving a 2.5cm (1 inch) border around the edges.

4. Combine cheeses, and sprinkle evenly over sauce. Top with Parma ham and tomatoes.

5. Bake until cheese is bubbly and base is browned around the edges, 12–15 minutes. Remove from oven, and distribute basil leaves evenly over pizza. Let pizza rest for 5 minutes. Cut into 8 slices, and serve immediately.

Serving size: 2 slices Calories 286; Fat 9.3g (sat 3.4g, mono 1.1g, poly 0.2g); Cholesterol 18mg; Protein 17g; Carbohydrate 38g; Sugars 5g; Fibre 6g; RS 2g; Sodium 699mg

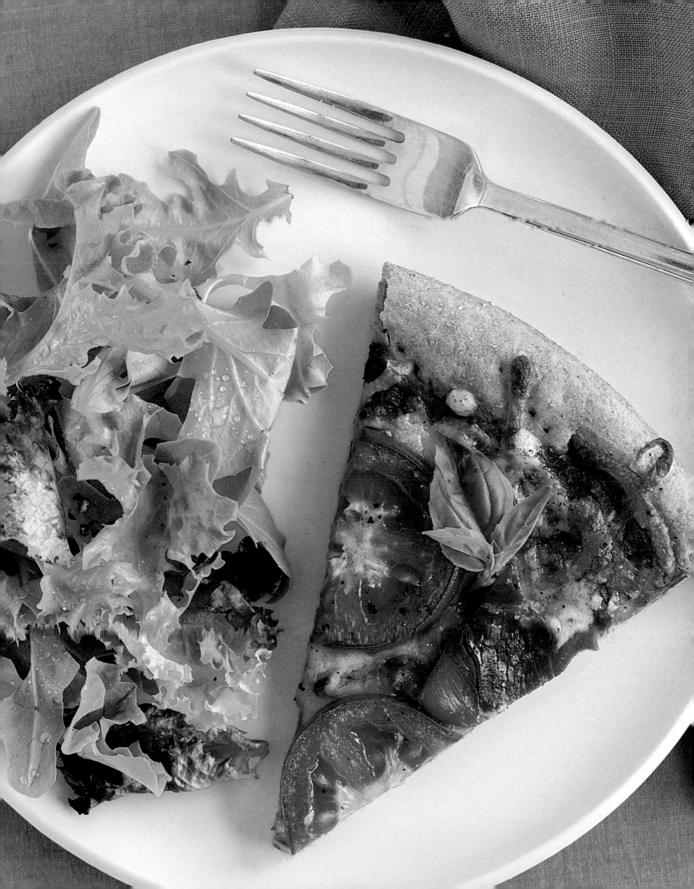

RS
1g

Mini Mediterranean Pizzas

Prep: *10 minutes* | **Cook:** *10 minutes* | **Total time:** *20 minutes* | **Makes:** *4 servings*

A quick lunch or dinner is just 20 minutes away with these delicious mini pizzas.

250g (8oz) cherry tomatoes
1 garlic clove, sliced
¼ teaspoon freshly ground black
  pepper
4 x 15 cm (6 inch) wholemeal pittas
1 tablespoon olive oil, plus more for
  drizzling
65g (2½oz) feta cheese, crumbled
4 tablespoons halved, pitted
  kalamata olives
4 tablespoons roasted peppers, sliced
40g (1½oz) baby rocket

1. Preheat oven to 230°C/450°F/gas mark 8.

2. Crush tomatoes with garlic and pepper in a small bowl.

3. Arrange 4 pittas on a large rimmed baking sheet; brush both sides of pittaa with oil. Top pittas with equal amounts of the tomato mixture, feta, olives and peppers.

4. Bake 7–8 minutes or until edges are golden.

5. Remove pittas from oven; top each with ¼ of the rocket.

6. Drizzle with additional oil, if liked. Serve.

Serving size: 1 pizza Calories 274; Fat 8.9g (sat 3.5g, mono 4.5g, poly 0.7g); Cholesterol 17mg; Protein 10g; Carbohydrate 29g; Sugars 5g; Fibre 1g; RS 1g; Sodium 608mg

> **TIP:**
> If you aren't a fan of rocket, you
> can top the pizzas with baby spinach
> or other favourite ingredients.

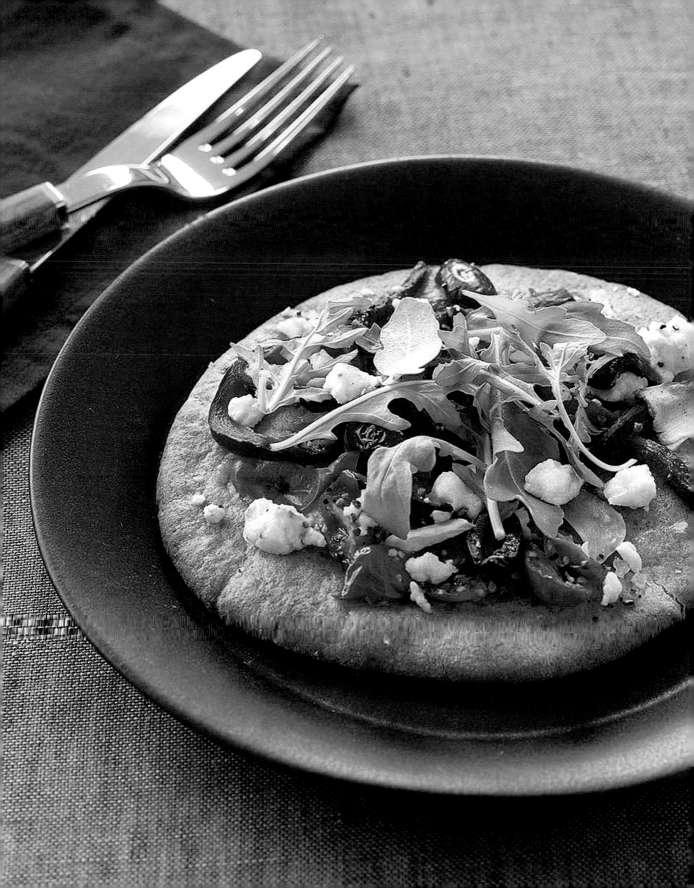

Spinach-Tomato Pasta Shells

Prep: *5 minutes* | **Cook:** *15 minutes* | **Total time:** *20 minutes* | **Makes:** *4 servings*

RS
3.3g

"I'm a pasta junkie. If you're going to indulge in the greatest of carbs, at least fortify it with a little baby spinach. Not only is this dish healthy, but with the colour from the tomatoes and spinach, it looks great as well." Guy Fieri, TV chef

375g (12oz) wholemeal pasta shells
15g (½oz) butter
1 shallot, thinly sliced
¼ teaspoon dried chilli flakes
150g (5oz) baby spinach
125ml (4fl oz) low-sodium chicken
  stock
4 tablespoons single cream
25g (1oz) Pecorino Romano cheese,
  grated
½ teaspoon freshly ground black
pepper
250g (8oz) cherry tomatoes,
  halved lengthways
1 tablespoon chopped flat-leaf
  parsley

1. Cook pasta according to packet instructions.

2. Meanwhile, heat butter in a large frying pan over medium-high heat. Add shallot and chilli flakes; reduce heat to medium-low, and cook for 1–2 minutes or until translucent. Add spinach and stock; cover and cook for 1 minute. Add cream, ¾ of the cheese and the black pepper. Stir to combine; cook for 3 minutes. Remove from heat.

3. Add tomatoes and the cooked pasta; toss. Garnish with parsley and remaining cheese. Serve.

Serving size: about 300g (10oz) Calories 402; Fat 7.8g (sat 4.4g, mono 2g, poly 0.7g); Cholesterol 21mg; Protein 17g; Carbohydrate 72g; Sugars 5g; Fibre 9g; Iron 4mg; RS 3.3g; Sodium 165mg

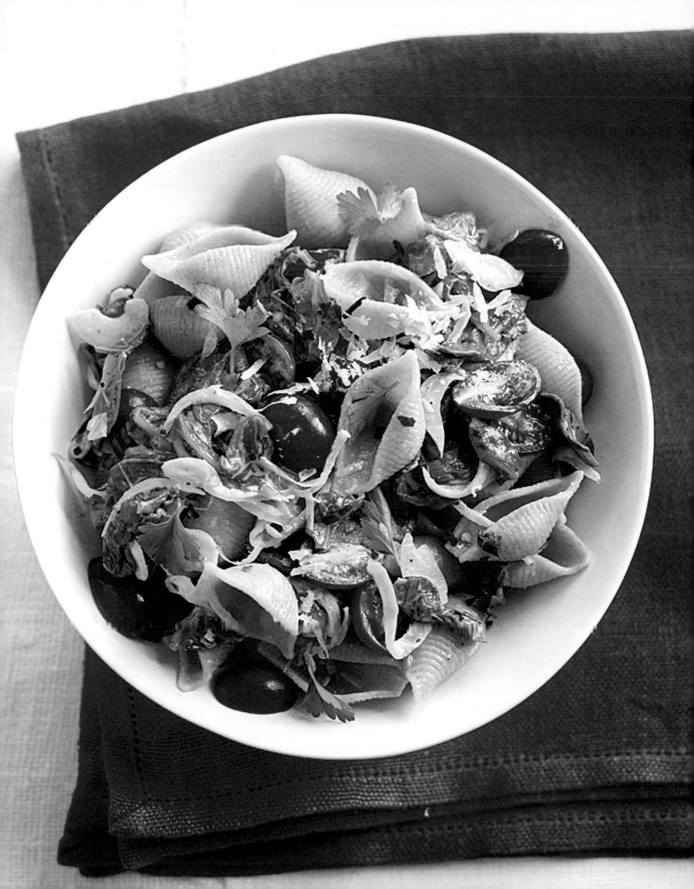

RS
2.6g

Barbecue Chicken Pizza

Prep: 10 minutes | **Cook:** 15 minutes | **Total time:** 25 minutes | **Makes:** 5 servings

"I like this recipe because you can add grilled or sautéed vegetables to the toppings. Or try spinach, Swiss chard, or kale. Blanch in boiling salted water first, then drain, squeeze dry, chop, and top the pizza." Wolfgang Puck, chef

2 teaspoons olive oil

175g (6oz) yellow and red
  peppers, thinly sliced

Plain flour for rolling

500g (1lb) refrigerated pizza dough

50g (2oz) mozzarella cheese, grated

50g (2oz) fontina cheese, sliced

175g (6oz) cooked chicken breast, cut
  into 2.5cm (1 inch) pieces

4 tablespoons barbecue sauce, warmed

¼ teaspoon salt

¼ teaspoon pepper

4 tablespoons chopped flat-leaf parsley

1. Preheat oven to 240°C/ 465°F/gas mark 9.

2. Heat oil in a medium frying pan over medium-high heat; sauté peppers for 2 minutes. Set aside. Roll out pizza dough to a 37cm (15 inch) round on a lightly floured surface; top with cheeses and sautéed peppers. Transfer to a baking sheet. Bake pizza for about 12 minutes or until crust is golden brown.

3. Meanwhile, warm up chicken. Toss warm chicken pieces with barbecue sauce. Remove pizza from the oven; evenly arrange chicken on top. Sprinkle with salt and pepper, and top with parsley. Cut pizza into slices; serve.

Serving size: ⅕ of pizza Calories 414; Fat 10.7g (sat 4g, mono 3.3g, poly 0.8g); Cholesterol 54mg; Protein 27g; Carbohydrate 49g; Sugars 6g; Fibre 7g; Iron 2mg; RS 2.6g; Sodium 804mg

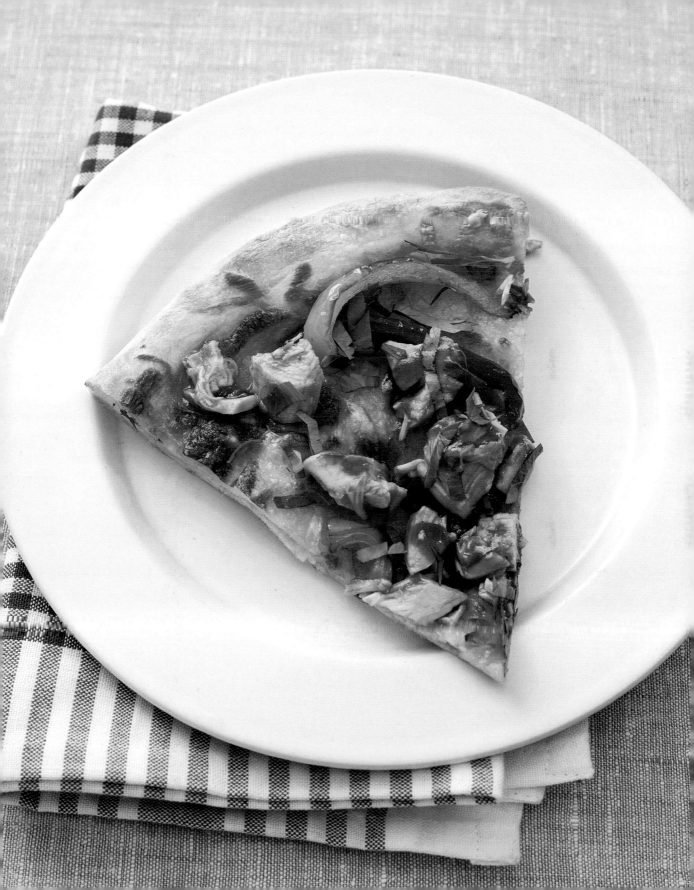

Fusilli Michelangelo with Roasted Chicken

Prep: *10 minutes* | **Cook:** *20 minutes* | **Total time:** *30 minutes* | **Makes:** *6 servings*

"This dish is one of my all-time favorites. It's tasty, simple, and full of flavour."
Michael Chiarello, chef and winemaker

7 sun-dried tomatoes
1½ tablespoons balsamic vinegar
1½ teaspoons sugar
250g (8oz) whole wheat fusilli
2 tablespoons olive oil
300g (10oz) mushrooms, sliced
2 minced garlic cloves
8 tablespoons finely chopped fresh basil
  leaves
350ml (12fl oz) tomato sauce
75g (3oz) Parmesan cheese, grated
1 rotisserie chicken, meat removed
(skin discarded)
150g (5oz) rocket
2 tablespoons toasted pine nuts

1. Place sun-dried tomatoes in a bowl. Bring balsamic vinegar, sugar and 3 tablespoons water to the boil. Pour over tomatoes; let stand 10 minutes. Drain and slice.

2. Cook pasta according to packet instructions; reserve 125ml (4fl oz) cooking water and drain.

3. Heat oil in a nonstick frying pan over medium heat. Add mushrooms. Cook 1 minute without stirring, then cook, stirring, 5 minutes or until browned. Add garlic; cook 1 minute. Add basil and reserved tomatoes; cook 1 minute. Add tomato sauce; bring to a simmer. Add pasta, 50g (2oz) grated Parmesan, reserved cooking water, chicken; toss, and transfer to serving bowl. Add rocket, pine nuts and remaining Parmesan. Serve.

Serving size: 200g (7oz) Calories 431; Fat 16.9g (sat 4.6g, mono 7.2g, poly 3.4g); Cholesterol 81mg; Protein 37g; Carbohydrate 36g; Sugars 6g; Fibre 5g; Iron 4mg; RS 1.5g; Sodium 620mg

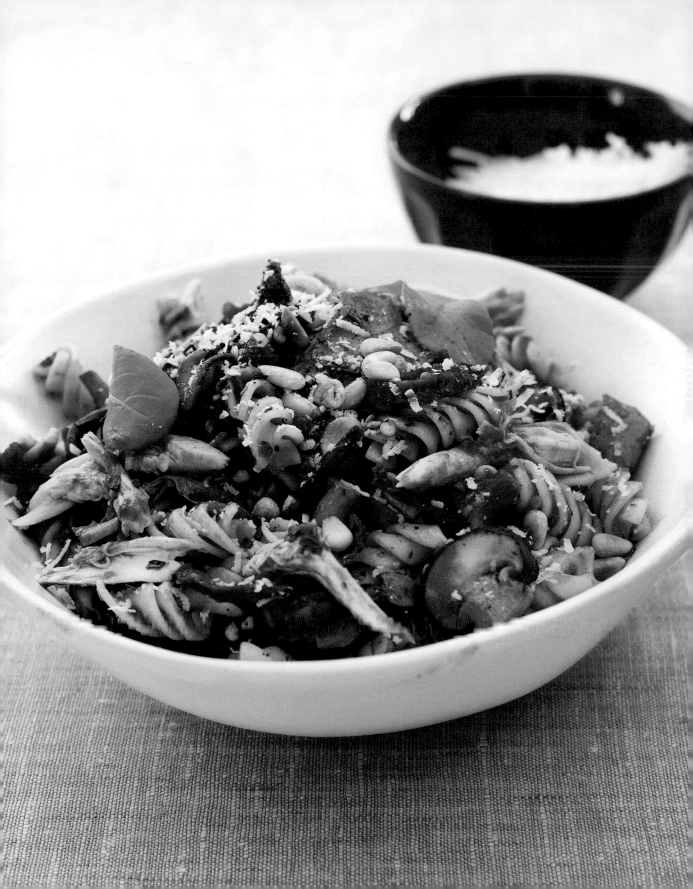

Scoglio (Seafood Pasta)

Prep: *5 minutes* | **Cook:** *47 minutes* | **Total Time:** *52 minutes* | **Makes:** *6 servings*

"Carbs – especially pasta – are the fuel my body needs to maintain an athletic lifestyle. This classic Italian dish, loaded with delicious iron-rich shellfish, is both sustaining and satisfying." Joe Bastianich, restaurateur, winemaker and author

FOR SAUCE:

2 tablespoons olive oil
2 garlic cloves, crushed
500g (1lb) can whole Italian tomatoes
Salt and freshly ground black pepper,
  to taste
1 teaspoon Sicilian oregano
  (optional)

FOR PASTA:

500g (1lb) dry spaghetti
2 tablespoons plus 2 teaspoons
  olive oil
4–6 medium scallops
¼ teaspoon salt
¼ teaspoon pepper
8 medium peeled prawns
1 sprig fresh oregano
1 sprig fresh thyme
8 mussels
8 clams
125ml (4fl oz) white wine

MAKE SAUCE:

1. Heat oil in a saucepan over medium heat. Add garlic to oil and cook, stirring, until golden brown. While garlic browns, pour tomatoes into a bowl; break them up using clean hands. Once garlic is browned, add tomatoes and their juices. Add salt and pepper (and oregano if using).

2. Simmer over low heat for 45 minutes, adding water to keep the sauce from becoming too thick. The sauce should be a rich red color. If it turns brick red, it's too thick.

MAKE PASTA:

1. Cook pasta according to packet instructions. Drain, reserving 250ml (8fl oz) cooking water.

2. Heat 2 tablespoons oil in a large frying pan. Season scallops with salt and pepper; cook over medium high heat, about 2–3 minutes per side, until golden brown on each side. Remove and set aside.

3. In the same pan, cook prawn until they just turn pink, about 1–2 minutes. Remove and set aside.

4. Add reserved pasta water to pan along with oregano and thyme. Simmer for 10 minutes to

CONTINUED ON PAGE 150

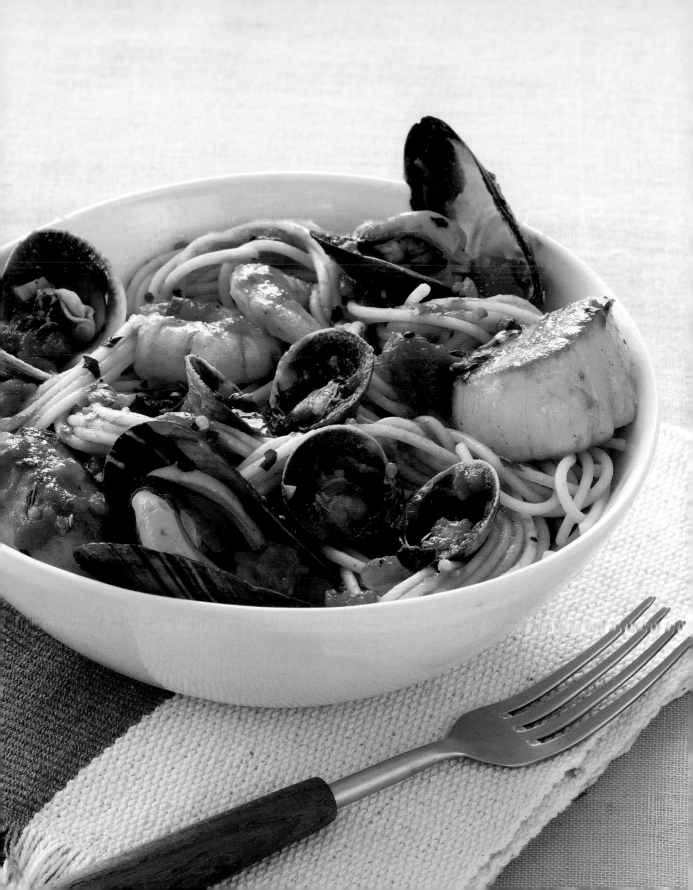

Scoglio (Seafood Pasta)

...create a fish stock, scraping the bottom of the pan with a spatula to release the caramelized bits left over from sautéing into the stock.

5. Once the stock is ready, add mussels with remaining 2 teaspoons oil and cover. Cook 2–3 minutes, removing mussels as soon as they open. Set aside. Repeat with the clams, cooking about 4 minutes. Remove and set aside.

6. Strain the remaining fish stock through a sieve and return to the same pan. Add wine and simmer over medium heat, 2–3 minutes, to burn off the alcohol. Add scallops back to the pan. Then add 125ml (4fl oz) pomodoro sauce. Add prawns and a little more pomodoro sauce. Add pasta to the saucepan, stirring to coat with pomodoro sauce. Simmer 2–3 minutes and fold clams and mussels into the pasta. Serve immediately.

Serving size: about 475ml (16fl oz) Calories 433; Fat 10.4g (sat 1.6g, mono 6.1g, poly 1.6g); Cholesterol 25mg; Protein 19g; Carbohydrate 61g; Sugars 2g; Fibre 4g; Iron 4mg; RS 2g; Sodium 491mg

TIP:
Keep shellfish and fresh fish cold before you start cooking. Place in a bowl, cover with a damp towel, and let chill in the coldest part of the fridge.

Individual Spinach and Mushroom Pizzas with Wholemeal Crust

Prep: 35 minutes | *Cook:* 35 minutes | *Total Time:* 2 hours 30 minutes | *Makes:* 6 servings

"Pizza is one of those foods I could never give up. The combination of crispy crust, tangy sauce, and fresh mozzarella is always so satisfying. I also love adding chile flakes before serving for a little extra little kick." Gail Simmon, food writer and chef

FOR BASE:

1 sachet fast-action yeast
250ml (8fl oz) very warm water
 38–43°C/100°–110°F
½ teaspoon sugar
175g (6oz) wholemeal flour
175g (6oz) unbleached plain flour
 plus more for kneading
1 teaspoon fine sea salt
4 tablespoons olive oil

FOR TOPPINGS:

1 tablespoon olive oil, plus
more for drizzling (optional)
250g (8oz) chestnuti mushrooms,
 cleaned well and patted dry, thinly
sliced
175g (6oz) baby spinach
Pinch of coarse sea salt, plus more
for sprinkling on top (optional)
875g (1³/₄lb) canned whole tomatoes,
 juices drained
4 ounces fresh, salted mozzarella,
 thinly sliced
2 large garlic cloves, thinly sliced
Dried chilli flakes (optional)

MAKE BASE:

1. Put yeast in a small bowl; add water and sugar. Gently whisk to combine. Let stand until foamy, about 5 minutes.

2. Mix together flours and salt in a large bowl. Form a well in centre of flour. Pour oil into the well and, with clean hands, rub oil into flour. Add yeast mixture to flour; mix to combine. Knead dough on a lightly floured work surface until smooth and elastic, about 6 minutes. Form dough into a ball, place in an oiled bowl, cover with clingfilm and a clean tea towel, and let dough rise at room temperature for 90 minutes.

3. About 30 minutes before dough is ready, preheat oven to 240°C/475°F/gas mark 9 with rack in centre and pizza stone on rack. Once the oven reaches temperature, heat stone for at least 30 minutes.

MAKE TOPPINGS:

1. Heat ½ tablespoon oil in a large frying pan over medium-high heat. Add mushrooms; cook until tender, about 2 minutes. Transfer to a small colander set over a bowl to drain excess liquid. Add remaining oil to skillet, and add spinach;

CONTINUED ON PAGE 152

Individual Spinach and Mushroom Pizzas with Wholemeal Crust

cook until wilted and deep green, about 2 minutes. Transfer to a plate. Place tomatoes in a bowl and, with clean hands, break up into small pieces. Season sauce with salt.

2. When dough is ready, gently remove from bowl and cut into 6 pieces. Work with 1 piece of dough at a time, keeping unused dough covered with clingfilm. Using both hands, roll into a ball, then press into a flat round, about 10cm (4 inches) in diameter. Using a floured rolling pin, roll out dough on a lightly floured surface to an 18cm (7 inch) round; transfer to a floured pizza peel.

3. Spread about 4 tablespoons sauce onto dough, leaving a 5mm (¼ inch) border at edge. Working quickly, sprinkle with some of garlic, then add ⅙ of the mozzarella. Top with ⅙ of the spinach and ⅙ of the mushrooms. If liked, lightly drizzle pizza with additional oil and sprinkle with salt. Slide pizza off of peel onto stone and bake until edges are puffed and golden, about 5–6 minutes.

4. Transfer pizza to a chopping board; cut into 6 slices and serve immediately, with chilli flakes, if liked. Repeat with remaining ingredients.

Serving size: 1 pizza Calories 418; Fat 16.1g (sat 3.3g, mono 5.6g, poly 0.9g); Cholesterol 15mg; Protein 14g; Carbohydrate 56g; Sugars 4g; Fibre 7g; Iron 5mg; RS 3.2g; Sodium 811mg;

TIP:
Make these pizzas a healthy, satisfying meal by adding a crisp green salad and a glass of red wine.

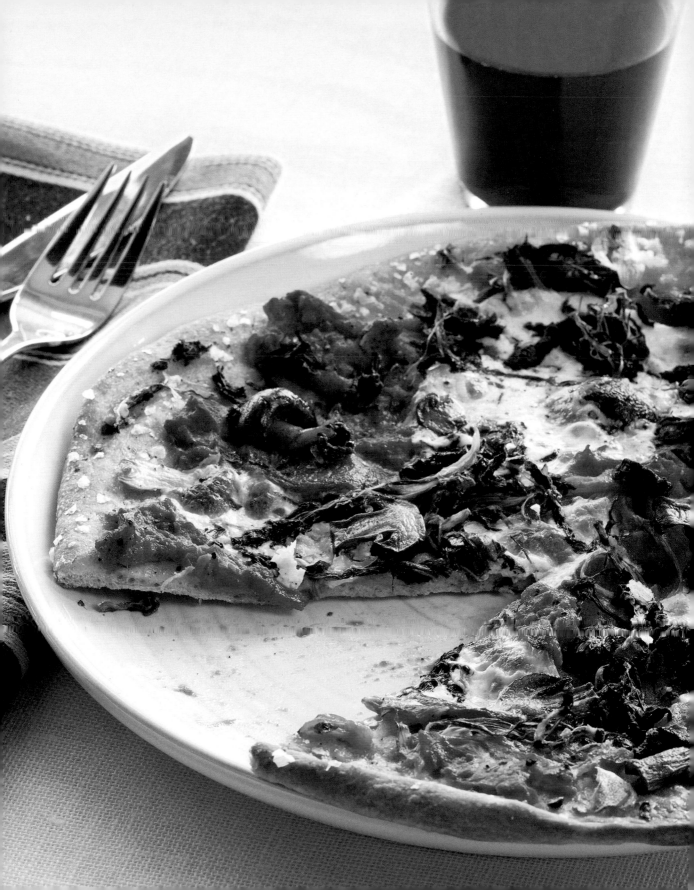

Seafood, Meat & Poultry

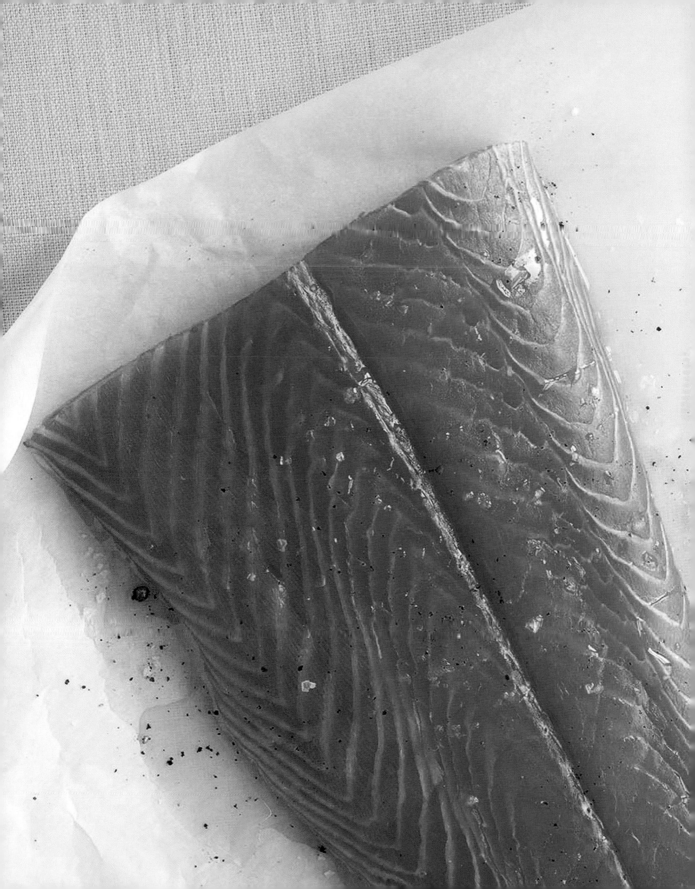

Maple-Glazed Cod with Baby Pak Choi

Prep: *5 minutes* | ***Cook:*** *10 minutes* | ***Total time:*** *15 minutes* | ***Makes:*** *4 servings*

Meaty and slightly sweet, heart-healthy cod lends itself to Asian-inspired dishes like this one. Serve it with brown rice for a complete meal and added Resistant Starch.

2 tablespoons maple syrup
2 tablespoons low-sodium soy sauce
1 teaspoon sesame oil
¼ teaspoon dried red chilli flakes
4 x 175g (6 oz) skinless cod fillets
1 tablespoon rapeseed oil
3 garlic cloves, finely chopped
1 tablespoon chopped fresh ginger
6 heads baby pak choi, halved
2 tablespoons mirin
2 tablespoon rice wine vinegar
4 teaspoons chopped spring onion
2 teaspoons lightly toasted sesame seeds

1. Make cod: Combine maple syrup, 1 tablespoon soy sauce, sesame oil and chilli flakes. Place fish in a glass baking dish and pour marinade over fish; refrigerate for 30 minutes or up to 2 hours.

2. Preheat oven to 240°C/475°F/gas mark 9. Transfer fillets to a foil-lined baking sheet and roast until fish is cooked through and slightly browned, 9–10 minutes.

3. Meanwhile, make pak choi: Heat rapeseed oil in a very large frying pan over medium-high heat. Add garlic and ginger and cook, stirring, until fragrant but not browned, 1 minute. Add pak choi, then follow immediately with mirin, remaining soy sauce and vinegar. Cook, stirring, until greens are wilted and stalks are tender-crisp, 3–4 minutes.

4. Remove fish from oven. Sprinkle each fillet with 1 teaspoon chopped spring onion and ½ teaspoon toasted sesame seeds. Serve with pak choi.

Serving size: 175g (6oz) cod and 1½ pak choi Calories 256; Fat 7.1g (sat 0.8g, mono 3.3g, poly 2.5g); Cholesterol 65mg; Protein 31g; Carbohydrate 16g; Sugars 11g; Fibre 3g; RS 0g; Sodium 509mg

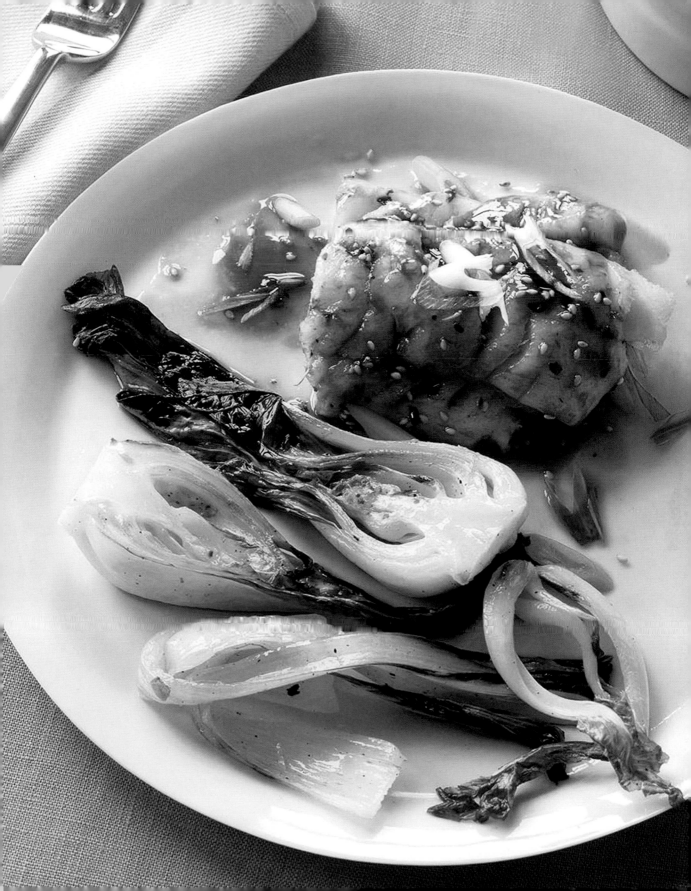

Parma Ham, Pear and Blue Cheese Sushi

Prep: 20 minutes | *Total time:* 20 minutes | *Makes:* 4 servings

"Eating a balanced diet including complex carbohydrates such as brown rice keeps me going both in and out of the kitchen. This delicious, unique twist on sushi keeps me energized." Cat Cora, chef and author

400g (13oz) cooked brown rice
4 tablespoons rice vinegar
½ teaspoon sea salt
3 tablespoons pine nuts
4 sheets nori (seaweed)
4 slices Parma ham
2 tablespoons blue cheese
8 tablespoons peeled julienned pear
2 tablespoons balsamic glaze

1. Combine cooked rice, vinegar and salt in a medium bowl; set aside. Toast and crush pine nuts; set aside.

2. Cover a sheet of aluminium foil with clingfilm; top with 1 sheet nori. Press(¼ of the seasoned rice onto nori, leaving a 5mm(¼ inch) border at the top and bottom. Press ½ tablespoon crushed pine nuts into the rice; top with 1 slice Parma ham, ½ tablespoon blue cheese and 2 table-spoons pear.

3. Roll foil tightly towards you; remove foil and clingfilm. Cut roll into 2.5cm (1 inch) pieces with a sharp, wet knife.

4. Repeat steps with 3 more rolls. Drizzle pieces of each sushi roll evenly with 1½ teaspoons balsamic glaze.

Serving size: 1 roll Calories 280; Fat 8.4g (sat 1.9g, mono 2g, poly 2.7g); Cholesterol 14mg; Protein 11g; Carbohydrate 40g; Sugars 4g; Fibre 4g; Iron 1mg; RS 2.5g; Sodium 686mg

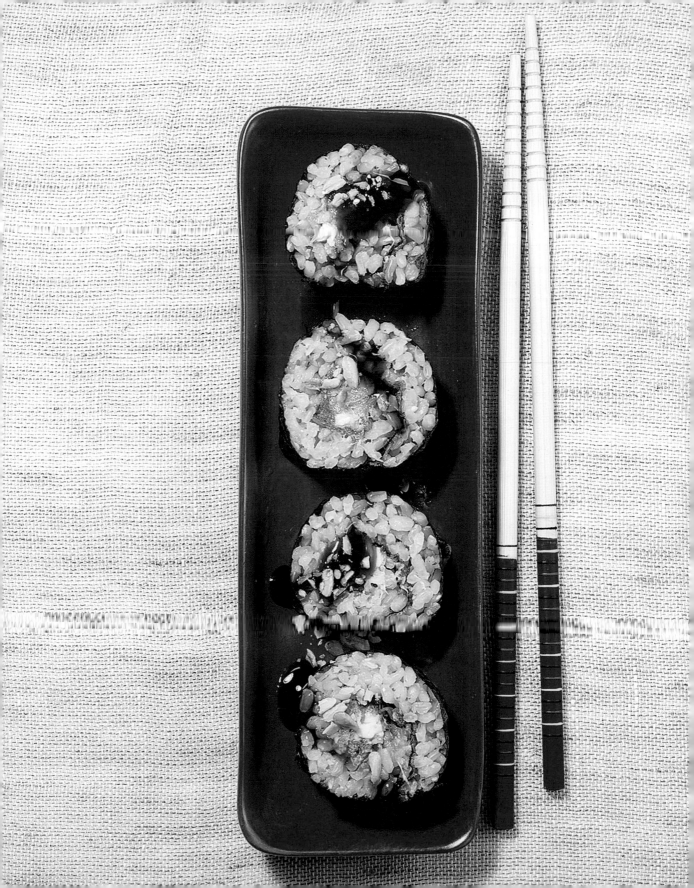

RS
2.1g

Polenta-Crusted Tilapia with Sautéed Greens and Whipped Honey Yams

Prep: 20 minutes | **Cook:** 45 minutes | **Total time:** 1 hour 5 minutes | **Makes:** 4 servings

This complete meal is Southern food at its finest–and skinniest!

1kg (2lb) yams, peeled and cut into
  5cm (2inch) chunks
250ml (8fl oz) vegetable or chicken
  broth, divided
1 tablespoon honey
Cooking spray
2 tablespoons vegetable oil
1 small onion, chopped
3 garlic cloves, sliced
500g (1lb) spring greens, greens
  separated from stems, then
  sliced, stems chopped
¾ teaspoon smoked paprika
¼ teaspoon dried red chilli flakes
¼ teaspoon salt
½ teaspooon pepper
1 egg white, beaten
4 tablespoons polenta
4 x 175g (6oz) tilapia fillets
4 tablespoons flour

1. Place yams and 125ml (4fl oz) stock in a saucepan; bring to the boil. Reduce heat, cover and cook until yams are fork-tender, about 20 minutes. Remove from heat, transfer to a bowl, and add honey.

2. Whip yams with a hand mixer, 2 minutes. Cover to keep warm.

3. Add 2 teaspoons oil to a large nonstick frying pan coated with cooking spray; heat over medium-high heat. Add onion and cook, stirring, until lightly browned, 7–8 minutes. Add garlic, greens, remaining stock, ½ teaspoon paprika, chilli flakes and half of the salt and pepper; cook until stems are slightly softened, 2–3 minutes. Add greens and cook 1–2 minutes until wilted. Remove from heat and cover with foil.

4. Place egg white in a shallow dish. Combine polenta and remaining salt and pepper in another shallow dish. Combine flour and remaining ¼ teaspoon paprika in a plastic bag. Dredge fish in flour, then moisten with egg white. Press into polenta mixture on both sides. Heat 2 teaspoons oil in a nonstick frying pan over medium-high heat. Place 2 fish fillets in pan and cook until browned, 3 minutes. Flip fish and cook until cooked through, 3–4 minutes more. Repeat with remaining oil and fish.

Serving size: 1 piece fish, 250g (8oz) yams and 125g (4oz) sautéed greens Calories 502; Fat 12.2g (sat 2.3g, mono 2g, poly 5g); Cholesterol 114mg; Protein 41g; Carbohydrate 60g; Sugars 17g; Fibre 10g; RS 2.1g; Sodium 513mg

Honey and Sesame-Glazed Salmon with Confetti Barley Salad

Prep: 10 minutes | **Cook:** 30 minutes | **Total time:** 40 minutes | **Makes:** 4 servings

This is truly a power meal! Omega-3-packed salmon helps boost your metabolism. And the barley kicks in Resistant Starch and fibre.

150g (5oz) pearl barley
500g (1lb) frozen stir-fry
  vegetables, thawed and chopped
1 tablespoon toasted sesame seeds
4 x 125g (4oz) skinless salmon fillets
3 tablespoons honey
4 tablespoons low-sodium soy sauce
1½ teaspoons toasted sesame oil
¼ teaspoon dried chilli flakes
4 tablespoons chopped spring onions

1. Preheat oven to 200°C/400°F/gas mark 6.

2. Bring a large pan of salted water to the boil.

3. Add barley, return to the boil, and boil until tender, 30 minutes. Add vegetables during last 3 minutes of cooking. Drain, cool slightly, and toss with 2 teaspoons sesame seeds; set aside.

4. While barley is cooking, make salmon: Combine honey, soy sauce, sesame oil and chili flakes. Reserve 4 tablespoons of mixture. Place salmon on a baking sheet, and brush with honey-soy mixture. Bake until salmon is flaky, 15 minutes. Place reserved sauce in a small saucepan over low heat, and keep warm.

5. Divide barley mixture between 4 plates, top with 1 salmon fillet and 1 tablespoon warmed sauce, and sprinkle with spring onions and remaining sesame seeds.

Serving size: 150g (5oz) barley-vegetable mixture, 125g (4oz) salmon and 1 tablespoon additional sauce
Calories 435; Fat 8.8g (sat 0.3g, mono 2.2g, poly 2.3g), Cholesterol 72mg; Protein 33g; Carbohydrate 53g; Sugars 16g; Fibre 9g; RS 0.3g; Sodium 615mg

Prawn Tacos with Lime Crema

Prep: *10 minutes* | **Cook:** *5 minutes* | **Total:** *15 minutes* | **Makes:** *4 servings*

Tacos de camarones (prawn tacos) originated in Baja California in Mexico. We love them because they're outrageously good – and take less than 20 minutes to make.

500g (1lb) medium shrimp, peeled and deveined

¼teaspoon chilli powder

¼teaspoon cumin

⅛teaspoon black pepper

1teaspoon olive oil

2tablespoons lime juice

125ml (4fl oz) reduced-fat soured cream

8 (6inch) corn tortillas, warmed according to packet instructions

4 tablespoons finely diced red onion, for serving

150g (6oz) shredded lettuce, for serving

1. Toss prawns with chilli powder, cumin and pepper in a medium bowl. Heat oil in a large nonstick frying pan over medium heat. Add prawns; sauté 3 minutes, turning once, or until done. Remove from heat. Season with 1 tablespoon lime juice.

2. Stir together soured cream and remaining lime juice in a small bowl. To serve, fill tortillas with lettuce, top with prawn mixture and red onion, and drizzle with lime crema.

Serving size: 2 tortillas, 1 tablespoon onion, 40g (1½ oz) lettuce, 125g (4oz) prawns, 2 tablespoons crema
Calories 258; Fat 7.3g (sat 2.7g, mono 2.3g, poly 1g); Cholesterol 155mg; Protein 20g; Carbohydrate 29g; Sugars 1g; Fibre 4g; RS 1.5g; Sodium 665mg

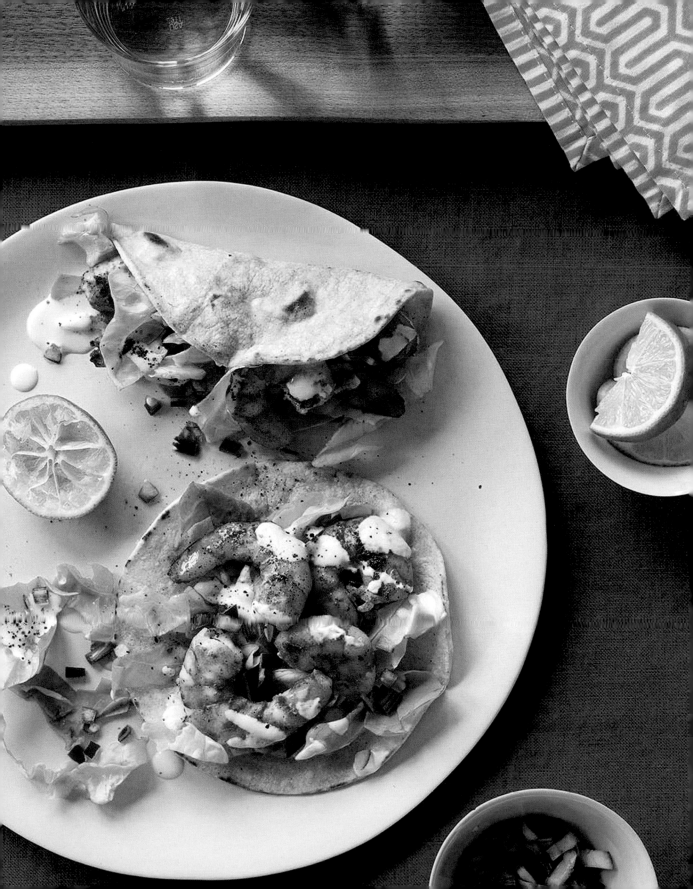

RS
1.7g

Seared Scallops with Asian Slaw

Prep: 10 minutes | **Cook:** 5 minutes | **Total time:** 15 minutes | **Makes:** 4 servings

Superlight and very quick cooking, scallops are a busy dieter's dream. We love the combination of the tangy slaw and the sweet, meaty scallops.

1 tablespoon finely grated ginger

2 tablespoons rice wine vinegar

1 teaspoon fish sauce (optional)

1½ teaspoons sugar

4 baby pak choi, thinly sliced

2 spring onions, thinly sliced

1 teaspoon black or white sesame
    seeds

500g (1lb) scallops (about 16)

¼ teaspoon sea salt

¼ teaspoon freshly ground black
    pepper

275g (9oz) cooked brown rice

1. Whisk together ginger, vinegar, fish sauce (if using) and sugar in a medium bowl. Toss with pak choi, spring onions, and sesame seeds. Set aside.

2. Season scallops with salt and pepper. Heat a large nonstick frying pan over medium-high heat. Place 1 scallop in centre of pan. When scallop sizzles, arrange remaining scallops in pan, flat sides down (make sure they aren't touching or they will steam and not sear properly). Cook 2–3 minutes on each side until lightly browned and opaque in the centre. Place ¼ of the slaw on each of 4 plates. Add ¼ of the cooked brown rice and top with 4 scallops each. Serve immediately.

Serving size: 125g (4oz) slaw, 65g (2 ½oz rice, and 4 scallops   Calories 217; Fat 1.9g (sat 0.4g, mono 0.6g, poly 0.7g); Cholesterol 27mg; Protein 18g; Carbohydrate 32g; Sugars 4g; Fibre 4g; RS 1.7g; Sodium 625mg

Grilled Spice-Rubbed Pork Fillet

Prep: *10 minutes* | **Cook:** *25 Minutes* | **Total time:** *35 minutes* | **Makes:** *4 servings*

The slightly bitter bite of broccoli rabe pairs well with the mild flavour of pork fillet. And the spice rub is absolutely delicious.

4 teaspoons olive oil

¼ teaspoon salt

1 teaspoon smoked paprika

1 teaspoon oregano

½ teaspoon pepper

1 teaspoon cumin

½ teaspoon sugar

625g (1¼lb) pork fillet

3 garlic cloves, thinly sliced

750g (1½lb) broccoli rabe, or Swiss chard (including leaves and stalks), trimmed, stalks chopped

1. Combine 2 teaspoons oil, ¼ teaspoon salt and next 5 ingredients (through to sugar) in a small bowl. Pat pork dry and rub with spice mixture.

2. Preheat a griddle pan over medium-high heat. Grill pork until a thermometer inserted into the thickest part of the meat reads 68°C/155°F, about 8 minutes per side. Remove from heat and let rest.

3. While meat is resting, heat remaining oil over medium heat in a very large frying pan. Add garlic and cook until softened and slightly browned, 2 minutes. In 2 batches add broccoli rabe and cook until crisp-tender, 3–4 minutes total, adding water by the tablespoon if the pan gets dry. Remove from heat. Slice meat against grain. Divide pork and broccoli rabe between 4 plates.

Serving size: 125g (4oz) pork and 150g (6oz) broccoli rabe   Calories 244; Fat 9.8g (sat 2.2g, mono 5g, poly 1.4g); Cholesterol 78mg; Protein 33g; Carbohydrate 7g; Sugars 1g; Fibre 5g; RS 0g; Sodium 409mg

Bison Sliders with Guacamole

Prep: 20 minutes | **Cook:** 5 minutes | **Total time:** 25 minutes | **Makes:** 4 servings

These juicy sliders are addictive! Make them for a party or an easy weeknight dinner.

1 large avocado
1 tablespoon reduced-fat soured cream
Juice and zest of 1 lime
1 tablespoon finely chopped jalapeño
  chilli
2 tablespoons chopped coriander
¾ teaspoon salt
½ teaspoon pepper
500g (1lb) ground bison, or lean
  minced beef
1 minced garlic clove, finely chopped
1 small head round lettuce, inner leaves
  separated
2 plum tomatoes, thinly sliced
½ small red onion, sliced into rings
8 wholemeal burger buns

1. Mash avocado, soured cream, lime juice and zest, jalapeño, coriander, ½ teaspoon salt and ¼ teaspoon pepper in a medium bowl until chunky. Press clingfilm onto surface of guacamole, and refrigerate.

2. Combine meat, garlic and remaining salt and pepper in a small bowl. Form into eight 50g (2oz) burgers, transfer to a plate, and set aside.

3. Preheat a griddle pan over medium-high heat. Grill sliders until thoroughly cooked; 4 minutes per side for medium.

4. Layer one lettuce leaf, a slice of tomato and an onion ring on bottom half of each bun, and top with 2 tablespoons guacamole. Add a slider and top with other half of bun.

Serving size: 2 sliders   Calories 444; Fat 24.2g (sat 7.6g, mono 11g, poly 2.9g); Cholesterol 61mg; Protein 23g; Carbohydrate 38g; Sugars 7g; Fibre 9g; RS 0.2g; Sodium 544mg

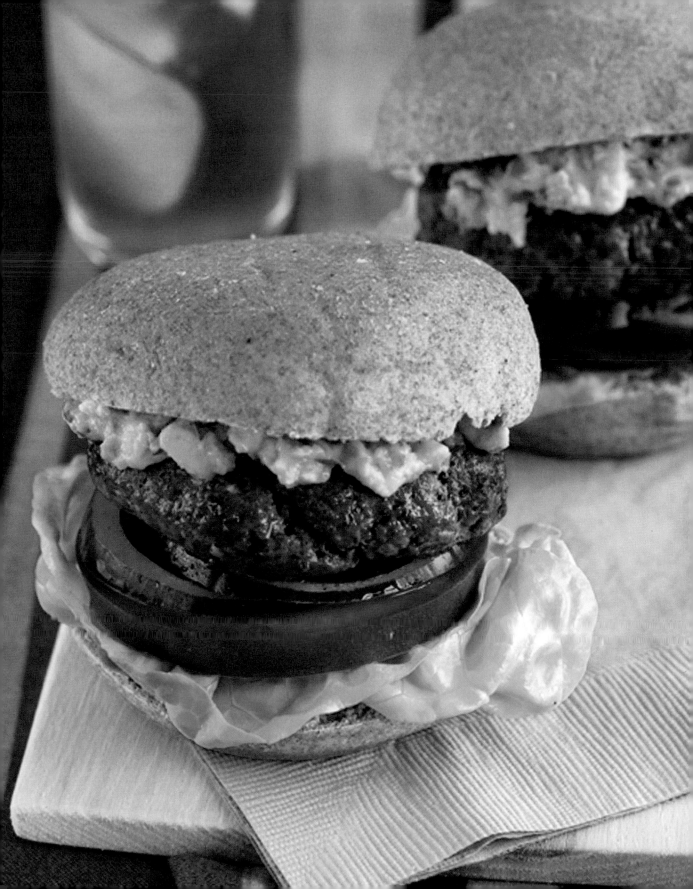

RS
2.9g

Grilled Steak Fajitas

Prep: 15 minutes | **Cook:** 30 minutes | **Total time:** 45 minutes | **Makes:** 4 servings

Fajitas make a perfectly balanced meal. You get vegetables, lean meat, beans and Resistant Starch–packed tortillas. Plus they're incredibly fun to eat!

4 tablespoons fresh lime juice plus
  2 teaspoons lime zest
4 tablespoons chopped fresh coriander
2 garlic cloves, finely chopped
2 teaspoons finely chopped jalapeño
  chilli
500g (1lb) beef skirt
15 oz) can reduced-salt pinto beans,
  rinsed and drained
4 tablespoons low-sodium chicken
  stock
½ teaspoon cumin
½ teaspoon coriander
¼ teaspoon chili powder
¼ teaspoon salt
¼ teaspoon pepper
1 tablespoon vegetable oil
½ red onion, sliced into wedges
1 red pepper, cut into strips
1 yellow squash, sliced
8 corn tortillas, warmed
Cilantro leaves and lime wedges
  for garnish

1. Combine lime juice and zest, cilantro, garlic and jalapeño in a large resealable plastic bag. Add steak and shake to coat; marinate in refrigerator for 1 hour and up to 8. Remove from refrigerator, scrape off excess marinade and set aside.

2. Place beans and spices (through to pepper) in a small saucepan and bring to the boil. Reduce heat and simmer 2 minutes. Remove from heat and mash until chunky. Cover and keep warm.

3. Heat a cast-iron frying over high heat. Add steak and cook until a crust forms and meat is medium-rare, 6–7 minutes per side. Remove from heat and let rest. Slice into 5mm (¼inch) thick slices and keep warm. Heat oil in a frying pan over high heat, add onion and cook, stirring, until charred, 4–5 minutes. Add pepper and cook, stirring occasionally, until charred, 5–6 minutes.

4. Divide vegetables and steak 4 plates and serve with 5 tablespoons refried beans and 2 tortillas. Garnish with coriander leaves and lime wedges.

Serving size: 2 tortillas, 125g (4oz) steak, 50g (2oz) veggies and 5 tablespoons refried beans Calories 414; Fat 11.3g (sat 2.8g, mono 3.3g, poly 3.1g); Cholesterol 70mg; Protein 33g; Carbohydrate 45g; Sugars 3g; Fibre 9g; RS 2.9g; Sodium 236mg

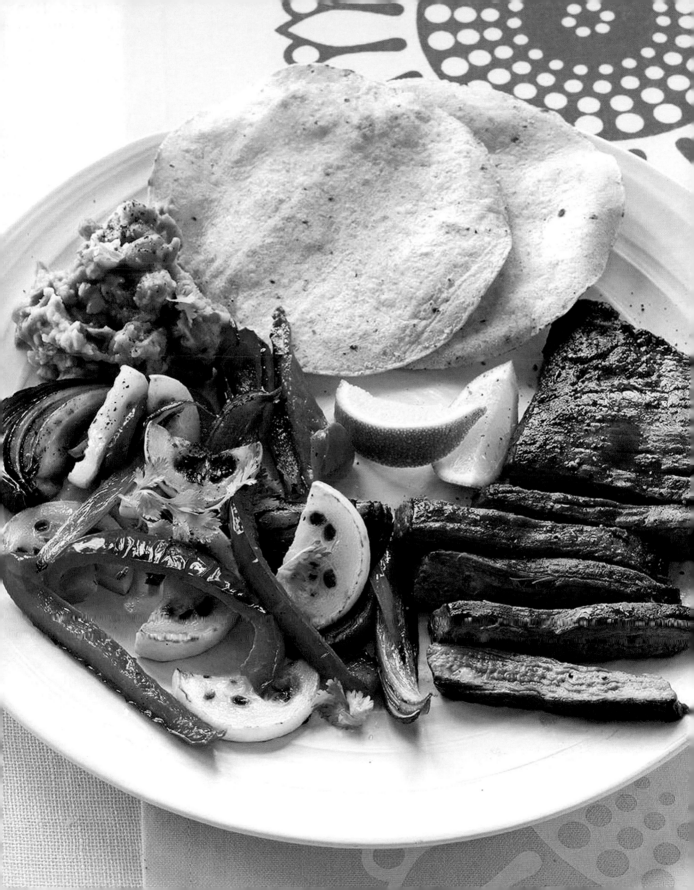

RS
2.6g

Steak Frites

Prep: *10 minutes* | **Cook:** *35 minutes* | **Total time:** *45 minutes* | **Makes:** *4 servings*

We love the simplicity of brasserie-style fare, and it doesn't get much better than steak and chips. We kept the skin on our frites *for extra fibre and nutrients.*

1kg (2lb) potatoes, skin-on
2 tablespoons olive oil
¾ teaspoon salt
750g (1½lb) skirt steak,
  trimmed of additional fat
1 teaspoon cracked black pepper
4 teaspoons chopped parsley

1. Preheat oven to 240°F/475°/gas mark 9. Cut potatoes into 8mm (⅓ inch) thick fries. Toss in a bowl with oil and ¼ teaspoon salt. Arrange in a single layer on a large rimmed baking sheet and bake for 20 minutes. Remove from oven. Using a metal spatula, turn chips, lifting carefully so as not to separate crisped parts from potatoes. Return to oven and roast until crisp and golden brown, an additional 15 minutes.

2. While chips are baking, preheat a griddle pan over medium-high heat. Season steak with ¼ teaspoon salt and the cracked pepper; grill until medium-rare, 7–8 minutes per side. Remove from heat, let rest and slice into 4 equal portions

3. Arrange each steak on a dinner plate. Remove chips from oven and season with remaining ¼ teaspoon salt. Place ¼ of chips on each plate and sprinkle with 1 teaspoon chopped parsley.

Serving size: 125g (4oz) steak and about 15 chips
Calories 463; Fat 18.4g (sat 5.4g, mono 10.9g, poly 1.2g); Cholesterol 96mg; Protein 34g; Carbohydrate 40g; Sugars 2g; Fibre 4g; RS 2.6g; Sodium 531mg

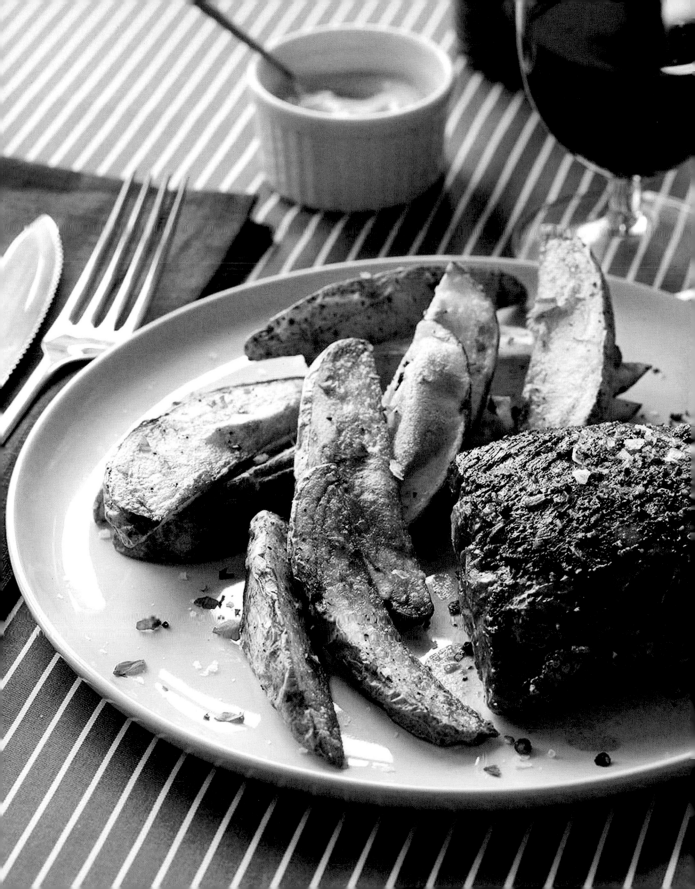

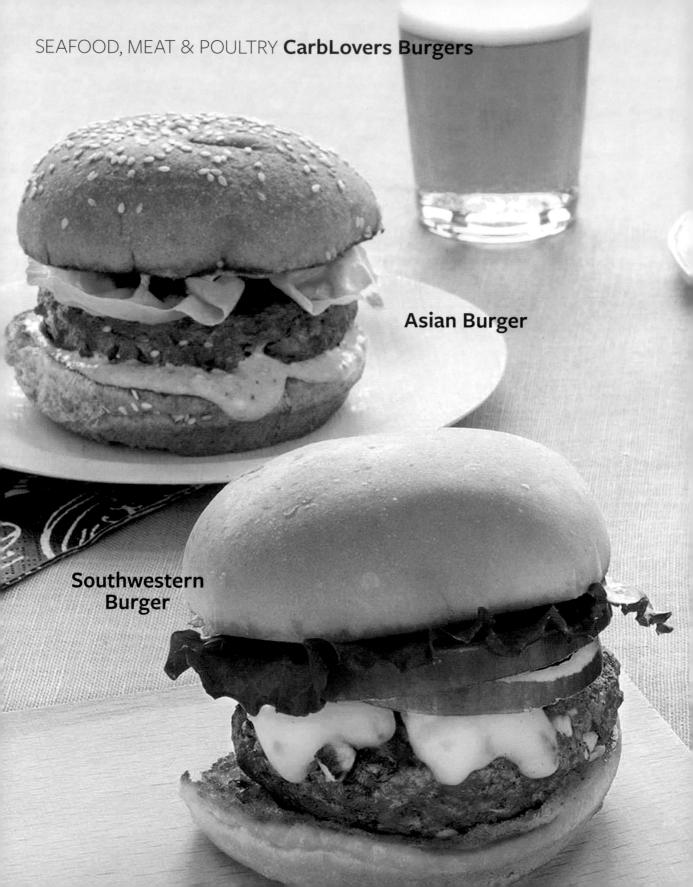

Asian Burger

Southwestern Burger

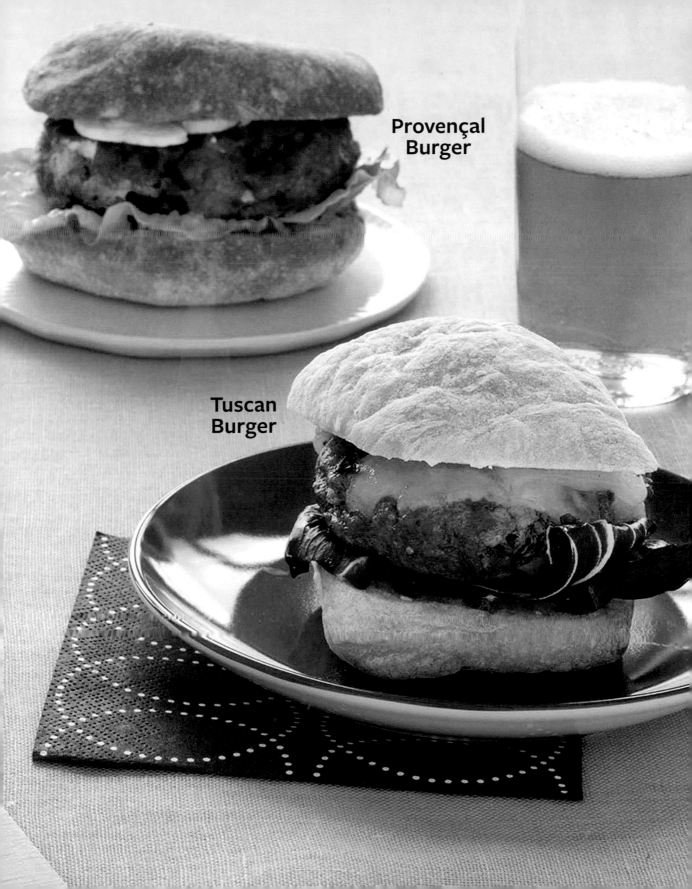

Provençal
Burger

Tuscan
Burger

RS
0.2–2.5g

Dressed-Up Burgers

Prep: 15 minutes | *Cook:* 10–12 minutes | *Total time:* 25 minutes | *Makes:* 4 servings

There's nothing like sinking your teeth into a juicy burger. To keep it interesting during grilling season, we came up with variations to please every palate, from mild to wild.

BURGER BASE:

500g (1lb) extra-lean minced beef
1 egg
4 tablespoons finely chopped red onion
2 teaspoons finely chopped garlic

Serving size: 1 burger, 1 bun and ¼ toppings

SOUTHWESTERN MIX-INS

75g (3 oz) frozen sweetcorn kernels
2 tablespoons chopped fresh coriander
¼ teaspoon chipotle chilli powder
Cheese: 4 (20g/¾ oz) slices Pepper Jack
Lettuce: 4 red-leaf lettuce leaves
Garnish: 8 red onion rings
Bun: 4 plain burger buns

Serving size: 1 burger, 1 bun and ¼ toppings Calories 399; Fat 15.4g (sat 7.1g, mono 3.2g, poly 1.4g); Cholesterol 131mg; Protein 34g; Carbohydrate 31g; Sugars 5g; Fibre 2g; RS 0.2g; Sodium 414mg

ASIAN MIX-INS

4 tablespoons chopped scallion
1 tablespoon toasted sesame seeds
2 teaspoons toasted sesame oil

1 teaspoon Sriracha (chilli-garlic sauce

SRIRACHA MAYO FOR BUNS

4 tablespoons light mayo
2 teaspoons Sriracha sauce
Lettuce: 4 round lettuce leaves
Bun: 4 sesame seed buns

Serving size: 1 burger, 1 bun and ¼ toppings Calories 428; Fat 18g (sat 5.1g, mono 5.2g, poly 4.6g); Cholesterol 114mg; Protein 30g; Carbohydrate 36g; Sugars 6g; Fibre 2g; RS 0.5g; Sodium 560mg

TUSCAN MIX-INS

125g (4oz) drained, rinsed, canned cannellini beans
2 tablespoons chopped sun-dried tomatoes
2 tablespoons finely chopped rosemary
25g (1 oz) chopped rocket
Lettuce for bun: 4 radicchio leaves
Cheese: 4 (20g/¾oz) slices Fontina
Bun: 4 square rolls

Serving size: 1 burger, 1 bun and ¼ toppings Calories 467; Fat 14.4g (sat 7g, mono 4.6g, poly 1g); Cholesterol 133mg; Protein 37g;

Carbohydrates 45g; Sugars 3g; Fibre 4g; RS 2.5g; Sodium 685mg

PROVENÇAL MIX-INS

1 tablespoon chopped Niçoise olives
2 teaspoons dried herbes de Provence
Cheese: 65g (2½oz) goat cheese
Lettuce: 4 Romaine lettuce leaves
Bun: 4 sourdough rolls

Serving size: 1 burger, 1 bun, and ¼ toppings Calories 447; Fat 11g (sat 4.4g, mono 4g, poly 1.4g); Cholesterol 112mg; Protein 35g; Carbohydrate 51g; Sugars 3g; Fiber 3g; RS 1.8g; Sodium 625mg

1. With clean hands, combine base plus mix-in ingredients in a large bowl, then form into 4 equal-size burgers. Heat a griddle pan over medium-high heat and grill burgers until medium-rare, 5–6 minutes per side. Transfer to a large plate.

2. If recipe calls for cheese, immediately place on top of cooked burger. Place on bun and add additional toppings.

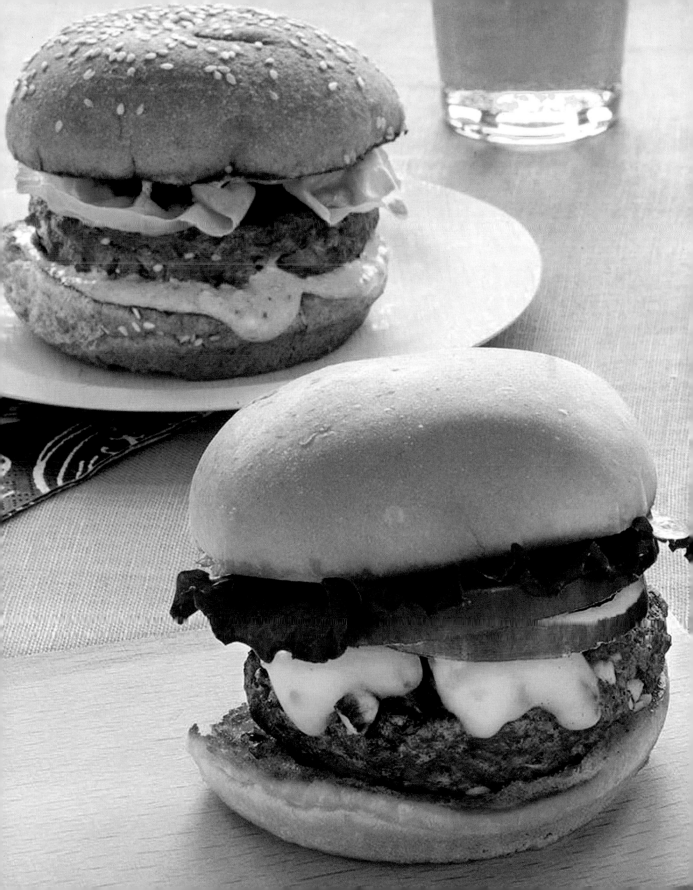

Roast Beef Fillet with Rosemary Roasted Potatoes

Prep: *15 minutes* | **Cook:** *1 hour* | **Total time:** *1 hour 15 minutes* | **Makes:** *8 servings*

Classic and satisfying, a Sunday roast fills your house with the most amazing aroma. We promise that this will become a family favourite.

1kg (2lb) baby potatoes, halved

1 tablespoon plus 1 teaspoon olive oil

1 tablespoon chopped rosemary

1¾ teaspoons sea salt

½ plus ⅛ teaspoon freshly ground black pepper

2 garlic cloves

1.25 kg (2½lb) centre-cut beef fillet, trimmed

450ml (¾pint) reduced-sodium beef stock

1 tablespoon cornflour

125ml (4fl oz) dry red wine

15g (½oz) cold butter

1. Preheat oven to 200°C/400°F/gas mark 6. Toss potatoes with 1 tablespoon oil and rosemary on a rimmed baking sheet; season with 1 teaspoon salt and ¼ teaspoon pepper. Roast 10 minutes.

2. Meanwhile, finely chop garlic; sprinkle with ½ teaspoon salt. Using flat edge of knife, smash salt and garlic to form a paste. Transfer to a bowl; combine with 1 teaspoon oil and ¼ teaspoon pepper. Rub beef with mixture.

3. Heat a large frying over high heat. Add beef to frying pan, turning occasionally, until browned all over, 5–8 minutes. Remove baking sheet from oven; nestle beef among potatoes. (Reserve pan.) Roast beef with potatoes until internal temperature reaches 52°C/125°F, about 30–35 minutes. Transfer to a carving board to rest; continue roasting potatoes until tender, about 10 minutes.

4. Return reserved pan to heat; add stock, stirring to loosen browned bits. Simmer until reduced by half, 5–8 minutes. Whisk together cornflour and red wine; add to pan. Simmer until thickened, 2 minutes. Remove from heat and swirl in butter; season with remaining ¼ teaspoon salt and ⅛ teaspoon pepper. Slice roast and serve with potatoes and sauce.

Serving size: 125g (4oz) beef, 65g (2½oz) potatoes, 2 tablespoons sauce Calories 335; Fat 11.7g (sat 4.3g, mono 5.2g, poly 0.6g); Cholesterol 81mg; Protein 30g; Carbohydrate 23g; Sugars 2g; Fibre 2g; RS 1g; Sodium 581mg

Slow-Baked BBQ Ribs

Prep: *10 minutes* | **Cook:** *3 hours 10 minutes* | **Total time:** *3 hours 20 minutes*
Makes: *6 appetizer-size servings*

Succulent, juicy, and super-saucy, our BBQ ribs are much lower in fat than a traditional version. Definitely don't wear white when you eat them!

4 tablespoons no-salt-added tomato
   sauce
1 tablespoon mustard
1 tablespoon brown sugar
1 tablespoon chilli powder
1 teaspoon cider vinegar
½ teaspoon cumin
¼ teaspoon salt
½ teaspoon smoked paprika
¼ teaspoon cayenne pepper
750g (1½lb), 7cm (3 inch) beef spare
   ribs (about 6 pieces), trimmed of
   visible fat

1. Combine first 9 ingredients (through cayenne) in a small bowl; reserve barbecue sauce.

2. Preheat grill. Place ribs on a rimmed baking sheet and grill until browned, 5 minutes per side. Remove ribs from oven and tip fat from baking sheet; discard. Cool ribs for 15 minutes. Meanwhile, preheat oven to 150°C/300°F/ gas mark 2.

3. Place ribs in a square baking dish and spread barbecue sauce on ribs. Wrap tightly in foil and bake until fork-tender, about 3 hours. Drain additional fat from baking dish and serve ribs while hot.

Serving size: 1 spare rib Calories 306; Fat 23.1g (sat 9.3g, mono 9.8g, poly 1g); Cholesterol 70mg; Protein 19g; Carbohydrate 4g; Sugars 3g; Fibre 1g; RS 0g; Sodium 205mg

RS
1.3g

Chilli Dogs

Prep: *15 minutes* | **Cook:** *19 minutes* | **Total time:** *34 minutes* | **Makes:** *4 servings*

Break out the extra napkins! Our loaded chilli dogs are absolutely packed with toppings – and totally delicious. You'll have chilli left over, which is great on its own or served over a baked potato.

CHILLI:

2 teaspoons olive oil
1 small onion, diced
2 garlic cloves, finely chopped
475g (15oz) can reduced-salt
  kidney beans, rinsed and drained
250ml (8fl oz) can low sodium
  tomato sauce
1 teaspoon chilli powder
¼ teaspoon salt
¼ teaspoon pepper
4 low-fat hot dogs, grilled
4 hot dog rolls

TOPPINGS:

4 tablespoons diced tomato
4 tablespoons diced red onion
4 tablespoons coarsely grated reduced-fat
  Cheddar cheese
4 tablespoons diced green chillies

1. Make chilli: Heat oil in a small saucepan over medium-high heat. Add onion and cook, stirring, until soft and translucent, 6–7 minutes, Add garlic and cook 1 minute. Add beans, tomato sauce, 4 tablespoons water, chilli powder, salt and pepper. Bring to boil, then reduce heat and cook, stirring occasionally, until beans absorb some of the liquid and chilli has thickened, 12–15 minutes.

2. Place a hot dog on a hot dog roll. Top with 4 tablespoons chilli, and 1 tablespoon each of tomato, onion, cheese and chillies.

Serving size: 1 hot dog, 4 tablespoons chilli, 1 tablespoon each tomato, onion, cheese and chillies   Calories 340; Fat 13g (sat 4.3g, mono 0.8g, poly 0.2g); Cholesterol 35mg; Protein 17g; Carbohydrate 38g; Sugars 9g; Fibre 7g; RS 1.3g; Sodium 811mg

{
TIP:
To lower the risk of choking, please be sure to cut hot dogs into small pieces for young children.
}

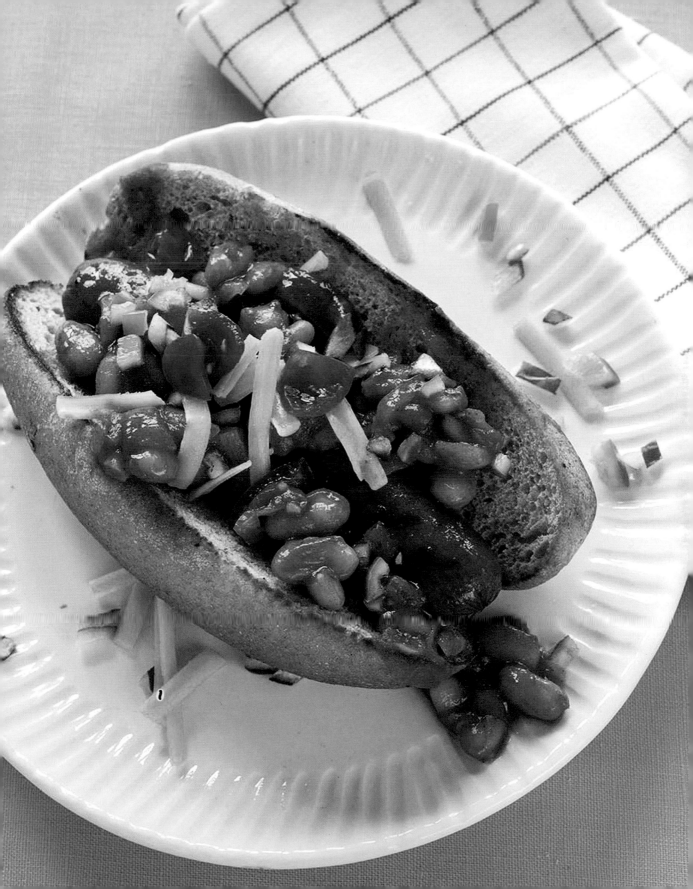

RS
0.6g

Grilled Chicken Escalopes with Summer Succotash

Prep time: 1 minute | *Cook time:* 4 minutes | *Total time:* 5 minutes | *Makes:* 4 servings

A main dish in 5 minutes flat? It's do-able when you use frozen vegetables and ultra-thin chicken escalopes.

4 chicken escalopes (500g/1lb in total)
¼ teaspoon sea salt
¼ teaspoon freshly ground
   black pepper
1 tablespoon olive oil
75g (3oz) frozen sweetcorn, thawed
175g (6oz) frozen baby broad beans,
   thawed
225g (8oz) cherry tomatoes
1 tablespoon grated Parmesan
8 tablespoons fresh basil leaves, torn if
   large
Lemon wedges for serving

1. Heat a griddle pan over high heat; season chicken escalopes with salt and pepper. Cook chicken escalopes until cooked through, 3–4 minutes, turning once.

2. Meanwhile, heat oil in a large frying pan over medium-high heat. Add corn, broad beans, and cherry tomatoes to pan. Cook, tossing occasionally, until tomatoes begin to burst, 3–4 minutes. Stir Parmesan and basil into pan and divide mixture between plates. Top with cooked chicken; serve with lemon wedges.

Serving size: 1 chicken escalope and 125g (4oz) vegetables Calories 265; Fat 7.1g (sat1.6g, mono 3.7g, poly 1.2g); Cholesterol 73mg; Protein 31g; Carbohydrate 18g; Sugars 4g; Fibre 4g; RS 0.6g; Sodium 216mg

TIP:
Pump up the Resistant Starch
in this meal by adding a
wholemeal or rye roll.

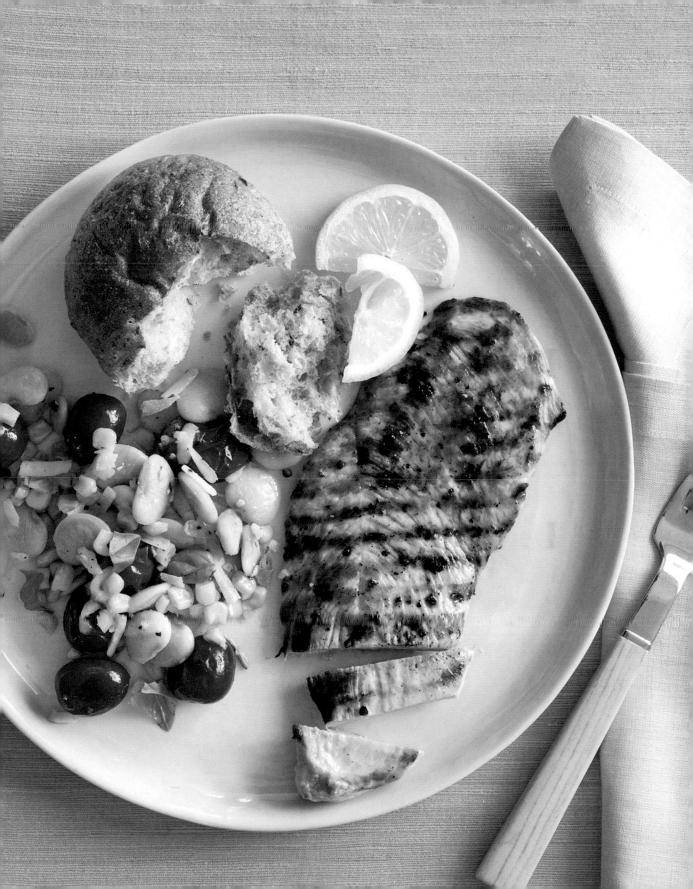

RS
0.9g

Cornflake-Crusted Chicken Strips

Prep: *25 minutes* | **Cook:** *12 minutes* | **Total time:** *37 minutes* | **Makes:** *4 servings*

Kids of all ages love fried chicken fingers. We lightened up this recipe by using Resistant Starch–filled cornflakes to coat the chicken, and then baked them to cut the fat. Go on—they're not just for kids anymore!

125g (4oz) cornflakes
1 tablespoon sesame seeds
½ teaspoon paprika
¼ teaspoon salt
½ teaspoon pepper
¼ teaspoon cayenne pepper
4 tablespoons plain flour
4 x 125g (4oz) boneless, skinless
   chicken breasts, pounded to
   ½ inch (1cm) thickness
2 egg whites, lightly beaten
Olive oil cooking spray

1. Preheat oven to 200°C/400°F/gas mark 6.

2. Place cornflakes in a food processor and pulse to make crumbs, 20–30 seconds. Combine cornflake crumbs, sesame seeds, ¼ teaspoon each paprika, salt and pepper, and cayenne in a shallow dish.

3. Place flour and remaining paprika and pepper in a resealable plastic bag and shake gently to mix.

4. Place egg whites in another shallow dish.

5. Slice each chicken breast into 6 strips and place in bag with flour and shake well to coat.

6. In batches, place coated chicken strips in egg whites. Remove, shaking off excess, and roll in cornflake-crumb mixture.

7. Arrange coated strips on a baking sheet and coat tops of strips lightly with cooking spray.

8. Bake until crisp and golden, 11–12 minutes.

Serving size: 6 strips Calories 284; Fat 4.7g (sat 0.9g, mono 1.5g, poly 1.2g); Cholesterol 73mg; Protein 29g; Carbohydrate 31g; Sugars 3g; Fibre 1g; RS 0.9g; Sodium 508mg

Lemon-Herb Roasted Turkey Breast

Prep: 10 minutes | *Cook:* 1 hour 30 minutes + resting | *Total time:* 1 hour 40 minutes | *Makes:* 6 servings

There's no reason to spend hours cooking a whole turkey when you can make this juicy turkey breast in half the time. Serve with roasted new potatoes or our Herb and Olive Oil Mashed Potatoes on page 194.

2 tablespoons olive oil
1 tablespoon chopped rosemary
1 tablespoon chopped thyme
1 tablespoon chopped oregano
1 lemon, zested; reserve zest and
  lemon
1 large garlic clove, finely chopped
½ teaspoon salt
½ teaspoon cracked black pepper
1.25kg/ 2½lb) bone-in skinless
  turkey breast, patted dry
⅓ cup dry white wine

1. Preheat oven to 180°C/350°F/gas mark 4.

2. Combine oil, rosemary, thyme, oregano, zest, garlic, salt, and pepper in a small bowl to form a paste. Spread evenly over turkey breast. Place in a roasting pan and gently pour wine into bottom of pan.

3. Slice zested lemon into wedges and place in bottom of pan. Tent with foil and roast for 1 hour. Remove foil and continue roasting until an instant-read thermometer reads 74°C/165°F, about 30–40 minutes. Remove from oven and let turkey rest for 10 minutes.

4. Transfer to a carving board and slice off the bone into 1cm(½ inch) thick slices. Squeeze roasted lemon wedges into pan juices and pour 2 tablespoons pan juices onto each portion.

Serving size: 125g (4oz) turkey and 2 tablespoons sauce
Calories 236; Fat 5.6g (sat 1g, mono 3.5g, poly 0.8g); Cholesterol 110mg; Protein 40g; Carbohydrate 3g; Sugars 0g; Fibre 1g; RS 0g; Sodium 264mg

Individual Chicken Pot Pies

Prep time: *20 minutes* | **Cook Time:** *1 hour 15 minutes* | **Total:** *1 hour 35 minutes* | **Makes:** *4 servings*

RS
1.6g

The flaky crust on our chicken pot pie is so inviting, you'll hardly be able to resist digging in. This may be the ultimate comfort recipe.

---

1 tablespoon olive oil

1 small onion, chopped

2 garlic cloves, finely chopped

1 tablespoon chopped thyme

125g (4oz) celery, diced

150g (5oz) carrots, diced

500g (1lb) boneless, skinless chicken breasts, diced

4 tablespoons white wine

40g (1½oz) flour

750ml (1¼ pints) milk

250ml (8fl oz) low-sodium chicken stock

2 teaspoons Worcestershire sauce

¼ teaspoon salt

¼ teaspoon pepper

150g (5oz) frozen peas

6 sheets frozen filo pastry, thawed

Olive oil cooking spray

1. Preheat oven to 200°C/400°F/gas mark 6.

2. Heat oil in a medium saucepan over medium-high heat and cook onion, stirring occasionally, until soft and translucent, 6–7 minutes. Add garlic and thyme and cook 1 minute. Add celery and carrots and cook until crisp-tender, 2–3 minutes. Add chicken and cook, stirring occasionally, until no longer pink and cooked through, 5–6 minutes.

3. Add wine; cook until mostly absorbed, 2–3 minutes. Add flour to pan; cook, stirring, for 2 minutes. Whisk in milk, stock, Worcestershire sauce, salt and pepper. Bring to boil, reduce heat, and cook, whisking, until mixture thickens, 15 minutes. Add peas during last minute. Remove from heat and reserve.

4. Arrange 6 sheets of stacked filo pastry on a surface. Place a 12cm (5 inch) bowl on the bottom right quarter of the stacked sheets. Using a pizza cutter, cut around the bowl to form a circle. Coat on top and in between layers lightly with cooking spray. Using the pizza cutter, cut 3 1cm (½inch) slits into the filo round. Repeat with remaining pastry. Place four 12cm (5 inch) ovenproof bowls on a rimmed baking sheet. Divide the mixture between bowls; transfer filo rounds to cover, pressing gently. Bake until tops are brown, 35–40 minutes. Serve hot.

Serving size: 1 pot pie Calories 455; Fat 9.8g (sat 2.8g, mono 4.7g, poly 1.4g); Cholesterol 76mg; Protein 39g; Carbohydrate 49g; Sugars 16g; Fibre 7g; RS 1.6g; Sodium 551mg

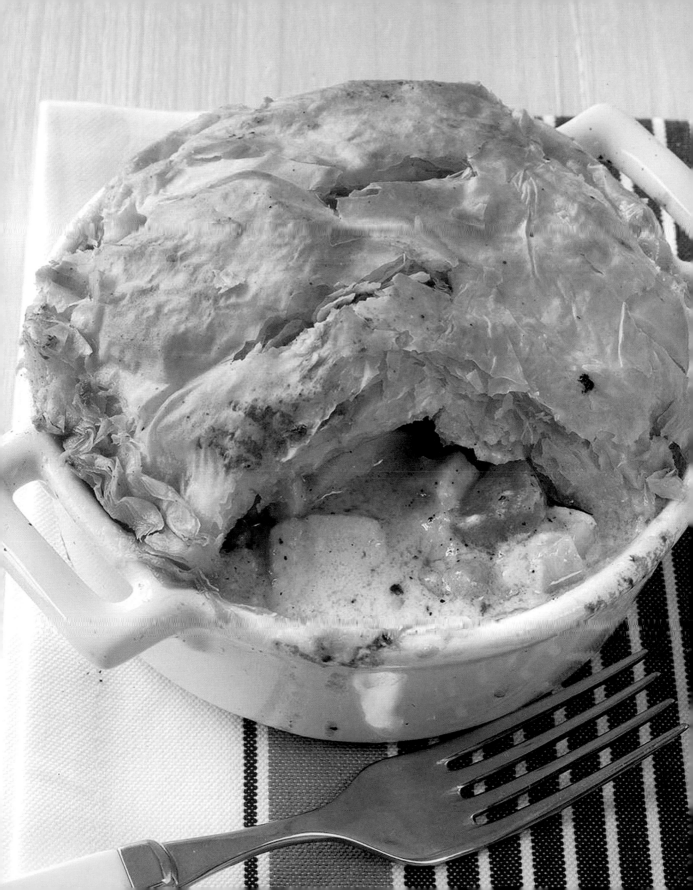

RS
2.7g

Orange Chicken Stir-Fry

Prep: *10 minutes* | **Cook:** *35 minutes* | **Total:** *45 minutes* | **Makes:** *4 servings*

If you're a fan of Chinese takeaways, give this healthy, superlow-sodium version a spin. It will probably be on the table faster than your local retaurant can deliver.

2 navel oranges, cut into segments,
  membranes squeezed to
  make 4 tablespoons juice
2 tablespoons rice wine vinegar
1 teaspoon finely grated ginger
1 garlic clove, finely grated
¼ teaspoon dried chilli flakes
2 spring onions, sliced, whites and greens
  separated
2 x 175g (6oz) boneless, skinless
  chicken breasts, thinly sliced
200g (7oz) brown rice
2 teaspoons vegetable oil
4 tablespoons flaked almonds
2 bunches watercress (300g/10 oz),
  thick stems removed
1 teaspoon sesame oil

1. Whisk together orange juice, vinegar, ginger, garlic, chilli flakes, and spring onions in a large shallow bowl. Add chicken and marinate in the refrigerator for at least 20 minutes and up to 1 hour.

2. Meanwhile, cook rice according to packet instructions.

3. Heat oil in a large heavy frying pan over medium-high heat. With a slotted spoon, remove chicken from marinade and transfer to hot pan. Cook chicken about 3 minutes or until partially cooked through; stir in almonds and watercress. Cook, stirring, until watercress is wilted and chicken is cooked, 1 minute more. Gently toss orange segments and sesame oil into stir-fry; serve over rice.

Serving size: About 125g (4oz) stir-fry, 65g (2½oz) cooked rice Calories 378; Fat 10.1g (sat 1.3g, mono 3.9g, poly 3.6g); Cholesterol 54mg; Protein 26g; Carbohydrate 47g; Sugars 7g; Fibre 6g; RS 2.7g; Sodium 135mg

Herbed Turkey-Feta Burgers

RS 0.4g

*Prep: 15 minutes | **Cook:** 15 minutes (including assembly) | **Total time:** 30 minutes | **Makes:** 4 servings*

Greek spices, feta cheese and zesty yogurt dip make this the tastiest turkey burger you've ever tried. Use minced turkey breast to lower the fat even more.

500g (1lb) minced turkey
½ teaspoon freshly ground black pepper
4 tablespoons crumbled feta cheese
4 tablespoons diced roasted red pepper
4 tablespoons diced red onion
2 tablespoons finely chopped parsley
2 teaspoons finely chopped oregano
4 x 1cm (½ inch) onion ring slices
125ml (4fl oz) low-fat Greek yogurt
2 tablespoons lemon juice
1 teaspoon lemon zest
⅛ teaspoon salt
⅛ teaspoon pepper
4 wholegrain burger buns, split
4 lettuce leaves

1. Combine turkey, pepper, feta, roasted red pepper, red onion, parsley, and oregano in a large bowl; form into 4 equal-sized burgers. Chill until ready to use.

2. Coat a griddle pan with cooking spray and heat over medium-high heat. Grill burgers until cooked through, 5 minutes per side. When cooking second side of burgers, grill onions until charred, about 5 minutes. Whisk together yogurt, lemon juice, zest, salt and pepper. Spread 2 tablespoons yogurt dressing on the bottom of a bun. Place one lettuce leaf and one grilled onion ring on it. Top with a burger and other half of bun.

Serving size: 1 bun, 1 burger, 1 lettuce leaf and 1 grilled onion ring Calories 370; Fat 13.7g (sat 4.4g, mono 4.1g, poly 3.4g); Cholesterol 85mg; Protein 31g; Carbohydrate 34g; Sugars 9g; Fibre 5g; RS 0.4g; Sodium 441mg

Quick Chicken Mole

Prep: *5 minutes* | **Cook:** *20 minutes* | **Total time:** *25 minutes* | **Makes:** *6 servings*

"Mole is the perfect solution for chocolate lovers to have chocolate before dessert, not to mention packing in the healthful antioxidants that chocolate possesses. Besides chicken, try the mole on beef, seasoned tofu, drizzled over rice and beans, and even as a condiment." Carla Hall

1 tablespoon vegetable oil

1 medium onion, finely chopped

2 garlic cloves, minced

1½ teaspoons ground cumin

1 teaspoon ground cinnamon

½ teaspoon salt

¼ teaspoon freshly ground black
  pepper

875g (1¾ diced tomatoes

125g (4oz) diced green chillies

1 teaspoon tahini

75g (3oz) chopped dark chocolate

1 tablespoon chopped fresh coriander

  1   rotisserie chicken, divided into 6
pieces, warmed

½ avocado, stoned and sliced

1 tomato, diced

1. Heat oil over medium heat in a large saucepan. Add onion; cook for 3 minutes or until translucent. Add garlic; cook for 1 minute. Stir in cumin, cinnamon, salt and pepper; cook for 1 minute.

2. Add canned diced tomatoes and chilies to saucepan; simmer for 10 minutes. Stir in tahini and chocolate until melted. Stir in chopped coriander; remove from heat and cool slightly. Process in a blender or food processor for 30 seconds or until smooth. (Add some water if sauce is too thick.) Spoon sauce over chicken. Serve with avocado and tomato.

Serving size: ⅙ chicken with sauce Calories 354; Fat 17.2g (sat 5.7g, mono 6.2g, poly 3.6g); Cholesterol 85mg; Protein 31g; Carbohydrate 19g; Sugars 11g; Fibre 5g; Iron 3mg; RS 0g; Sodium 648mg

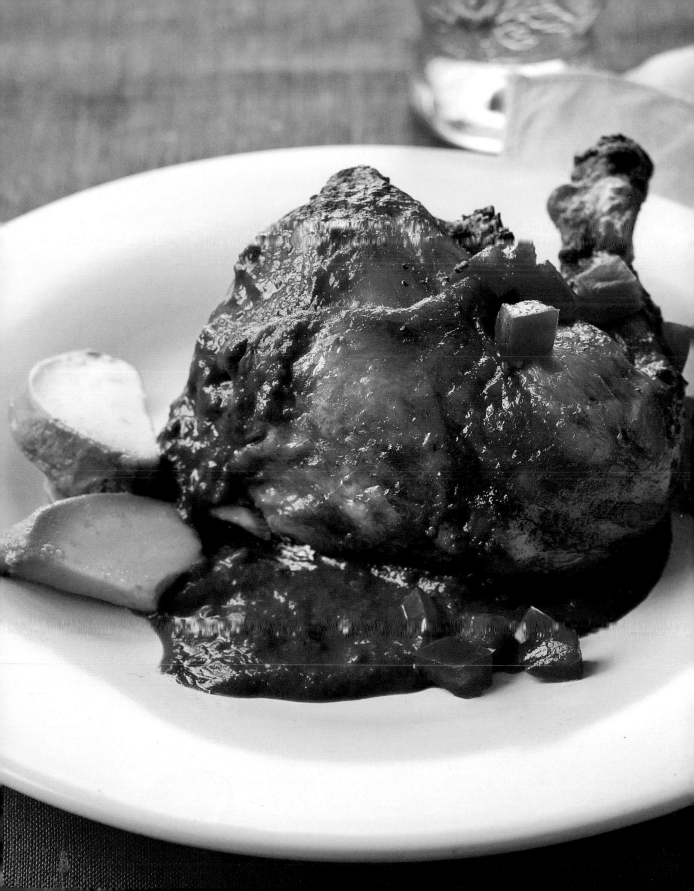

Sides & Salads

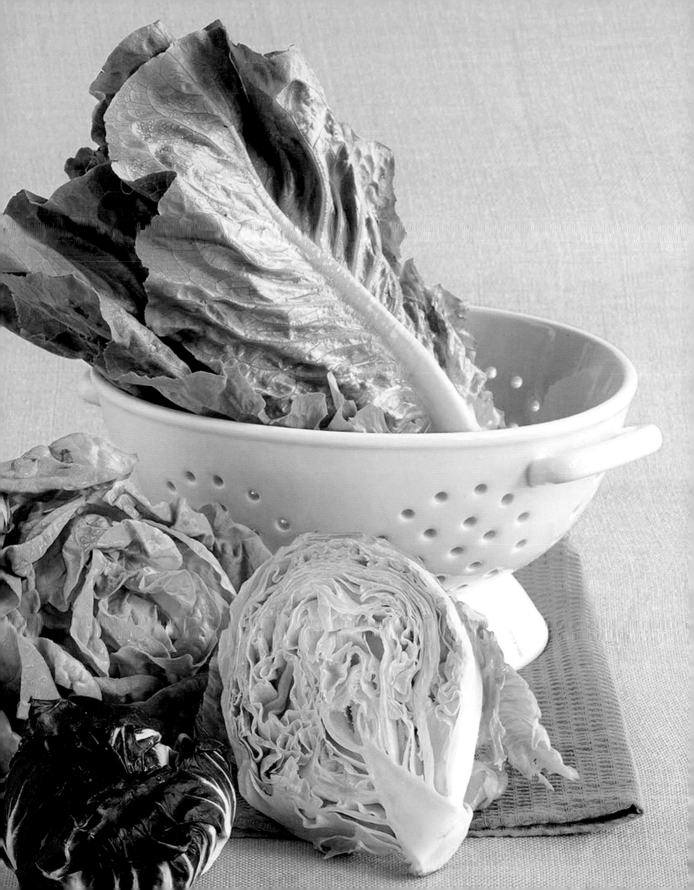

RS
3g

Barley Salad with Corn, Feta, Basil and Charred Tomatoes

Prep: 5 minutes | **Cook:** 20 minutes | **Total time:** 25 minutes | **Makes:** 4 servings

Flavourful, colourful and full of Resistant Starch, this healthy salad is a wonderful side dish for chicken or steak, and makes a fantastic vegetarian main course.

200g (7oz) pearl barley
175g (6oz) frozen sweetcorn
225g (8oz) cherry tomatoes
3 tablespoons olive oil
1 tablespoon white wine vinegar
½ teaspoon salt
¼ teaspoon freshly ground black pepper
50g (2oz) feta cheese, crumbled
4 tablespoons sliced basil leaves

1. Preheat grill with rack in highest position. Cover barley with salted water in a medium saucepan and cook over medium heat until just tender, about 15 minutes. Add corn; remove from heat. Let stand 1 minute; drain and run under cold water until cooled.

2. Meanwhile, toss tomatoes with 1 tablespoon oil; season with ¼ teaspoon salt and pepper. Grill, tossing occasionally, until tomatoes become charred and they burst, about 8 minutes.

3. Whisk together vinegar and remaining 2 tablespoons oil in a medium bowl; season with remaining ¼ teaspoon salt. Add barley and corn to bowl and toss with dressing; fold in tomatoes, feta and basil.

Serving size: 1¼ cups salad Calories 340; Fat 14.9g (sat 4.4g, mono 8.4g, poly 1.6g); Cholesterol 17mg; Protein 7g; Carbohydrate 46g; Sugars 5g; Fibre 6g; RS 3g; Sodium 562mg

TIP
Barley is loaded with Resistant Starch and makes a delicious, filling side dish. Cook extra and refrigerate for up to 4 days or freeze for up to 3 months in a freezer-safe bag or container. Squeeze out all the air before freezing, and mark with the cook date.

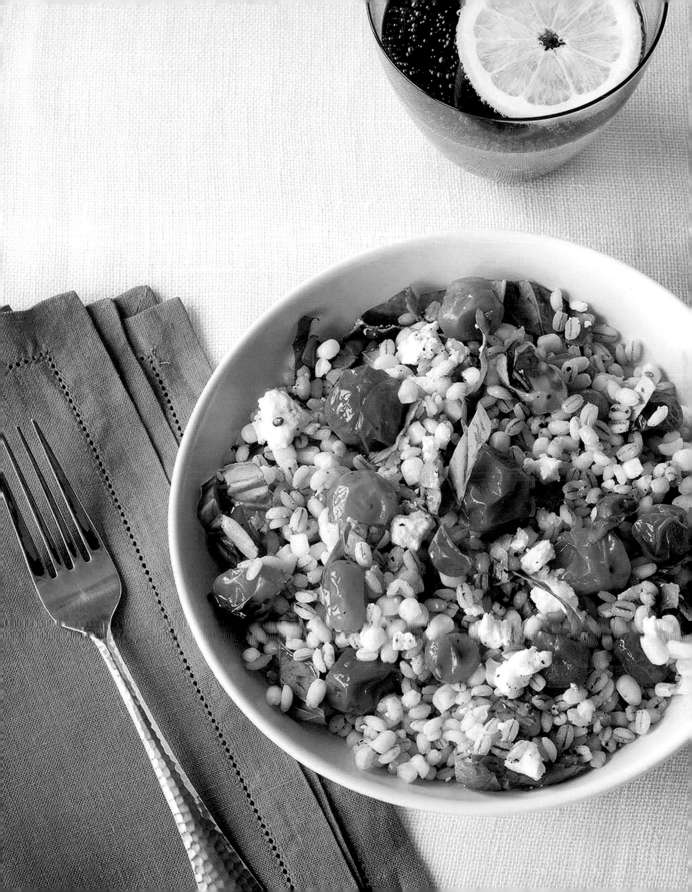

Thai Green Mango Salad with Rotisserie Chicken

Prep: *10 minutes* | **Total time:** *10 minutes* | **Makes:** *4 servings*

Refreshing and light, this salad is perfect for warm summer nights. And it's a great way to use leftover chicken.

1 tablespoon chilli-garlic sauce
  (such as Sriracha)
4 tablespoons fresh lime juice
1 tablespoon fish sauce
2 tablespoons brown sugar
1 unripe mango (about 500g/1lb),
  peeled and thinly sliced
50g (2oz) carrots, cut into matchsticks
250g (8oz) rotisserie chicken,
  shredded
25g (1oz) coriander leaves
250g (8oz) cherry tomatoes, halved
2 tablespoons peanuts, chopped

Whisk together chilli-garlic sauce, lime juice, fish sauce and sugar in a large bowl. Add mango, carrots, chicken, coriander and tomatoes; toss. Sprinkle with peanuts before serving.

Serving size: 275g (9oz) Calories 265; Fat 7.7g (sat 1.8g, mono 3.1g, poly 1.9g); Cholesterol 63mg; Protein 23g; Carbohydrate 28g; Sugars 22g; Fibre 3g; RS 0g;Sodium 352mg

ASK CARBLOVERS

Q: Can I eat all the veggies and salads I want on *CarbLovers*?

A: We love veggies and salads on this diet! Feel free to add a green side salad with a tablespoon of vinaigrette to any meal. Vegetables are high in fibre and water and help you feel full between meals, but you can overdo the calories once you start adding toppings and dressing.

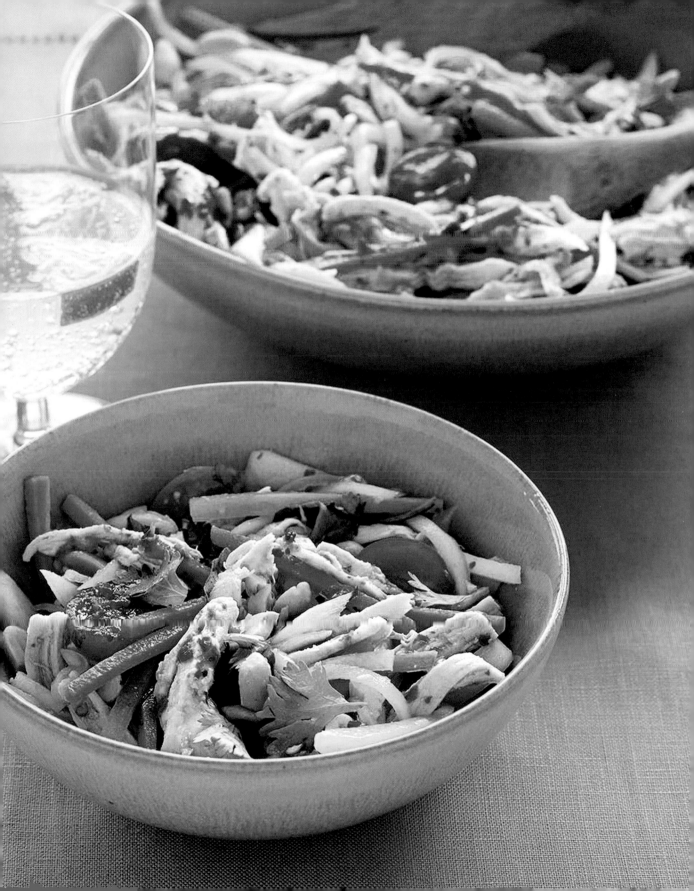

RS
3.7g

Pearl Barley with Peas and Edamame

Prep: 5 minutes | **Cook:** 30 minutes | **Total Time:** 35 minutes | **Makes:** 4 servings

"Carbs are the ultimate food in my book. I will never – mark my words – cut them from my diet! My day is filled with them, from my morning muesli to a late-night pizza with the girls." Candice Kumai, chef and author

200g (7oz) dry pearl barley
175g (6oz) shelled frozen edamame
  (soya beans)
150g (5oz) frozen peas
50g (2oz) fresh spinach, chopped
2¼ teaspoons Worcestershire sauce
1½ teaspoons lemon zest
1½ tablespoons fresh lemon juice
¼ teaspoon sea salt

1. Place barley and 1 litre (1¾ pints) water in a medium saucepan; bring to the boil. Cover, reduce heat to low, and cook until water is nearly absorbed, 25–30 minutes. Stir in edamame and peas and cook, uncovered, until barley absorbs all of the remaining water, 5–10 minutes. Remove from heat.

2. Stir in spinach; set aside. Combine Worcestershire sauce, lemon zest, lemon juice and sea salt in a small bowl, whisking well. Pour vinaigrette over barley; stir to combine. Serve warm or at room temperature.

Serving size: About 150g (5oz) Calories 227; Fat 2.4g (sat 0.3g, mono 0.6g, poly 1.1g); Cholesterol 0mg; Protein 10g; Carbohydrate 43g; Sugars 4g; Fibre 9g; Iron 4mg; RS 3.7g; Sodium 213mg

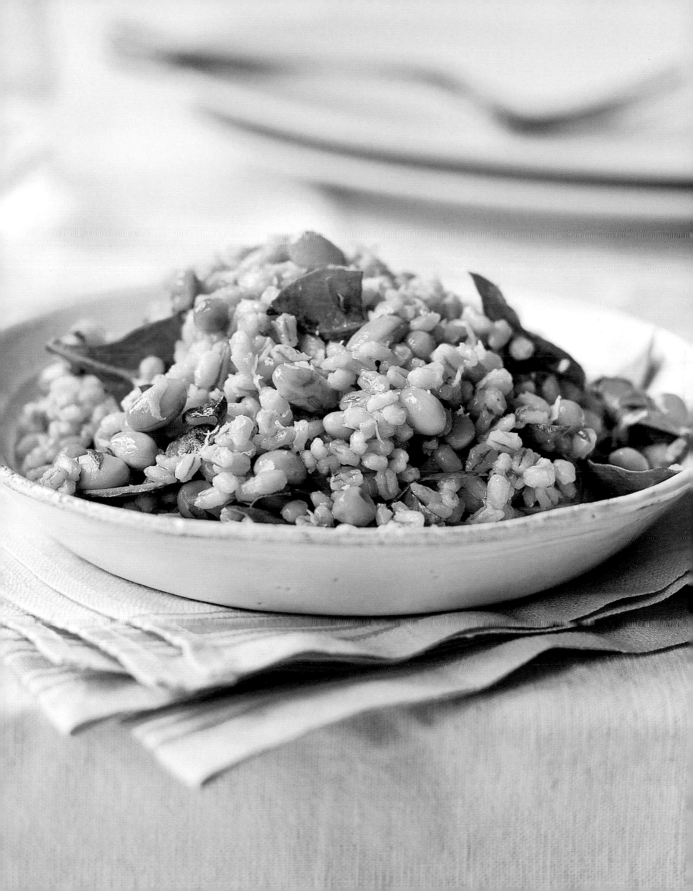

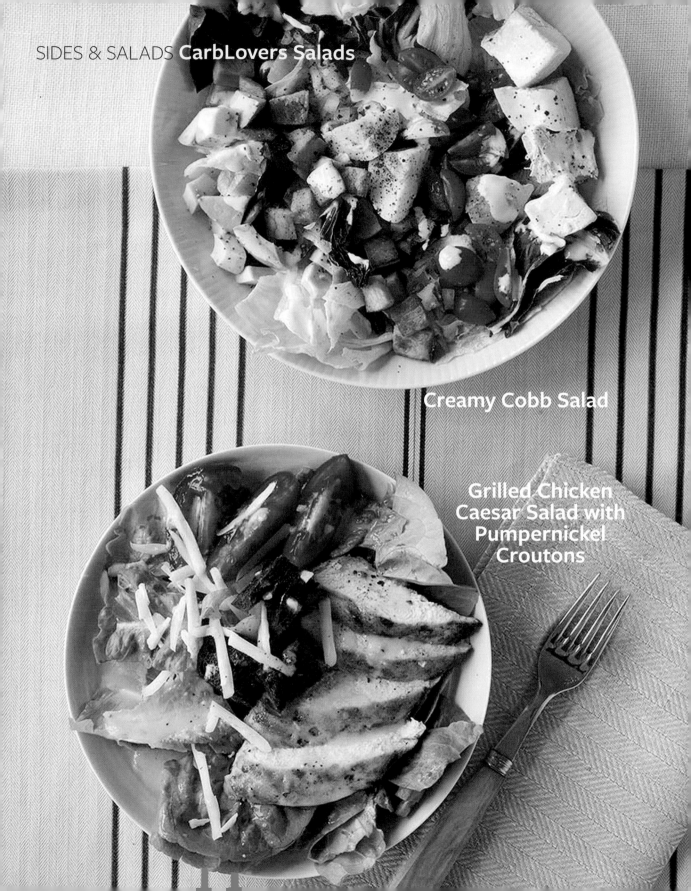

Creamy Cobb Salad

Grilled Chicken
Caesar Salad with
Pumpernickel
Croutons

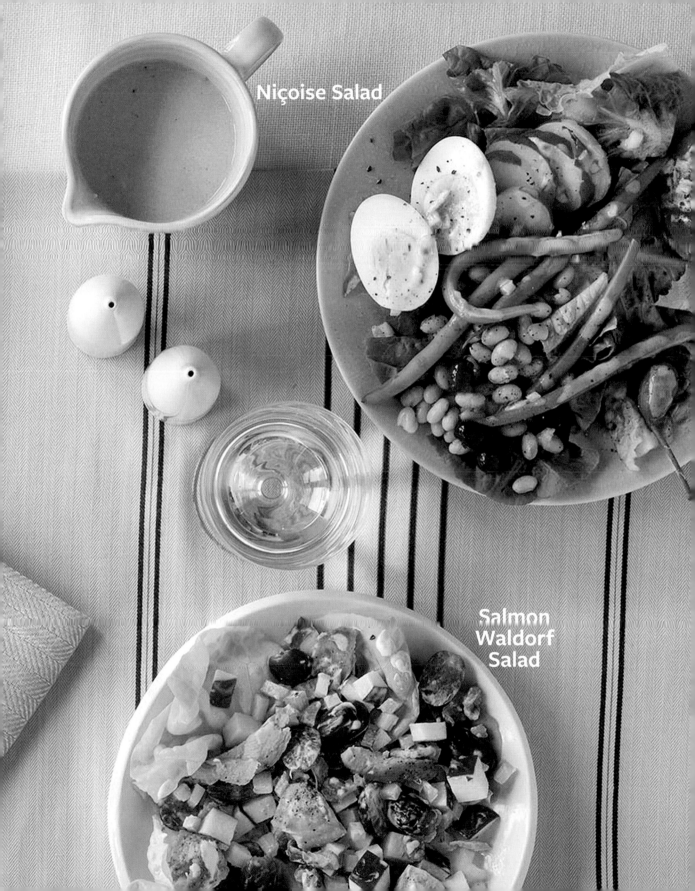

Niçoise Salad

Salmon
Waldorf
Salad

Creamy Cobb Salad

Prep: *15 minutes* | **Cook:** *5 minutes* | **Total time:** *20 minutes* | **Makes:** *4 servings*

Salads can sometimes taste a bit boring. Not this one. We've taken a traditional Cobb and lightened it up, but it's still packed with flavour.

FOR DRESSING:

75ml (3fl oz) low-fat buttermilk

3 tablespoons light soured cream

2 tablespoons light
  mayonnaise

1 tablespoon red wine
  vinegar

1 teaspoon Dijon mustard

1 teaspoon freshly ground black
  pepper

FOR SALAD:

4 rashers (75g/3oz) smoked back
  bacon, diced

375g (12oz) iceberg lettuce, chopped

250g (8oz) radicchio, chopped

250g (8oz) thick-cut roasted
  turkey breast, diced

500g (1lb) cherry tomatoes, halved

½ avocado, diced

4 tablespoons chopped red onion

2 hard-boiled eggs, chopped

MAKE DRESSING:

Whisk together dressing ingredients in a small bowl. Cover and refrigerate until ready to use.

MAKE SALAD:

1. Coat a large nonstick pan with cooking spray and heat over medium-high heat. Add bacon and cook until crisp, 4–5 minutes. Remove from pan and reserve.

2. Toss together lettuce and radicchio in a large bowl; divide between 4 salad bowls. Top each with ¼ of the bacon, turkey, tomatoes, avocado, onion and eggs. Drizzle each salad with about 2½ tablespoons dressing; toss and serve.

Serving size: 1 salad Calories 279; Fat 12.1g (sat 3.1g, mono 4.4g, poly 2.6g); Cholesterol 158mg; Protein 29g; Carbohydrate 15g; Sugars 7g; Fibre 4g; RS 0g; Sodium 499mg

TIP
If you follow a gluten-free diet, check the ingredients on your mayo; some contain gluten. Go to coeliac.org.uk for more info.

Grilled Chicken Caesar Salad with Pumpernickel Croutons

Prep: 20 minutes | **Cook:** 10 minutes | **Total time:** 30 minutes | **Makes:** 4 servings

We took a basic Caesar salad and put our CarbLovers *spin on it by adding homemade pumpernickel croutons for more Resistant Starch.*

FOR CROUTONS:

2 thick slices pumpernickel
  bread, cubed
1 tablespoon olive oil
1 small garlic clove, finely chopped
¼ teaspoon pepper

FOR CHICKEN BREASTS:

4 thin-cut skinless boneless chicken
  breasts (500g/1lb)
¼ teaspoon salt
¼ teaspoon pepper
¼ teaspoon paprika

FOR DRESSING:

1 raw egg or 3 tablespoons
  pasteurized egg product
3 tablespoons lemon juice
1 tablespoon water
1 tablespoon finely chopped garlic
2 teaspoons Dijon mustard
¼ teaspoon cracked black pepper
2 anchovy fillets, drained and
  mashed (about 2 teaspoons)
4 tablespoons olive oil

FOR SALAD:

875g (1¾lb) romaine lettuce, chopped
2 vine-ripened tomatoes, cut into
  wedges
4 tablespoons coarsely grated
  Parmesan cheese

MAKE CROUTONS:

Preheat oven to 180°C/350°F/gas mark 4. Toss bread, oil, garlic and pepper in a bowl to coat. Transfer to a rimmed baking sheet; bake until lightly toasted, 8–9 minutes. Remove from oven and cool completely.

MAKE CHICKEN BREASTS:

Preheat a griddle over medium-high heat. Season chicken with salt, pepper and paprika; grill until cooked through, 3 minutes per side. Remove from heat, rest and slice into 1cm (½inch) slices on the diagonal.

MAKE DRESSING:

Combine first 7 dressing ingredients in a bowl and whisk to incorporate. Slowly whisk in oil until emulsified and creamy.

MAKE SALAD:

Divide the lettuce between 4 salad bowls. Add 1 sliced chicken breast, 1 tomato wedge, and ¼ of the croutons on top of each salad. Drizzle with 3 tablespoons dressing and garnish with 1 tablespoon Parmesan and additional cracked pepper, if liked.

Serving size: 1 salad Calories 423; Fat 23.7g (sat 4.6g, mono 14.5g, poly 3.3g); Cholesterol 115mg; Protein 32g; Carbohydrate 22g; Sugars 4g; Fibre 6g; RS 1.1g; Sodium 609mg

Salmon Waldorf Salad

Prep: *15 minutes* | **Cook:** *17 minutes* | **Total time:** *32 minutes* | **Makes:** *4 servings*

Creamy dressing and crunchy walnuts are the cornerstones of this main or side-dish salad. We added heart-healthy salmon to boost the good fats in this classic dish.

FOR DRESSING:

2 tablespoons light
  mayonnaise
2 tablespoons natural low-fat
  yogurt
2 tablespoons fresh lemon juice
½ teaspoon salt
½ teaspoon pepper

FOR SALAD:

500g (1lb) skinless salmon fillet
1 small red apple, diced
50g (2oz) seedless red grapes,
  halved
2 celery stalks, finely chopped
2 tablespoons walnuts, coarsely
  chopped
1 head round lettuce, leaves
  separated

Preheat oven to 180°C/350°F/gas mark 4.

MAKE DRESSING:

Whisk mayonnaise, yogurt, lemon juice and ¼ teaspoon each of salt and pepper together in a large bowl. Set aside.

MAKE SALAD:

1. Season salmon with remaining salt and pepper, place on a foil-lined baking sheet; bake until cooked through, 16–17 minutes. Remove from oven, cool and flake.

2. Add flaked salmon, apples, grapes, celery and half of the walnuts to the bowl with the dressing. Arrange 4 lettuce leaves in each of 4 shallow bowls and top with ¼ of the salad. Garnish with remaining walnuts.

Serving size: 1 salad Calories 268; Fat 13.3g (sat 2g, mono 3.7g, poly 6.4g); Cholesterol 75mg; Protein 27g; Carbohydrate 10g; Sugars 7g; Fibre 1g; RS 0g; Sodium 420m

Niçoise Salad

Prep: *30 minutes* | ***Total time:*** *30 minutes* | ***Makes:*** *4 servings*

This classic French recipe was popularized by Julia Child. Our version is vegetarian, but you could add a 175g (6oz) can of unsalted tuna back in if you'd like.

FOR DRESSING.

1 teaspoon finely chopped shallot
1 teaspoon Dijon mustard
¼ teaspoon salt
¼ teaspoon pepper
2 tablespoons fresh lemon juice
4 tablespoonsextra virgin olive oil

FOR SALAD:

750g (1½lb) romaine lettuce
 leaves, chopped
4 (125g/4oz) potatoes,
 steamed and sliced
250g (8oz) canned cannellini beans,
 rinsed and drained
4 hard-boiled eggs, halved
250g (8oz) green beans,
 lightly steamed
2 large vine-ripened
 tomatoes, cut into wedges
16 niçoise olives
4 large caperberries, rinsed
 and drained

MAKE DRESSING:

Whisk together first 5 dressing ingredients in a small bowl. Add oil in a slow stream and whisk to emulsify. Set aside.

MAKE SALAD:

Divide lettuce between 4 salad bowls. Evenly distribute potatoes, beans, eggs, green beans, tomatoes, olives and caperberries among bowls. Drizzle each salad with about 2½ tablespoons dressing.

Serving size: 1 salad Calories 433; Fat 23.1g (sat 4.1g, mono 14.8g, poly 3.2g); Cholesterol 186mg; Protein 16g; Carbohydrate 44g; Sugars 7g; Fibre 9g; RS 3.2g; Sodium 641mg

RS
2g

Sweet Potato and Black Bean Salad

Prep: 5 minutes | **Cook:** 25 minutes | **Total time:** 30 minutes | **Makes:** 4 servings

Sweet potatoes and black beans score sky-high in antioxidants. Combine them in this simple, filling salad, and you have a power pair!

2 medium sweet potatoes (500g/1lb),
  cut into 1cm (½inch) cubes
1 tablespoon olive oil
½ teaspoon paprika
¼ teaspoon sea salt
¼ teaspoon pepper
475g (15oz) can black beans,
  rinsed and drained
4 tablespoons chopped fresh coriander
1 tablespoon lime juice

1. Preheat oven to 200°C/400°F/gas mark 6. Toss potatoes with oil, paprika, salt and pepper on a large rimmed baking sheet. Roast 20 to 25 minutes, tossing once, or until potatoes are browned in spots and tender.

2. Transfer potatoes to a large bowl with beans, coriander and lime juice; toss to combine. Serve warm.

Serving size: 250g (8oz) Calories 184; Fat 3.9g (sat 0.6g, mono 2.5g, poly 0.6g); Cholesterol 0mg; Protein 7g; Carbohydrate 32g; Sugars 5g; Fibre 8g; RS 2g; Sodium 297mg

TIP:
Add 375g (12oz) grilled prawns or chicken to turn this into a delicious protein-packed meal for four.

Warm Potato and Spinach Salad

Prep: *5 minutes* | **Cook:** *20 minutes* | **Total time:** *25 minutes* | **Makes:** *6 servings*

This delicious side will become your new picnic standby. The salty Parma ham and tangy vinaigrette are a winning combination.

625g (1¼lb) new potatoes
2 tablespoons olive oil
2 tablespoons white balsamic
  vinegar
¼ teaspoon salt
¼ teaspoon pepper
150g (5oz) baby spinach
50g (2oz) Parma ham,
  pulled into pieces

1. Place potatoes in a medium saucepan and cover with water. Bring to the boil. Reduce heat and simmer 20 minutes. Cut potatoes into quarters.

2. Whisk oil and vinegar in a large bowl to combine; season with salt and pepper. Add warm potatoes, spinach and Parma ham to dressing; toss to combine and serve.

Serving size: about 200g (7oz) Calories 138; Fat 5.6g (sat 1g, mono 3.3g, poly 0.5g); Cholesterol 7mg; Protein 5g; Carbohydrate 19g; Sugars 1g; Fibre 2g; RS 1.1g; Sodium 374mg

Broccoli and Cheese-Stuffed Baked Potato

Prep: *10 minutes* | **Cook:** *13 minutes to 70 minutes, depending on method*
Total time: *23 minutes (microwave)* | **Makes:** *4 servings*

When was the last time you indulged in a cheesy baked potato? Well, it's on the menu again, and this one is nutrition-packed!

4 baking potatoes, scrubbed
175ml (6fl oz) skimmed milk
1 tablespoon flour
125g (4oz) reduced-fat mature
  Cheddar cheese, grated
½ teaspoon salt
¼ teaspoon pepper
⅛ teaspoon cayenne pepper
300g (10oz) frozen broccoli
  florets, defrosted

1. Cook potatoes:

OVEN: Preheat oven to 200°C/400°F/gas mark 6. Pierce potatoes with a fork, and wrap each in foil. Bake until tender, 1 hour.

MICROWAVE: Pierce potatoes with a fork, and wrap each in kitchen paper. Place in microwave, and cook on HIGH 8 minutes, until just tender (test with with a knife; potatoes will continue to cook when removed from microwave).

2. While potatoes are cooking, make sauce: Combine milk and flour in a small saucepan over high heat; bring to a simmer and cook, whisking, until thickened, 2–3 minutes. Add cheese, salt, pepper and cayenne; whisk until sauce is smooth. Continue to simmer, whisking, 2 minutes.

3. Place broccoli in a microwave-safe dish; microwave on HIGH 4–5 minutes, until hot.

4. Split cooked potatoes open with a knife. Spoon ¼ of the broccoli into each potato, and top with 4 tablespoons Cheddar sauce.

Serving size: 1 potato, 75g (3oz) broccoli, and 4 tablespoons Cheddar sauce Calories 377; Fat 5.8g (sat 3.4g, mono 1.4g, poly 0.4g); Cholesterol 17mg; Protein 18g; Carbohydrate 66g; Sugars 6g; Fibre 7g; RS 2.9g; Sodium 403mg

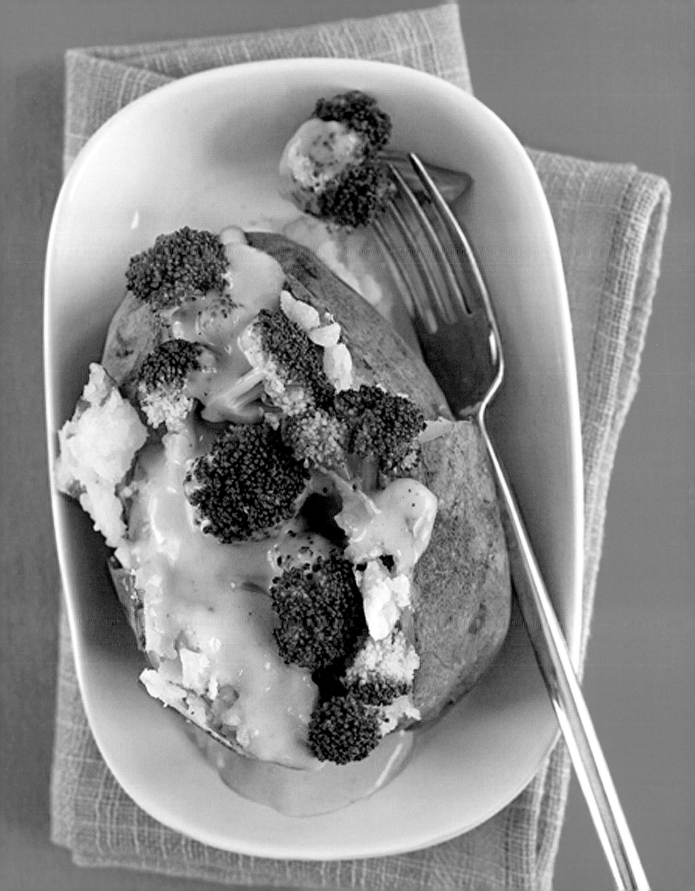

Sweet Potato Chips with Curried Ketchup

Prep: *10 minutes* | **Cook:** *30 minutes* | **Total time:** *40 minutes* | **Makes:** *4 servings*

Everyone loves chips, and our version can be enjoyed guilt-free! Not only are they delicious, but they also provide more than 100% of your daily vitamin A.

2 medium sweet potatoes, scrubbed
  and dried (about 500g/1lb), cut
  into long, 1cm (½ inch) thick wedges
1 tablespoon olive oil
½ teaspoon sea salt
¼ teaspoon freshly ground black
  pepper
1 tablespoon fresh lime juice
125ml (4fl oz) ketchup
2 teaspoons freshly grated ginger
1½ teaspoons curry powder
⅛ teaspoon cayenne pepper

1. Preheat oven to 200°C/400°F/gas mark 6. Toss potatoes on a large rimmed baking sheet with oil. Season potatoes with ¼ teaspoon of the salt and pepper. Roast 30–40 minutes, tossing once, until charred and tender. Toss potatoes with lime juice and remaining ¼ teaspoon salt.

2. While potatoes roast, stir together ketchup, ginger, curry powder and cayenne in a small bowl. Serve chips with ketchup.

Serving size: About 8 fries and 2 tablespoons ketchup
Calories 131; Fat 3.7g (sat 0.5g, mono 2.5g, poly 0.5g); Cholesterol 0mg; Protein 2g; Carbohydrate 24g; Sugars 12g; Fibre 3g; RS 1g; Sodium 599mg

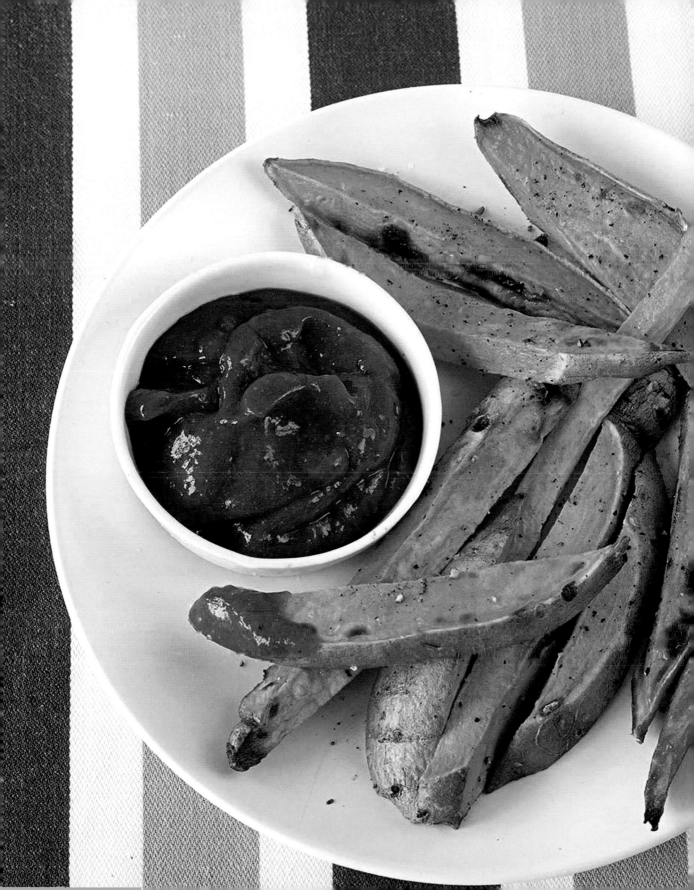

RS
1.9g

Potato Gratin Casserole

Prep: *10 minutes* | **Cook:** *25 minutes* | **Total time:** *35 minutes* | **Makes:** *8 servings*

Want to bring a Resistant Starch-filled dish to your next potluck or family gathering? This rustic casserole is super satisfying and an absolute crowd-pleaser.

1.5kg (3lb) potatoes, scrubbed
  and quartered
4 sprigs thyme plus 1 tablespoon
  thyme leaves
1 garlic clove, peeled
175ml (6fl oz) 2% fat milk
25g (1oz) unsalted butter
50g (2oz) Parmesan cheese, grated
⅛ teaspoon salt
¼ teaspoon pepper
8 tablespoons panko (Japanese
  breadcrumbs)

1. Place potatoes, thyme sprigs and garlic in a large saucepan and cover with cold water. Bring to the boil over high heat. Reduce heat; simmer, uncovered, about 20 minutes, until potatoes are tender (test with a knife). Reserve 125ml (4fl oz) cooking water; drain. Return potatoes to pan over low heat.

2. Add milk, reserved cooking water, butter, 4 tablespoons Parmesan, salt and pepper. Mash potatoes with a large fork or potato masher until smooth. Transfer potatoes to a shallow 1.5 litre (2½ pint) ovenproof casserole or baking dish.

3. Preheat grill. Combine panko, remaining Parmesan and thyme leaves; sprinkle over potatoes. Grill 10-12cm (4–5 inches) from heat source until cheese melts and starts to brown, 3–4 minutes. Serve warm.

Serving size: 175g (6oz) Calories 204; Fat 4.9g (sat 3g, mono 1.3g, poly 0.2g); Cholesterol 14mg; Protein 6g; Carbohydrate 35g; Sugars 3g; Fibre 3g; RS 1.9g; Sodium 138mg

TIP:
If you're bringing this to someone's house, make the casserole through step 2. Finish it under the grill before dinner is served.

German Potato Salad

Prep: *15 minutes* | ***Cook:*** *30 minutes* | ***Total time:*** *45 minutes* | ***Makes:*** *12 servings*

Tangy and just a bit sweet, this potato salad is a bacon lover's dream. It's yummy served warm or cold and is always a hit at summer picnics and barbecues.

1kg (2lb) potatoes
3 tablespoons olive oil
125g (4oz) turkey bacon, diced
2 celery stalks, thinly sliced
½ cup onion, finely chopped
125ml (4fl oz) cider vinegar
2 tablespoons wholegrain Dijon mustard
1 tablespoon sugar
½ teaspoon salt
½ teaspoon pepper
75g (3oz) dill pickle, chopped
3 hard-boiled eggs, chopped
3 tablespoons chopped fresh dill

1 Place potatoes in a saucepan and cover with cold water. Bring to the boil, reduce heat and cook until potatoes are fork-tender but not mushy, 20 minutes. Drain, cool, cut into 2.5cm (1 inch) cubes and place in a large bowl.

2. Heat 1 tablespoon oil in a large nonstick frying pan over medium-high heat. Add bacon and cook until crisp, 4–5 minutes. Carefully remove bacon from pan, reserving oil; drain bacon on kitchen paper. Add celery and onion to oil and cook until just softened, 2 minutes. Whisk together vinegar, 125ml (4fl oz) water, mustard, sugar, salt, pepper and remaining 2 tablespoons oil; add to frying pan.

3. Bring to the boil, reduce heat and simmer until partially reduced, 2 minutes. Pour over potatoes and add bacon, pickle, eggs and dill. Toss to fold gently. Chill or serve at room temperature.

Serving size: 75g (3oz) Calories 157; Fat 6.6g (sat 1.4g, mono 3.6g, poly 1.1g); Cholesterol 55mg; Protein 5g; Carbohydrate 19g; Sugars 3g; Fibre 2g; RS 0.8g; Sodium 353mg

Herb and Olive Oil Mashed Potatoes

Prep: 5 minutes | **Cook:** 20 minutes | **Total time:** 25 minutes | **Makes:** 4 servings

Mashed potatoes are a welcome sight on any dinner table. Our version gets extra flavour from cooking the potatoes with garlic, and then mashing them with thyme.

750g (1½lb) red potatoes,
  scrubbed and cubed
3 garlic cloves, peeled and thinly
  sliced
3 tablespoons olive oil
1 tablespoon thyme leaves
½ teaspoon salt
¼ teaspoon pepper
1 tablespoon chopped parsley

1. Place potatoes and garlic in a large saucepan and cover with cold water. Bring to the boil over high heat. Reduce heat; simmer, uncovered, about 20 minutes, until potatoes are tender (test with a knife). Reserve 125ml (4fl oz) cooking water; drain. Return potatoes to pan over low heat.

2. Meanwhile, heat oil and thyme in a small frying pan over medium heat. Cook until thyme sizzles, about 2 minutes.

3. Add 4 tablespoons of the reserved cooking water, oil with thyme, salt and pepper to potatoes. Mash with a potato masher to desired consistency (add more cooking water if necessary). Stir in parsley.

Serving size: 175g (6oz) Calories 221; Fat 10.3g (sat 1.4g, mono 7.4g, poly 1.1g); Cholesterol 0mg; Protein 3g; Carbohydrate 30g; Sugars 1g; Fibre 3g; RS 1.9g; Sodium 298mg

Savoury Cornbread Stuffing

Prep: *10 minutes* | **Cook:** *60 minutes* | **Total time:** *70 minutes* | **Makes:** *4 servings*

Warm and comforting, this stuffing is perfect. We love it with our Thanksgiving turkey, but it's a wonderful side dish with any autumn or winter meal.

400g (13oz) cornbread, cut into 2.5cm
  (1 inch) cubes
2 teaspoons olive oil
1 medium onion, chopped
2 garlic cloves, finely chopped
1 tablespoon dried sage
2 celery stalks, chopped
1 small apple, diced
40g (1½oz) dried cranberries
350ml (12fl oz) low-sodium chicken stock
1 egg
Cooking spray

1. Preheat oven to 180°C/350°F/gas mark 4. Place cornbread on a baking sheet and toast lightly, 8–10 minutes. Remove from oven and cool.

2. Heat oil in a large high-sided sauté pan; add onion and cook, stirring occasionally, until lightly browned, 8–9 minutes. Add garlic and sage and cook 1 minute. Add celery and apple and cook until crisp-tender, 2–3 minutes.

3. Add toasted stuffing and cranberries and stir gently to combine. Remove pan from heat and cool slightly.

4. Whisk together stock and egg; add to cornbread mixture. Gently stir until moistened. Coat a 20cm (8 inch) baking dish with cooking spray and transfer mixture to dish. Bake until top is browned, 35–40 minutes.

Serving size: 125g (4oz) stuffing Calories 270; Fat 8.5g (sat 1.7g, mono 3.7g, poly 2.5g); Cholesterol 69mg; Protein 7g; Carbohydrate 43g; Sugars 12g; Fiber 4g; RS 0g; Sodium 436mg

> **TIP:**
> Save time and pick up shop-bought cornbread instead of making your own. Or make one, cube it, and freeze it before the holidays!

Honey-Glazed Roasted Root Vegetables

Prep: *15 minutes* | **Cook:** *50 minutes* | **Total time:** *1 hour 5 minutes* | **Makes:** *6 servings*

The earthy flavours of autumn come together in this warming dish. It's a wonderful accompaniment to roast chicken or pork.

2 tablespoons olive oil
2 tablespoons honey
1 teaspoon salt
¼ teaspoon pepper
2 teaspoons chopped rosemary
500g (1lb) carrots (about 6 large),
  peeled and cut into 5cm (2 inch) chunks
500g (1lb) parsnips (about 1 large),
  peeled and cut into 5cm (2 inch)chunks
500g (1lb) yams (about 2 medium),
  skin-on, cut into 5cm (2 inch) chunks
1 large red onion, peeled and cut
  into 2.5cm (1 inch) wedges
15 garlic cloves, peeled

1. Preheat oven to 220°C/425°F/gas mark 7.

2. Whisk together oil, honey, salt, pepper and rosemary in a large bowl; add remaining ingredients and toss. Spread on a foil-lined baking sheet. Roast for 30 minutes until underside of vegetables is golden brown. Remove from oven. Using a spatula, turn vegetables and return to oven until golden brown and cooked through but not mushy, 20–30 minutes. Serve hot or at room temperature.

Serving size: 250g (8oz) Calories 215; Fat 5.1g (sat 0.7g, mono 3.4g, poly 0.7g); Cholesterol 0mg; Protein 3g; Carbohydrate 42g; Sugars 17g; Fibre 8g; RS 0.7g; Sodium 466mg

TIP:
If you have leftover roasted vegetables, you can use them to make a quick soup, or purée them in a food processor with a little olive oil for a delicious dip.

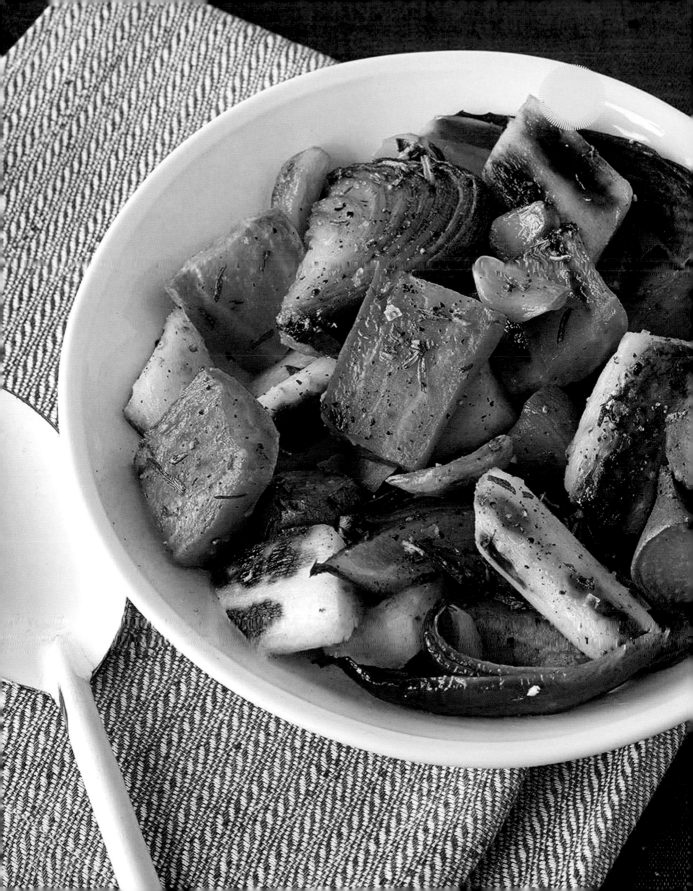

Crispy Onion Rings

Prep: 10 minutes | **Cook:** 15 minutes | **Total time:** 25 minutes | **Makes:** 4 servings

This bar-food favourite was begging for a CarbLovers makeover! Using cornflakes adds Resistant Starch, and baking instead of deep-frying helps slash the calories and

50g (2oz) cornflakes
20 cream crackers, coarsely crushed
1½ teaspoons olive oil
¼ teaspoon sea salt
¼ teaspoon freshly ground black pepper
1 large egg white
65g (2½oz) plain flour
½ teaspoon paprika
125ml (4fl oz) low-fat buttermilk
Cooking spray
1 large sweet onion (about 750g/1½lb), cut into 1.5cm (¾ inch) slices

1. Preheat oven to 230°C/450°F/gas mark 8. Combine cornflakes and crackers in a food processor; pulse until fine crumbs form. Add oil; pulse to distribute. Add salt and pepper; pulse. Transfer crumbs to a shallow dish. Whisk together egg white, flour, paprika, buttermilk and 2 tablespoons water in a medium bowl.

2. Coat 2 large rimmed baking sheets with cooking spray; transfer to oven to heat, 2 minutes. Separate onion slices into individual rings. Dip onion rings in batter, then crumb mixture; carefully transfer to hot baking sheets and arrange in a single layer. Bake, turning once, until onion rings are golden brown, about 15 minutes. Serve hot.

Serving size: 3–4 onion rings Calories 279; Fat 5.8g (sat 1.1g, mono 3.2g, poly 1.2g); Cholesterol 1mg; Protein 7g; Carbohydrate 50g; Sugars 12g; Fibre 3g; RS 0.5g; Sodium 450mg

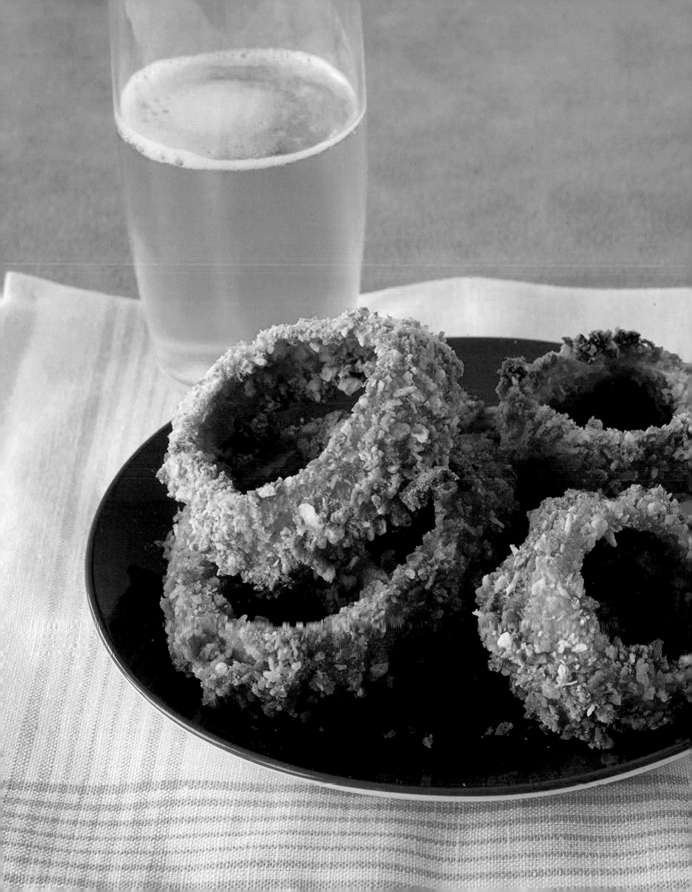

Fried Brown Rice with Edamame

Prep: *1 minute* | **Cook:** *4 minutes* | **Total time:** *5 minutes* | **Makes:** *4 servings*

No time to cook? As long as you have frozen or microwaveable rice to hand, this dish comes together in minutes.

2 tablespoons vegetable oil

275g (9oz) cooked brown rice

2 large eggs, lightly beaten

200g (7oz) coleslaw mix

175g (6oz) frozen shelled edamame (soya beans), thawed

2 tablespoons reduced-sodium soy sauce

1 tablespoon chili-garlic sauce (such as Sriracha)

4 tablespoons coriander leaves

4 tablespoonspeanuts, chopped

Heat oil in a large heavy-bottomed frying pan over high heat. Add rice; cook until heated through, about 1 minute. Stir eggs into rice; cook 30 seconds. Stir in coleslaw mix, edamame, soy sauce and chilli-garlic sauce; cook 2 minutes or until eggs are cooked and edamame are heated through. Serve rice topped with coriander and peanuts.

Serving size: 175g (6oz) fried rice Calories 318; Fat 16.3g (sat 2.1g, mono 5g, poly 6.6g);Cholesterol 93mg; Protein 14g; Carbohydrate 30g; Sugars 4g; Fibre 5g; RS 1.7g; Sodium 429mg

TIP:
Great for flexitarians! Add a handful of sautéed prawns to boost the protein in this quick dish.

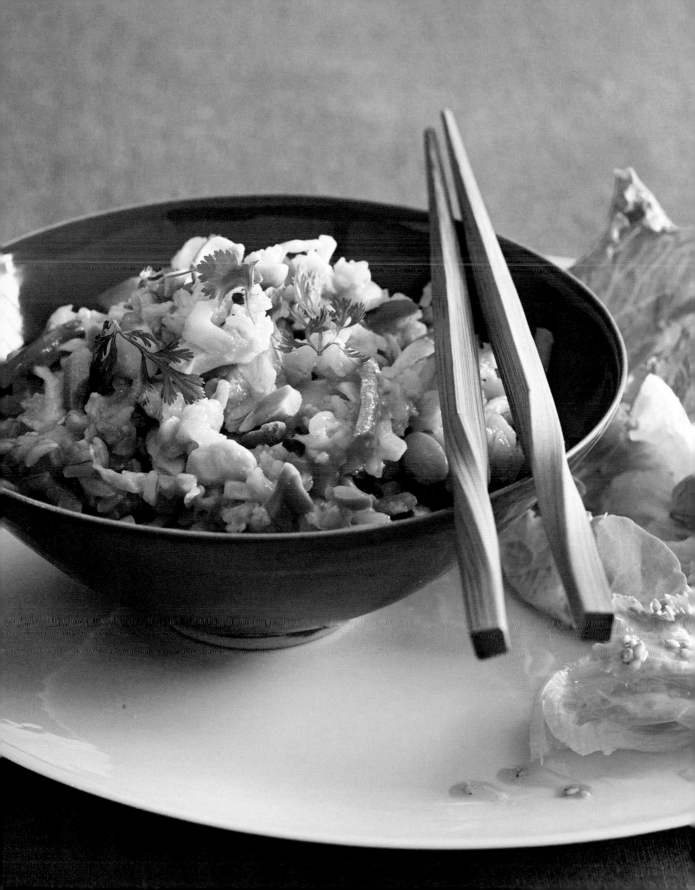

Hoppin' John

Prep: *10 minutes* | **Cook:** *20 minutes* | **Total time:** *30 minutes* | **Makes:** *4 servings*

RS
3.1g

Tradition says that if you start the New Year with a bowl of Hoppin' John, you'll have good luck all year long. All we know for sure is that this dish is a super tasty way to get your Resistant Starch!

50g (2oz) sliced pancetta, chopped
1 shallot, finely chopped
750g (1½lb) spring greens, chopped, thick stems discarded
250ml (4fl oz) low-sodium chicken stock
1 tablespoon cider vinegar
450g (14 ½oz) can diced tomatoes
¼ teaspoon crushed red pepper
475g (15oz) can black-eyed peas, rinsed and drained
550g (1lb 2oz) cooked brown rice, warmed

1. Heat a large sauté pan over medium heat. Add pancetta; cook, stirring, until browned and crisp, 4 to 6 minutes. Transfer pancetta with a slotted spoon to a kitchen paper–lined plate to drain; reserve fat in pan. Add shallot; cook over medium-high heat, stirring occasionally, until tender and golden, about 3 minutes.

2. Add greens, stock, vinegar, tomatoes and chilli flakes; bring to the boil. Simmer, covered, 5 minutes; stir in black-eyed peas. Cook 5 minutes or until greens and black-eyed peas are tender.

3. Serve greens and black-eyed peas over rice; sprinkle with reserved pancetta.

Serving size: 400g (13oz) Calories 364; Fat 6.9g (sat 2.5g, mono 2.6g, poly 1.9g); Cholesterol 10mg; Protein 15g; Carbohydrate 62g; Sugars 7g; Fibre 12g; RS 3.1g; Sodium 618mg

RS
1.4g

Wild Rice Pilaf with Pecans, Cranberries and Spring Onions

Prep: *10 minutes* | **Cook:** *45 minutes* | **Total time:** *55 minutes* | **Makes:** *12 servings*

This delicious dish has a wonderful blend of nutty rice, chewy cranberries and crunchy pecans. It makes a pretty addition to any holiday feast.

1 tablespoon olive oil

1 medium onion, chopped

1 teaspoon finely chopped garlic

500g (1lb) wild- and brown-rice mix, cooked according to packet instructions

40g (1½oz) dried cranberries

4 tablespoons toasted chopped pecans

4 spring onions, chopped

¾ teaspoon salt

½ teaspoon pepper

1. Heat oil in a large saucepan over medium-high heat. Add onion and cook, stirring occasionally, until tender and golden, 8–9 minutes. Add garlic and cook 1 minute.

2. Add rice and cook until heated through, 1–2 minutes. Transfer to serving dish and toss with cranberries, pecans, spring onions, salt and pepper. Serve warm.

Serving size: 65g (2½oz) Calories 181; Fat 3.7g (sat 0.5g, mono 2g, poly 1g); Cholesterol 0mg; Protein 5g; Carbohydrate 33g, Sugars 3g, Fibre 3g; RS 1.4g; Sodium 152mg

TIP:
Try substituting the cranberries with dried cherries, and experiment with different nuts.

Appetizers & Cocktails

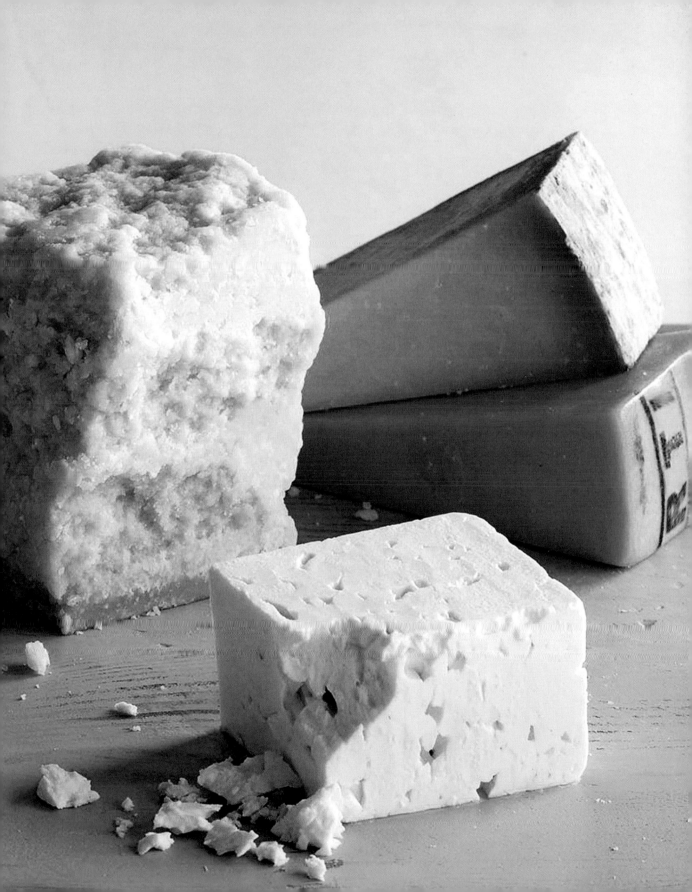

Ham and Cheddar Potato Skins

Prep: 10 minutes | **Cook:** 30 minutes | **Total time:** 40 minutes | **Makes:** 6 servings

We took this traditionally high-fat nibble and gave it a CarbLovers *makeover. Using smaller potatoes keeps these bites portion-controlled.*

6 small potatoes (750g/1½lb)
2 tablespoons reduced-fat
  soured cream
¼ teaspoon sea salt
¼ teaspoon freshly ground black
  pepper
2 spring onions, sliced (white and green
  parts separated)
50g (2oz) sliced deli ham, chopped
50g (2oz) mature Cheddar cheese,
  grated

1. Preheat oven to 180°C/350°F/gas mark 4.

2. Bake potatoes on baking sheet 25–30 minutes or until tender; set aside to cool. Preheat grill with rack in highest position.

3. Halve cooked potatoes lengthways. Scoop out flesh, leaving a 5mm (¼ inch) border; transfer potato flesh to a bowl. Mash potato with soured cream and 2 tablespoons water; season with salt and pepper. Fold in spring onion whites and ham; spoon filling into potato shells.

4. Arrange filled potato skins on a baking sheet; sprinkle evenly with cheese. Grill 5 minutes or until cheese is melted. Sprinkle with spring onion greens before serving, if liked.

Serving size: 2 potato skins Calories 186; Fat 4.3g (sat 2.5g, mono 1.2g, poly 0.2g); Cholesterol 16mg; Protein 7g; Carbohydrate 30g; Sugars 2g; Fibre 3g; RS 1.4g; Sodium 279mg

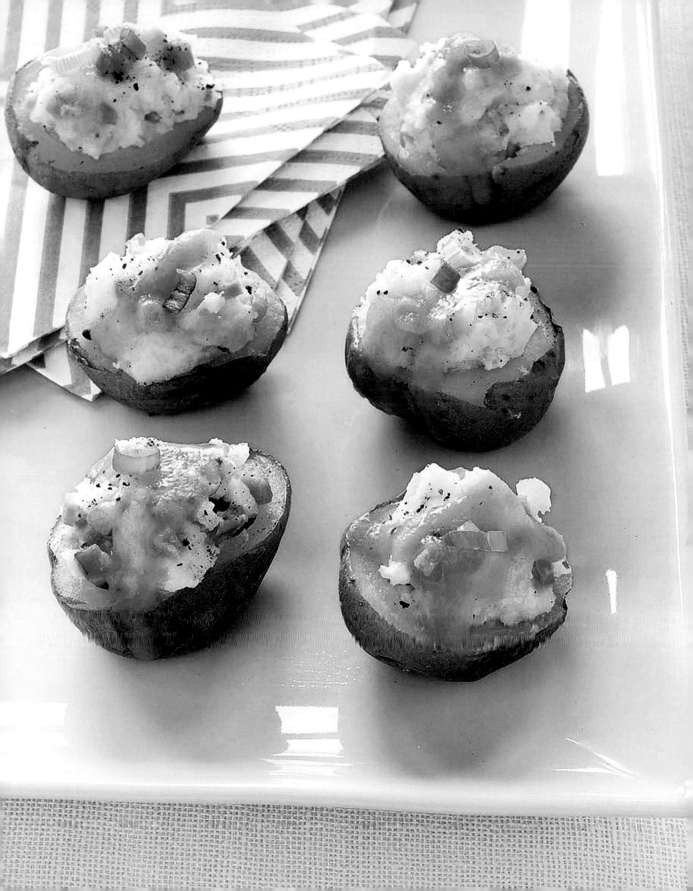

Layered Spicy Black Bean and Cheddar Dip

Prep: *20 minutes* | **Total time:** *20 minutes* | **Makes:** *8 servings*

This is the ultimate "wow" party dip! It's super-flavourful, filling, and makes for a stunning presentation.

1 medium avocado, stoned

1 tablespoon fresh lime juice

1 teaspoon lime zest

¼ teaspoon salt

¼ teaspoon pepper

475g (15oz) can reduced-salt black beans, rinsed and drained

1 teaspoon Tabasco

5 tablespoons chopped red onion

250ml (8 fl oz) jarred salsa

250ml (8 fl oz) reduced-fat soured cream

4 tablespoons chopped tomato

4 tablespoons chopped spring onion

Large bag of tortilla chips for serving

1. Mash avocado, lime juice, lime zest and half of the salt and pepper in a bowl; set aside.

2. Mash beans, Tabasco and remaining salt and pepper in another bowl.

3. Place black bean mixture on the bottom of a glass salad bowl. Layer avocado mash on top of beans, then sprinkle with 4 tablespoons of the red onion. Top with salsa, then with soured cream. Top with chopped tomato, spring onion and remaining red onion.

4. Serve dip with tortilla chips.

Serving size: 125ml (4fl oz) dip and 5 chips Calories 199; Fat 9.6g (sat 2.9g, mono 4.9g, poly 1.1g); Cholesterol 12mg; Protein 6g; Carbohydrate 23g; Sugars 2g; Fibre 6g; RS 0.7g; Sodium 345mg

ASK CARBLOVERS

Q: **What can I drink (besides plain water) when I'm out with friends?**

A: Unsweetened tea, coffee and water spiked with citrus fruit or cucumber slices can be enjoyed anytime. After the Kickstart, you can have a 150ml (5fl oz) glass of wine or 350ml (12fl oz) bottle of light beer as one of your daily snacks.

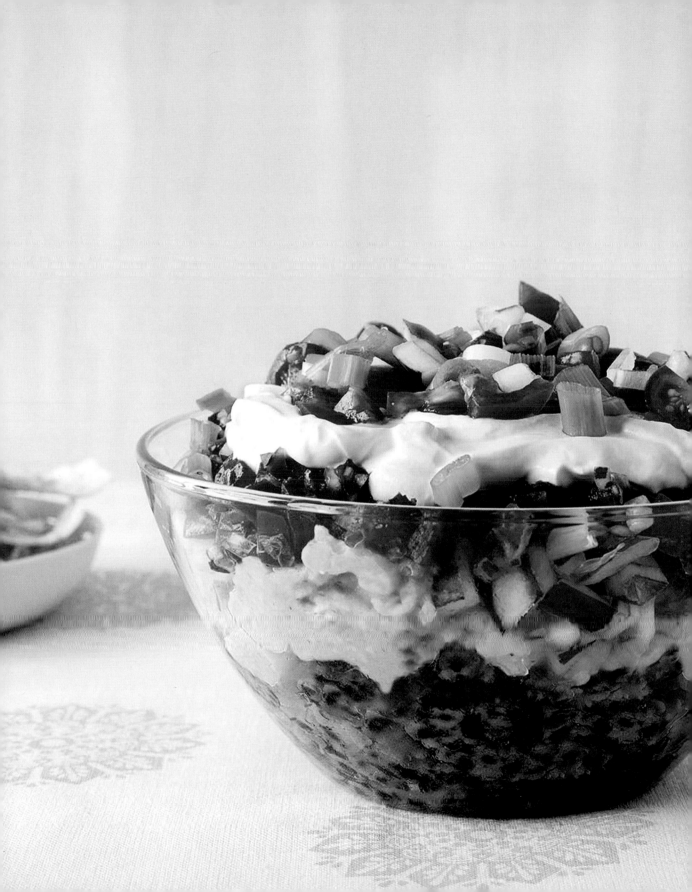

Pumpernickel Toasts with Smoked Salmon and Lemon-Chive Cream

Prep: 10 minutes | **Total time:** 10 minutes | **Makes:** 6 servings

The classic combination of pumpernickel and smoked salmon gets livened up with a dollop of our tangy lemon cream.

125ml (4fl oz) 2% Greek yogurt

2 tablespoons chopped chives, plus more for garnish

1 tablespoon olive oil

½ teaspoon finely grated lemon zest

50g (2oz) smoked salmon

18 small pumpernickel toasts

1. Stir together yogurt, chives, oil and zest in a small bowl.

2. Divide salmon between pumpernickel toasts; top each with about 1½ teaspoons yogurt mixture. Sprinkle with remaining chives and serve.

Serving size: 3 toasts Calories 119; Fat 4g (sat 0.8g, mono 2.1g, poly 0.7g); Cholesterol 3mg; Protein 6g; Carbohydrate 15g; Sugars 1g; Fibre 2g; RS 1.4g; Sodium 282mg

TIP:
Serve these bites for brunch with a crisp sparkling wine or the *CarbLovers* Fat-Flushing Cocktail, page 28.

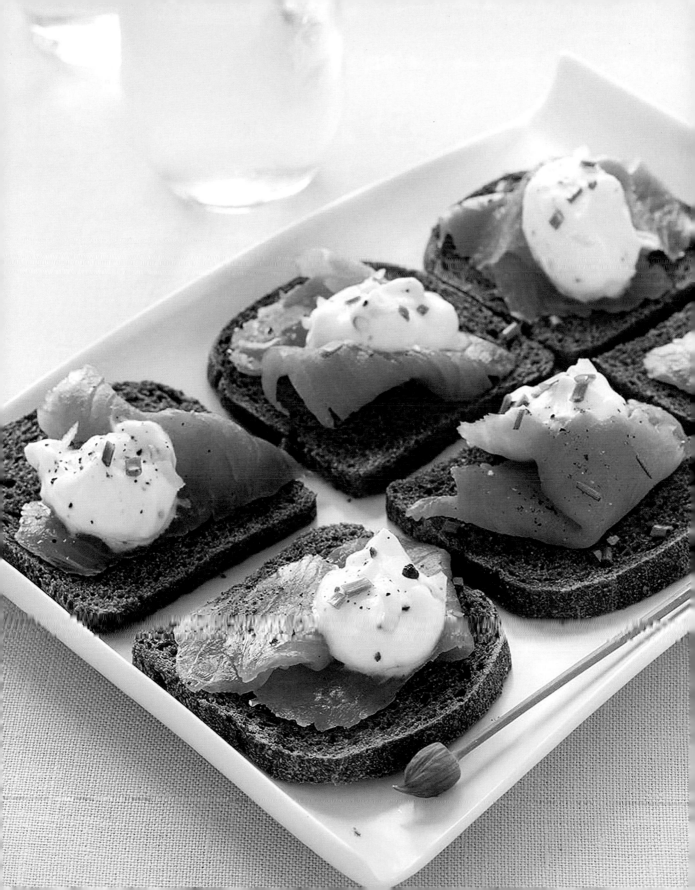

RS
0.6g

Edamame and Pear Crostini

Prep: *5 minutes* | **Cook:** *20 minutes* | **Total time:** *25 minutes* | **Makes:** *10 servings*

"Edamame and pear plays well on the traditional combination of broad beans and pear. It's healthy, sweet and crunchy with great texture and flavour. This light starter is perfect for a baby or bridal shower." Donatella Arpaia, restaurateur.

500g (16oz) frozen shelled
  edamame (soya beans)
4 tablespoons extra virgin olive oil
25g (1oz) mint, chopped, plus
  additional for garnish
50g (2oz) Pecorino Romano cheese,
  grated
½ teaspoon salt
¼ teaspoon freshly ground black
  pepper
1 baguette, thinly sliced
1–2 large pears, peeled and diced

1. Preheat oven to 190°C/375°F/gas mark 5.

2. Cook edamame in salted boiling water for 10 minutes. Remove with a slotted spoon and place in iced water; drain. Set aside 4 tablespoons whole edamame; process the remainder in a food processor until coarsely chopped. Combine mashed edamame with reserved whole edamame, 3 tablespoons oil, mint, cheese, salt and pepper.

3. Place baguette slices on a baking sheet, brush lightly with remaining 1 tablespoon oil, and bake for 10 minutes. Top each baguette slice with 1 tablespoon edamame mixture and 2 teaspoons pear. Garnish with additional mint, if liked.

Serving size: 3 crostini Calories 241; Fat 8.9g (sat 1.7g, mono 4.4g, poly 0.6g); Cholesterol 6mg; Protein 12g; Carbohydrate 29g; Sugars 2g; Fibre 4g; Iron 4mg; RS 0.6g; Sodium 445mg

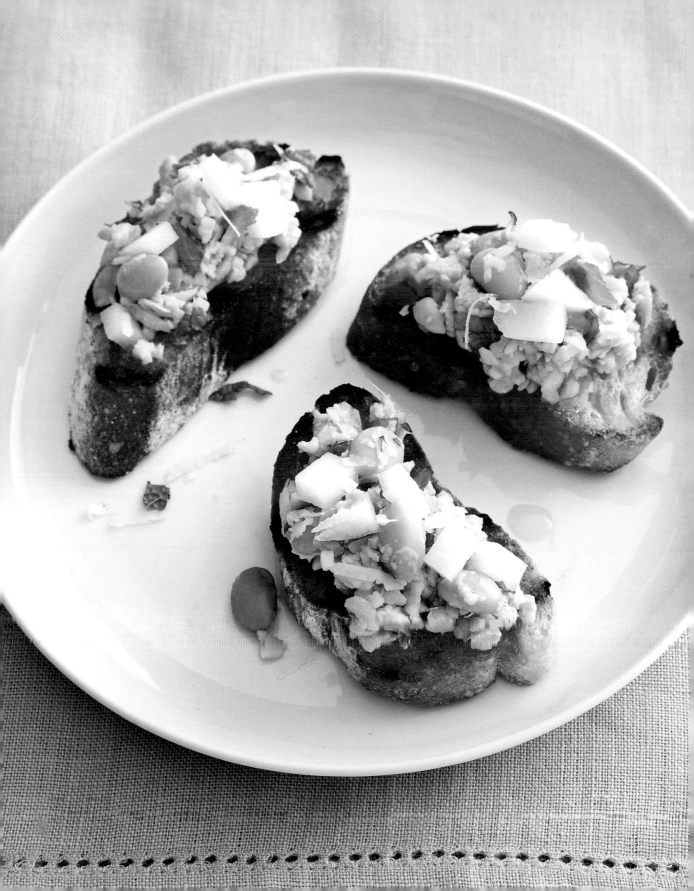

Grilled Polenta Cakes

Prep: *5 minutes* | **Cook:** *31 minutes* | **Total Time**: *36 minutes* | **Makes:** *10 servings*

"I keep ready-made polenta on hand for when I need a quick appetizer. I enjoy grilled polenta cakes plain or with a tomato bruschetta topping, brushed with pesto, or with a simple tomato sauce, like this recipe." Cristina Ferrare, author

500g (1lb) ready-made polenta
4 tablespoons extra virgin olive oil
Cooking spray
250ml (8fl oz) of your favourite
    tomato sauce
50g (2oz) Parmesan cheese, freshly
    grated (you may have some left over)
4 tablespoons whole basil leaves
Pinch of sea salt
⅛ teaspoon freshly ground black
        pepper

1. Cut polenta into ten 1cm (½ inch) slices (cakes), and pat dry with kitchen paper.

2. Brush both sides of polenta cakes with oil, and set aside.

3. Heat a griddle pan over high heat until hot. Lay polenta cakes in one layer on the pan; grill for 8–10 minutes on each side or until both sides are golden and crunchy and have grill marks.

4. Remove cakes from the grill pan and let cool on a wire rack. Preheat the oven to 180°C/350°F/ gas mark 4.

5. Coat a baking sheet with cooking spray. Arrange the grilled polenta cakes on the baking sheet. Place 1 tablespoon of tomato sauce on each slice, then add 1–2 teaspoons Parmesan to each. Bake for 15 minutes.

6. Garnish with basil, salt and pepper. Serve warm.

Serving size: 1 cake Calories 116; Fat 7g (sat 1.5g, mono 4.6g, poly 0.7g); Cholesterol 4mg; Protein 3g; Carbohydrate 10g; Sugars 1g; Fibre 1g; Iron 0mg; RS 0.3g; Sodium 387mg;

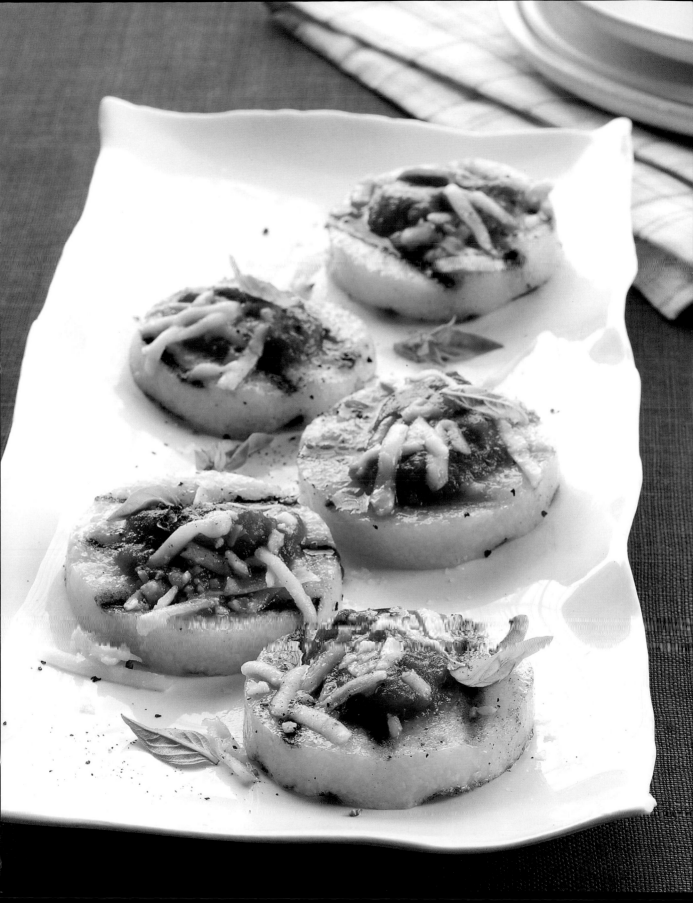

Mini Corn and Feta Muffins

Prep: *5 minutes* | **Cook:** *15 minutes* | **Total time:** *20 minutes* | **Makes:** *10 servings*

These savoury muffins get a flavor kick from feta cheese and buttermilk. They're easy to whip up on a weeknight and go perfectly with our Mexican Mole Chile on page 84.

65g (2½oz) plain flour
75g (3oz) polenta
1 tablespoon sugar
1 teaspoon baking powder
¼ teaspoon salt
¼ teaspoon ground pepper
75ml (3fl oz) buttermilk
25g (1oz) butter, melted
1 large egg white
40g (1½oz) feta cheese,
  crumbled
75g (3oz) thawed sweetcorn
  kernels
Cooking spray

1. Preheat oven to 220°C/425°F/gas mark 7.

2. Whisk together flour, polenta, sugar, baking powder, salt and pepper in a medium bowl; make a well in centre of mixture. Combine buttermilk, butter and egg white in a small bowl; add to flour mixture, stirring until just moist. Fold in feta and sweetcorn.

3. Coat a 20-hole mini muffin tin with cooking spray. Spoon batter into prepared pan; bake for 10–12 minutes or until muffins spring back when touched lightly in centre. Remove muffins from pan immediately; place on a wire rack. Serve warm.

Serving size: 2 muffins Calories 107; Fat 4g (sat 2.4g, mono 1.2g, poly 0.3g); Cholesterol 11mg; Protein 3g; Carbohydrate 15g; Sugars 2g; Fibre 1g; RS 0g; Sodium 178mg

TIP:
Make a double batch of these muffins, cool, and freeze in a resealable bag. Then, pop them in the microwave for 20–30 seconds before serving.

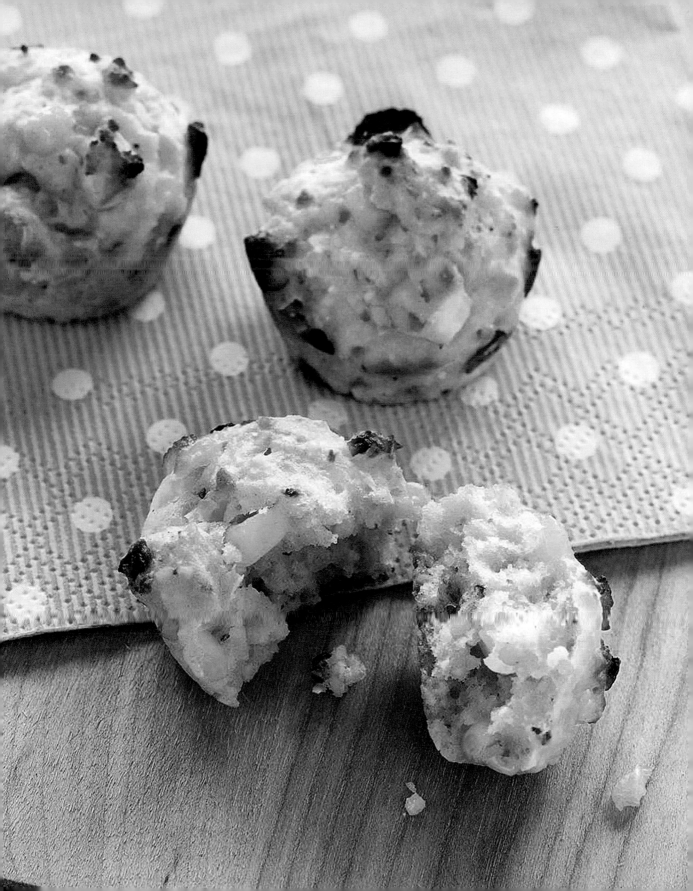

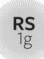

Smoky Oven-Baked Potato Crisps

Prep: *15 minutes* | **Cook:** *25 minutes* | **Total time:** *40 minutes* | **Makes:** *About 6 servings*

Potato crisps are back on the menu! These are lighter than most shop-bought varieties because we oven-bake them. Smoked paprika makes them even more flavourful.

2 baking potatoes (about 750g/1½lb),
 scrubbed
2 tablespoons olive oil
1 teaspoon smoked paprika
¾ teaspoon salt
¼ teaspoon pepper

1. Preheat oven to 200°C/400°F/gas mark 6.

2. Using a mandolin slicer or sharp knife, slice potatoes int0 2.5mm (⅛ inch) thick rounds. Pat dry on layers of kitchen paper to absorb as much moisture as possible.

3. Toss potato slices with oil in a large bowl, then toss with smoked paprika, ½ teaspoon salt and pepper; arrange in a single layer on baking sheets.

4. Bake until browned and potato edges lift slightly from baking sheets, 20–25 minutes. Remove from oven and sprinkle with remaining ¼ teaspoon salt.

5. Cool completely and store in an airtight container for up to 1 day.

Serving size: About 11 crisps Calories 130; Fat 4.7g (sat 0.7g, mono 3.3g, poly 0.5g); Cholesterol 0mg; Protein 2g; Carbohydrate 20g; Sugars 1g; Fibre 2g; RS 1g; Sodium 298mg

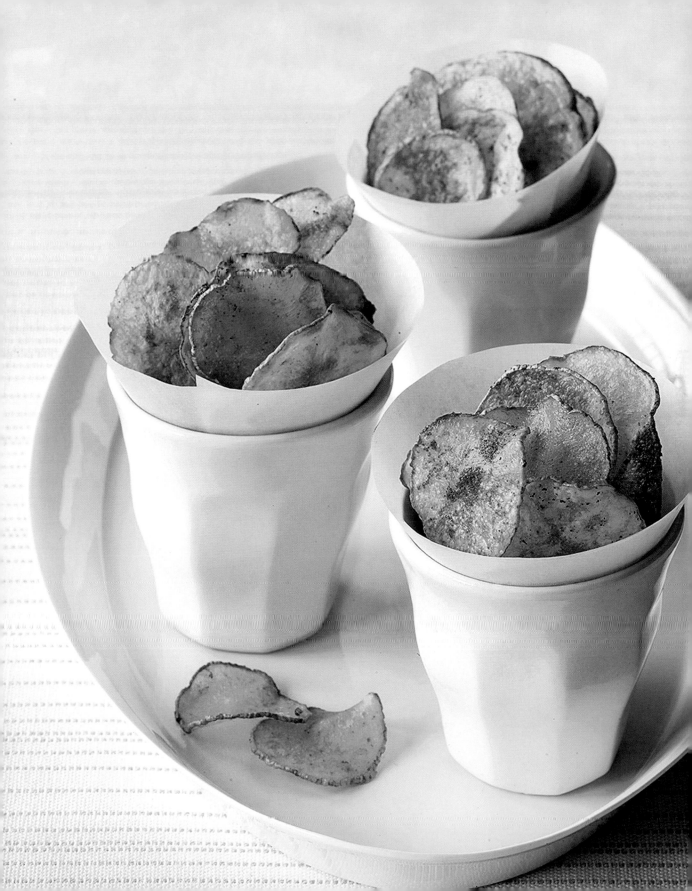

RS
0.5g

Edamame and Mushroom Potstickers

Prep: 35 minutes | *Cook:* 10 minutes | *Total time:* 45 minutes | *Makes:* 6 servings

Tasty and fun to eat, these bites make a perfect prelude to an Asian-themed meal.

1 tablespoon vegetable oil, divided
2 spring onions, greens sliced and
  whites finely chopped
1 tablespoon finely chopped ginger
2 garlic cloves, finely chopped
175g (6oz) shiitake mushrooms,
  halved
50g (2oz) frozen shelled edamame,
  (soya beans) thawed
4 tablespoons low-sodium soy sauce
2 teaspoons sesame oil
1 large egg white
¼ teaspoon sea salt
¼ teaspoon freshly ground pepper
18 (5 to 7cm/2 to 3 inch square)
  wonton wrappers

1. Heat 1 teaspoon vegetable oil in a large nonstick frying pan over medium heat. Add spring onion whites, ginger and garlic to pan; cook until fragrant, 1 minute. Add mushrooms to pan; cook, tossing occasionally, until browned, about 5 minutes. Transfer mushrooms to a food processor with edamame, 1 tablespoon soy sauce and sesame oil; pulse until finely chopped. Add egg white, salt and pepper; pulse to combine. (Wipe out pan and reserve.)

2. Arrange wontons. Use a dampened finger to trace around wonton edge; place about 2 teaspoons filling in each. Fold wonton over to cover filling; press to seal edge. Transfer dumplings to a plate; cover with damp kitchen paper until needed.

3. Heat 1 teaspoon oil in reserved pan over medium heat. Add half of wontons to pan; cook 2 minutes or until browned on one side. Add 4 tablespoons water to pan; cover and cook until cooked through, 3–4 minutes. Cook second batch of wontons in remaining 1 teaspoon of oil. Serve with remaining spring onion greens and soy sauce.

Serving size: 3 potstickers Calories 116; Fat 4.5g (sat 0.4g, mono 1.2g, poly 2.2g); Cholesterol 3mg; Protein 5g; Carbohydrate 14g; Sugars 1g; Fibre 2g; RS 0.5g; Sodium 608mg

TIP:
To store, freeze wontons on a greaseproof paper-lined plate until firm and store in a resealable freezer bag for up to 3 months.

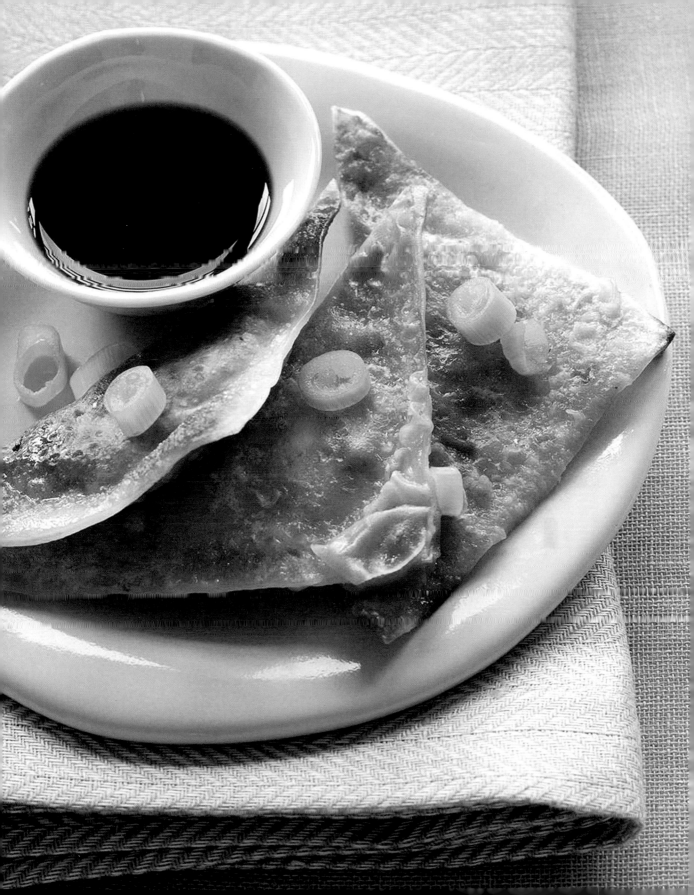

**RS
0.5g**

Chickpea and Artichoke Bruschetta

Prep: *5 minutes* | **Cook:** *20 minutes* | **Total time:** *25 minutes* | **Makes:** *6 servings*

Quick and versatile, bruschetta is one of our favourite appetizers to make. This one is packed with fibre and absolutely delicious.

½ French stick, sliced into 5mm
  (⅛ inch) rounds
425g (14oz) can artichokes in water,
drained and chopped
425g (14oz) can chickpeas, rinsed
  and drained
2 tablespoons olive oil
1 tablespoon fresh lemon juice
1 tablespoon chopped parsley
¼ teaspoon salt
¼ teaspoon pepper
1 garlic clove, peeled and halved

1. Preheat oven to 180°C/350°F/gas mark 4. Arrange bread slices in a single layer on baking sheet; bake about 20 minutes or until crispy. Set aside to cool completely.

2. Meanwhile, stir together artichokes, beans, oil, lemon juice, parsley, salt and pepper.

3. Rub tops of toasted bread slices with cut side of garlic; top with bean mixture and serve.

Serving size: About 4 bruschetta Calories 220; Fat 5.5g (sat 0.7g, mono 3.4g, poly 0.7g); Cholesterol 0mg; Protein 9g; Carbohydrate 34g; Sugars 1g; Fibre 6g; RS 0.5g; Sodium 631mg

RS
0.7g

Cinnamon-Sugar Tortilla Chips

Prep: *5 minutes* | **Cook:** *10 minutes* | **Total time:** *15 minutes* | **Makes:** *4 servings*

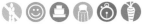

We love making homemade chips from tortillas, and this sweet spin is a fun change from the usual savoury ones.

4 (15cm/6 inch) corn tortillas
1 tablespoon vegetable oil
1 tablespoon sugar
½ teaspoon ground cinnamon
⅛ teaspoon salt

1. Preheat oven to 200°C/400°F/gas mark 6.

2. Brush both sides of tortillas with oil. Using a pizza cutter or clean kitchen scissors, cut each tortilla into 8 equal-sized triangles.

3. Combine sugar, cinnamon and salt in a large bowl. Add tortilla triangles and toss to coat.

4. Place on a baking sheet and bake until crisp, 10–12 minutes. Remove, cool and serve.

Serving size: 8 chips Calories 101; Fat 4g (sat 0.3g, mono 0.9g, poly 2.5g); Cholesterol 0mg; Protein 1g; Carbohydrate 16g; Sugars 3g; Fibre 2g; RS 0.7g; Sodium 76mg

TIP:
To make a dip to serve these with, just combine 250ml (8fl oz) low-fat vanilla yogurt with 2 teaspoons honey.

241

RS
0.2g

Roasted Red Pepper and Courgette Spread

Prep: *10 minutes* | **Cook:** *10 minutes* | **Total time:** *20 minutes* | **Makes:** *8 servings*

Zesty and bold, this richly textured spread is fabulous for parties, and also helps jazz up sandwiches and wraps.

500g (1lb) courgettes, sliced into 1cm (½ inch) rings
475g (15oz) jar roasted red peppers, rinsed, drained and patted dry
2 tablespoons olive oil
4 teaspoons red wine vinegar
3 tablespoons chopped parsley
2 teaspoons finely chopped garlic
50g (2oz) crumbled feta cheese
½ teaspoon black pepper
1 baguette, sliced into 5mm (¼ inch) rounds and toasted

1. Preheat grill. Arrange courgette slices in a single layer on a baking sheet and grill until tops are well charred and slices are slightly wilted, about 10 minutes.

2. Remove from oven and cool for 10 minutes.

3. Place cooled courgettes, peppers, oil, vinegar, parsley, garlic, feta and pepper in a food processor and pulse until incorporated but still chunky, 15–20 pulses.

4. Serve spread on toasted baguette slices.

Serving size: 4 tablespoons dip plus 3 baguette slices
Calories 94; Fat 5.4g (sat 1.6g, mono 2.8g, poly 0.6g); Cholesterol 6mg; Protein 3g; Carbohydrate 9g; Sugars 3g; Fibre 1g; RS 0.2g; Sodium 268mg

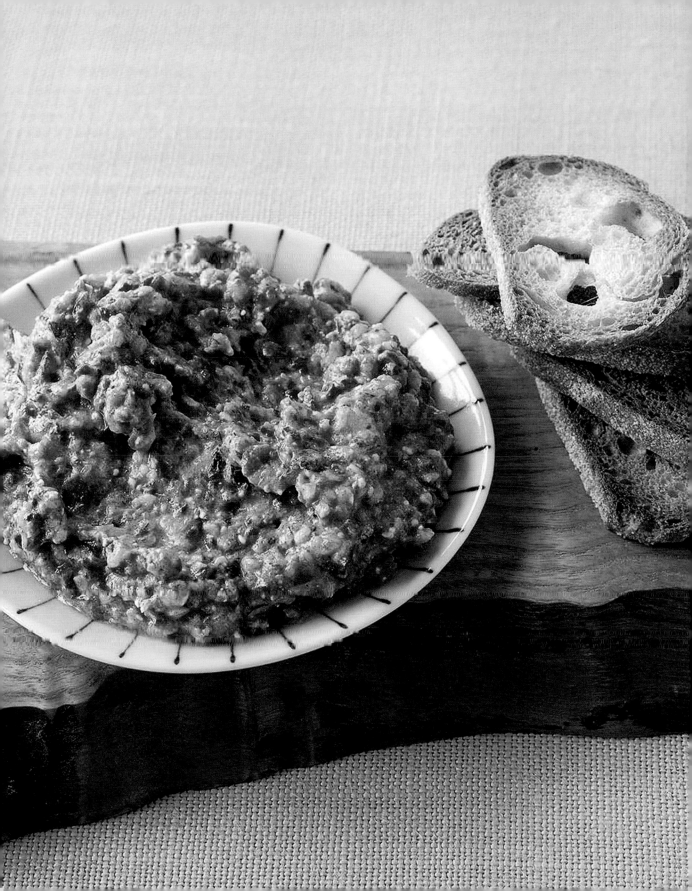

RS
0.5g

Creamy Spinach-Artichoke Dip

Prep: *5 minutes* | **Cook:** *5 minutes* | **Total time:** *10 minutes* | **Makes:** *8 servings*

This all-time favourite dip is typically packed with sodium and saturated fat. Our delicious version adds in Resistant Starch and slashes the salt and fat.

375g (12oz) jar water-packed
  artichokes, drained well and
  patted dry
300g (10oz) frozen spinach,
  thawed and water squeezed out
4 tablespoons light mayonnaise
4 tablespoons reduced-fat
  mayonnaise
125g (4oz) canned reduced-salt
  cannellini beans, rinsed and drained
50g (2oz) Parmesan cheese,
  freshly grated
2 tablespoons water
2 teaspoons finely chopped garlic
¼ teaspoon salt
½ teaspoon pepper
750g (1½lb) assorted raw vegetables,
  such as broccoli, courgettes and
  sugar snap peas

1. Combine all ingredients in a food processor and blend until smooth, 20 seconds. Serve with veggies or crisps.

Serving size: 4 tablespoons dip and 175g (6oz) assorted raw veggies   Calories 109; Fat 4.3g (sat 1g, mono 0.8g, poly 1.5g); Cholesterol 4mg; Protein 6g; Carbohydrate 14g; Sugars 2g; Fibre 4g; RS 0.5g; Sodium 528mg

Rosemary and Garlic White Bean Dip

Prep: *5 minutes* | ***Cook:*** *2 minutes* | ***Total time:*** *7 minutes* | ***Makes:*** *12 servings*

This creamy Tuscan dip and chip combo packs 2 grams of Resistant Starch into just 225 calories. Try the dip with chopped veggies too!

3 tablespoons olive oil, plus more
   for serving
4 garlic cloves, sliced
2 tablespoons rosemary leaves,
   plus more for garnish
2 x 475g (15oz) cans cannellini beans,
   rinsed and drained
2 tablespoons fresh lemon juice
300g (10oz) pitta chips, for serving

1. Heat oil in a small frying pan over medium heat; add garlic and rosemary. Cook until toasted, 1–2 minutes.

2. Transfer toasted garlic and beans to a food processor with lemon juice and 2 tablespoons water. Purée until smooth; drizzle with additional oil before serving, if liked, and garnish with rosemary. Serve with pitta chips.

Serving size: 3⅓ tablespoons dip and 25g (1oz) pitta chips Calories 225; Fat 7g (sat 0.4g, mono 1.7g, poly 0.3g); Cholesterol 0mg; Protein 7g; Carbohydrate 33g; Sugars 1g; Fibre 3g; RS 2g; Sodium 437mg

TIP:
This dip also works well as a Resistant Starch-packed sandwich spread. Make extra and refrigerate for up to 3 days.

RS
0.8g

Potato Canapés Stuffed with Soured Cream and Smoked Trout

Prep: 5 minutes | **Cook:** 20 minutes | **Total time:** 25 minutes | **Makes:** 16 canapés

Elegant enough for a fancy cocktail party, we love that these potatoes take less than 30 minutes to make. The trout filling is the perfect interplay of salty and creamy.

375g (12oz) baby potatoes
  (about 8)
75g (3oz) pepper-crusted smoked
  trout, flaked
2 tablespoons light mayonnaise
1 tablespoon reduced calorie
  soured cream
1 tablespoon fresh lemon juice
2 tablespoons chopped chives, plus
  more for garnish

1. Place potatoes in a steamer and steam until tender but not mushy, 18–20 minutes. Cool, then halve.

2. Using the small side of a melon baller, carefully scoop out the centres of the potato halves and discard or reserve for another use.

3. Combine trout, mayonnaise, soured cream, lemon juice and chives in a bowl.

4. Place potato halves on a large serving plate. Scoop about 1½ teaspoons trout mixture into each hollowed-out potato half and sprinkle with some chopped chives.

Serving size: 4 canapés Calories 136; Fat 5.7g (sat 1.5g, mono 0.7g, poly 1.4g); Cholesterol 29mg; Protein 8g; Carbohydrate 14g; Sugars 1g; Fibre 1g; RS 0.8g; Sodium 396mg

{ **TIP:**
Look for smoked trout in the fish aisle of your supermarket. It's usually right by the smoked salmon. }

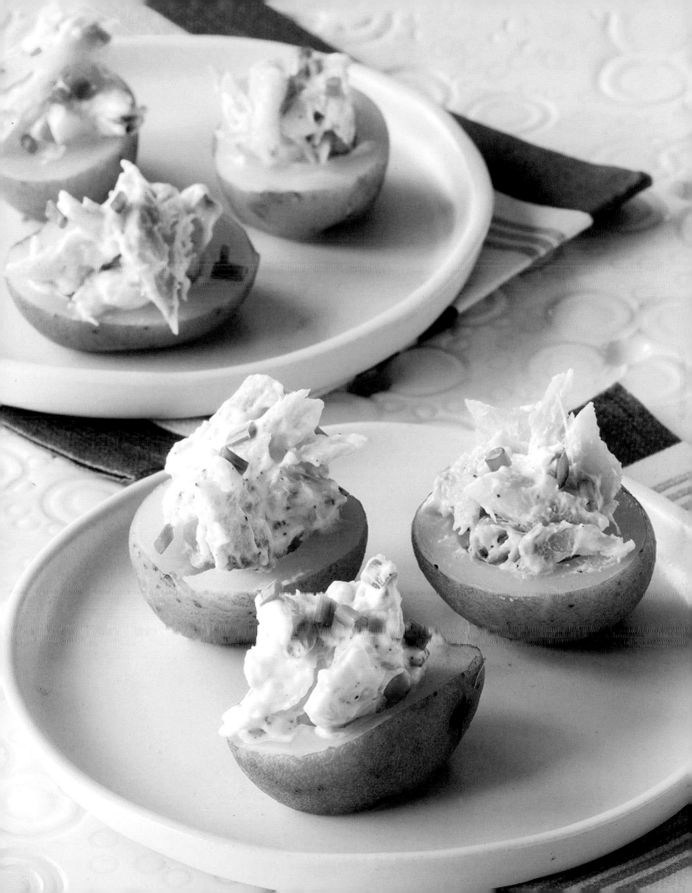

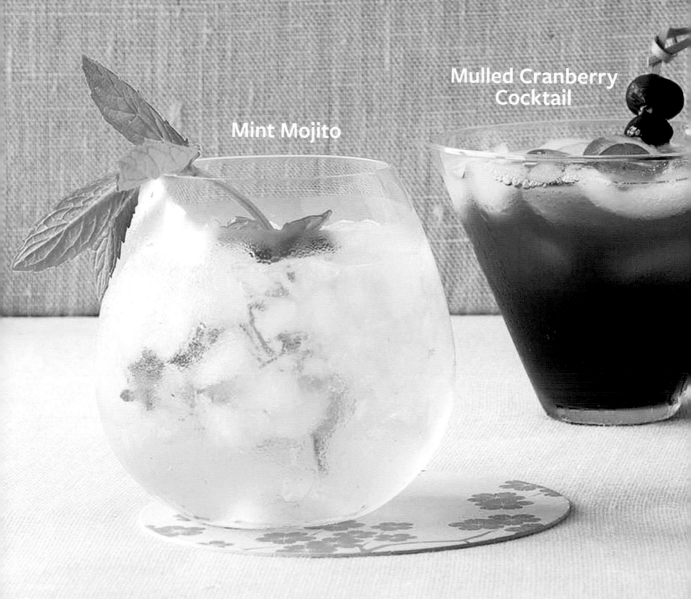

Mint Mojito

Mulled Cranberry Cocktail

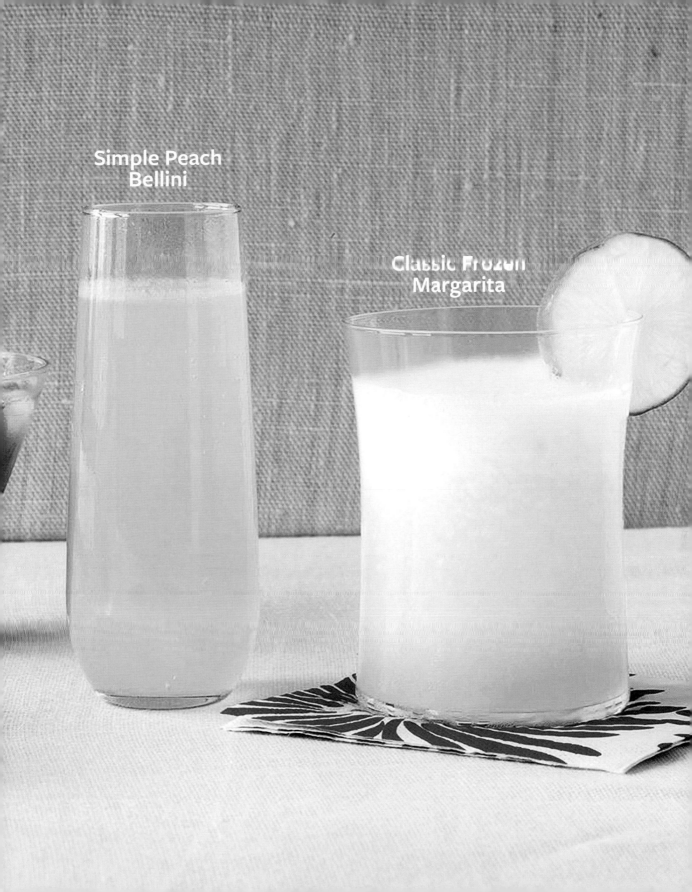

Simple Peach
Bellini

Classic Frozen
Margarita

Celebration Cocktails

Once you're on the 21-Day Immersion Plan, you can enjoy one of these cocktails.

Mulled Cranberry Cocktail

Prep: *5 minutes* **Cook:** *5 minutes*
Total Time: *40 minutes*
Makes: *5 servings*

1 litre (1¾ pints) cranberry juice, chilled
125g (4oz) brown sugar
2 strips orange zest
2 cinnamon sticks
4 cloves
½ teaspoon pure vanilla extract
175ml (6fl oz) rum
¼ teaspoon orange bitters, optional

1. Combine 475ml (16fl oz) cranberry juice, sugar, zest, cinnamon and cloves in a saucepan.

2. Simmer over medium heat until sugar dissolves. Let stand about 30 minutes.

3. Strain into a jug; stir in vanilla, rum, bitters (if using), and remaining cranberry juice. Divide between 5 ice-filled glasses.

Serving size: 250ml (8fl oz) Calories 234; Fat 0g (sat 0g, mono 0g, poly 0g); Cholesterol 0mg; Protein 1g; Carbohydrate 37g; Sugars 29g; Fibre 0g; RS 0g; Sodium 11mg

Classic Frozen Margarita

Prep: *10 minutes*
Total Time: *2 hours 10 minutes*
Makes: *5 servings*

4 tablespoons triple sec
175ml (6fl oz) lime juice
4 tablespoons water
125ml (4fl oz) orange juice
125ml (4fl oz) agave nectar
150ml (¼pint) tequila

1. Combine triple sec, lime juice, water, orange juice, and agave in a jug.

2. Pour into an ice cube tray; freeze until just firm. Transfer ice cubes and tequila to a blender; blend until smooth. Divide between 5 glasses.

Serving size: about 250ml (8fl oz)   Calories 219; Fat 0.1g (sat 0g, mono 0g, poly 0g); Cholesterol 0mg; Protein 0g; Carbohydrate 36g; Sugars 33g; Fibre 0g; RS 0g; Sodium 2mg

Mint Mojito

Prep: *5 minutes*
Total Time: *5 minutes*
Makes: *4 servings*

75g (3oz) mint leaves, plus more for garnish
75ml (3fl oz) agave nectar
175ml (6fl oz) white rum
250ml (8fl oz) ice cubes
250ml (8fl oz) fresh lime juice
250ml (8fl oz) sparkling water

1. Combine mint, agave, rum and ice cubes in jug.

2. Mash mint leaves, rum and agave together; stir in lime juice and water. Serve.

Serving size: 250ml (8fl oz) Calories 201; Fat 0.2g (sat 0.1g, mono 0g, poly 0.1g); Cholesterol 0mg; Protein 1g; Carbohydrate 28g; Sugars 22g; Fibre 2g; RS 0g; Sodium 8mg

Simple Peach Bellini

Prep: *3 minutes*
Total Time: *3 minutes*
Makes: *6 servings*

350ml (12fl oz) peach nectar, chilled
1 (750 ml/1¼) pint bottle Cava or other sparkling wine, chilled

1. Divide peach nectar between 6 glasses; top with Cava.

2. Serve immediately.

Serving size: 175ml (6fl oz) Calories 140; Fat 0g (sat 0g, mono 0g, poly 0g); Cholesterol 0mg; Protein 0g; Carbohydrate 12g; Sugars 10g; Fibre 1g; RS 0g; Sodium 3mg

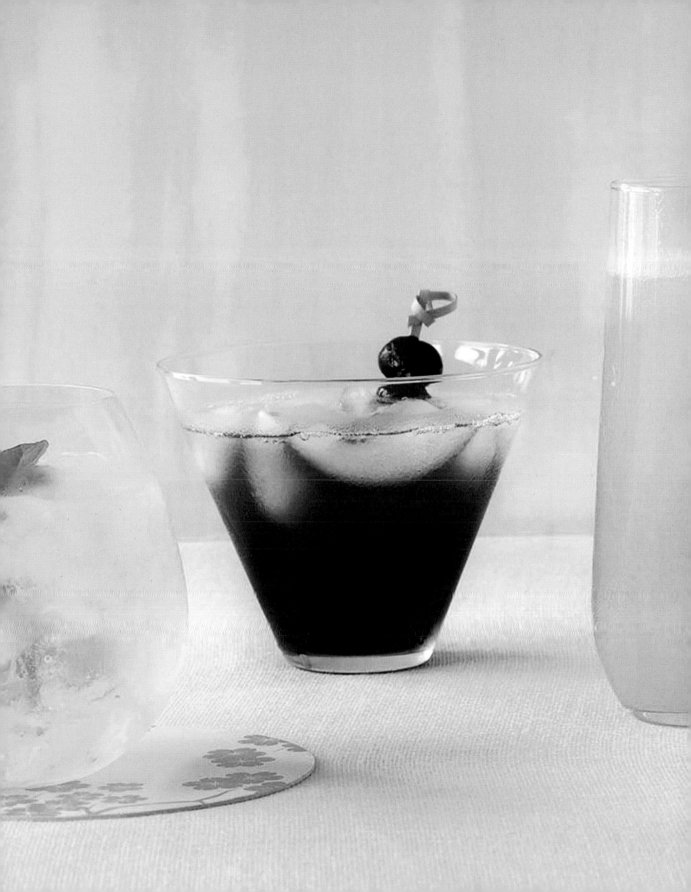

Dessert

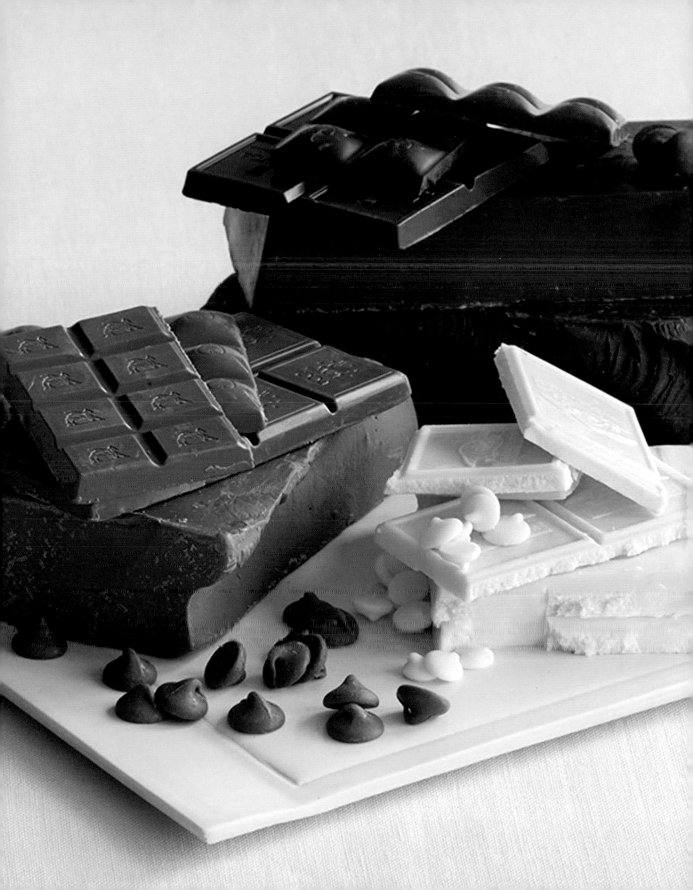

Rich Chocolate Pudding

Prep: *5 minutes* | **Cook:** *15 minutes* | **Total time:** *20 minutes + cooling time* | **Makes:** *4 servings*

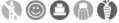

Chocolate pudding is the ultimate comfort food indulgence. Ours uses dark chocolate and unsweetened cocoa powder for a more intense chocolatey flavor.

50g (2oz) plain chocolate bar
150g (5oz) granulated sugar
4 tablespoons cornflour
2 tablespoons unsweetened
  cocoa powder
¼ teaspoon salt
600ml (1 pint) skimmed milk
1 teaspoon pure vanilla extract
15g (1½oz) butter

1. Using a vegetable peeler, shave 1 tablespoon curls from edge of chocolate bar (about 15g/½oz). Chop remaining chocolate.

2. Combine sugar, cornflour, cocoa and salt in a medium saucepan. Gradually whisk in milk; bring to the boil over medium heat, whisking constantly, then boil, whisking, 2 minutes. Remove from heat; whisk in vanilla, butter and chopped chocolate.

3. Divide pudding between 4 cups and cool for 30 minutes. Top with chocolate curls and serve.

Serving size: 175ml (6fl oz) Calories 333; Fat 8.4g (sat 5.3g, mono 0.8g, poly 0.1g); Cholesterol 11mg; Protein 7g; Carbohydrate 58g; Sugars 47g; Fibre 1g; RS 0g; Sodium 211mg

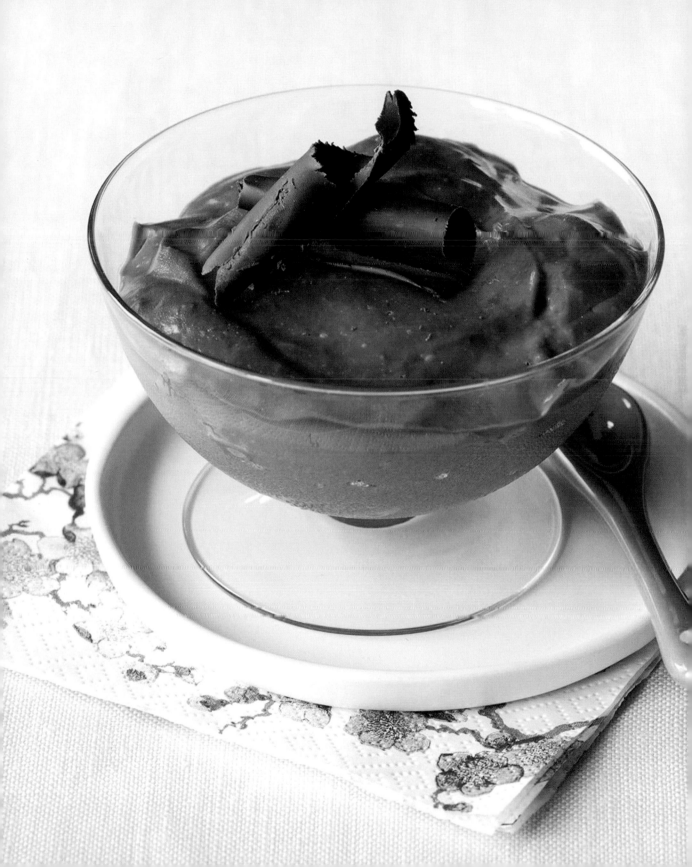

Old-Fashioned Banana Pudding

Prep: *10 minutes* | **Cook/Assembly:** *55 minutes* | **Total time:** *1 hour 5 minutes* | **Makes:** *8 servings*

RS
2g

This traditional Southern dessert is rich, creamy and downright decadent. We lightened up the custard and used a yogurt cream instead of the usual whipped cream, but it's still just as delicious.

4 tablespoons whipping cream
125ml (4fl oz) fat-free Greek yogurt
125g (4oz) sugar
750ml (1¼ pints) cold 1% fat milk
5 tablespoons cornflour
3 eggs
1 tablespoon pure vanilla extract
3 large bananas, sliced
9 sponge fingers, crumbled

1. Whip cream until soft peaks are formed, 2 minutes. Fold in yogurt and 1 tablespoon of the sugar and refrigerate until ready to use (you will have about 325ml (11fl oz) cream mixture). Whisk together milk, remaining sugar, cornflour, eggs and vanilla and pour into a saucepan. Bring to the boil, whisking often, then reduce the heat to a simmer and cook, whisking often, until custard has thickened, 9–10 minutes. Pour the custard into a 20 x 25cm (8 x 10 inch) glass dish, cover surface with clingfilm, and chill until cool, 40–45 minutes.

2. Reserve 8 banana slices and 1 crumbled sponge finger for garnish. Place about 4 tablespoons of the custard on the bottom of a small drinking glass or parfait glass. Layer 2 tablespoons of the bananas, 1½ tablespoons of the yogurt-cream mixture, then 1 crumbled sponge finger. Top with 2 tablespoons sliced bananas, 4 tablespoons custard and 1 tablespoon yogurt-cream mixture. Top with a few sponge finger crumbles and a banana slice.

Serving size: 1 pudding parfait   Calories 249; Fat 5.9g (sat 3g, mono 1.8g, poly 0.5g); Cholesterol 92mg; Protein 8g; Carbohydrate 42g; Sugars 27g; Fibre 2g; RS 2g; Sodium 92mg

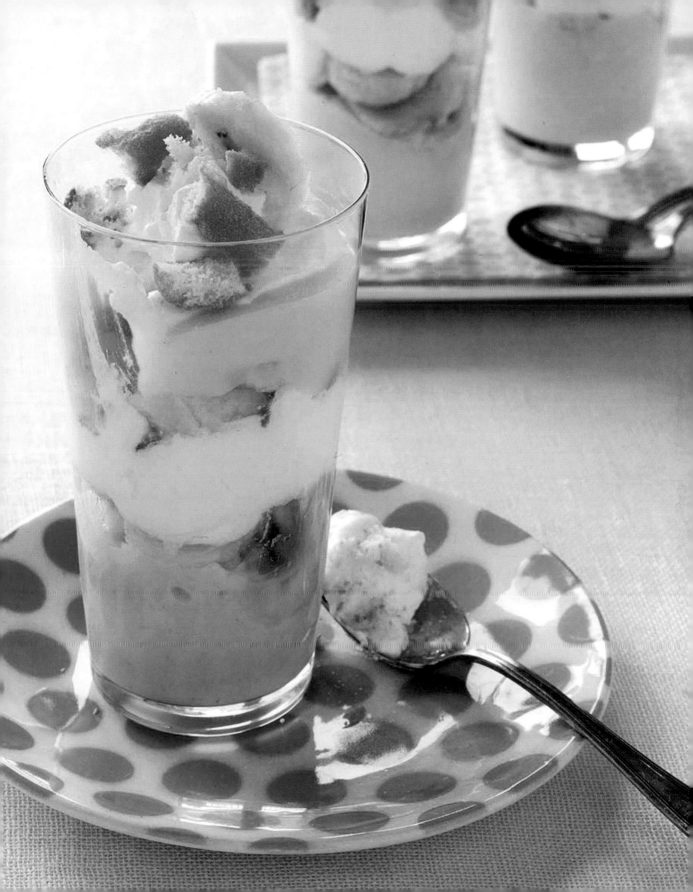

DESSERT

Banana-Walnut Loaf with Soured Cream Glaze

Prep: *15 minutes* | **Cook:** *55 minutes* | **Total:** *1 hour 5 minutes* | **Makes:** *14 slices*

Supermoist and packed full of toasty walnuts, this is no run-of-the-mill banana bread.
Enjoy it with your afternoon tea or coffee.

Cooking spray
100g (3½oz) plain flour
100g (3½oz) wholemeal flour
100g (3½oz) granulated sugar
1 teaspoon bicarbonate of soda
½ teaspoon baking powder
1 teaspoon cinnamon
½ teaspoon ground nutmeg
¼ teaspoon salt
3 large, very ripe bananas, peeled and
  mashed
5 tablespoons vegetable oil
6 tablespoons light soured cream
4 tablespoons unsweetened apple
  sauce
1 large egg
1 large egg white
1 teaspoon pure vanilla extract
5 tablespoons toasted chopped
  walnuts
4 tablespoons icing sugar

1. Preheat oven to 180°C/350°F/gas mark 4. Coat a 23 x 12cm (9 x 5 inch) loaf tin with cooking spray and set aside.

2. Whisk together flours, sugar, bicarbonate of soda, baking powder, cinnamon, nutmeg and salt in a medium bowl. Whisk together bananas, oil, 5 tablespoons soured cream, apple sauce, eggs and vanilla in a separate bowl.

3. Add wet ingredients to dry ingredients and mix until combined, then stir in walnuts until incorporated. Pour into prepared tin and bake for 55–60 minutes, or until a wooden skewer comes out clean. Cool completely.

4. Combine icing sugar and remaining 1 tablespoon soured cream and whisk until smooth. Drizzle over banana bread and cut into 14 equal slices.

Serving size: 1 slice banana bread Calories 186; Fat 8.7g (sat 1.3g, mono 2g, poly 4.9g); Cholesterol 16mg; Protein 3.3g; Carbohydrate 25g; Sugars 11g; Fibre 2g; RS 1.2g; Sodium 166mg

ASK CARBLOVERS

Q: I love sweets! How can I indulge in dessert without going overboard?

A: Here are some tricks to help you practise moderation. First, make sure to put away any extra biscuits, pudding, cake, etc. that haven't been eaten. And put freezable items in the back of the freezer (and out of sight!).

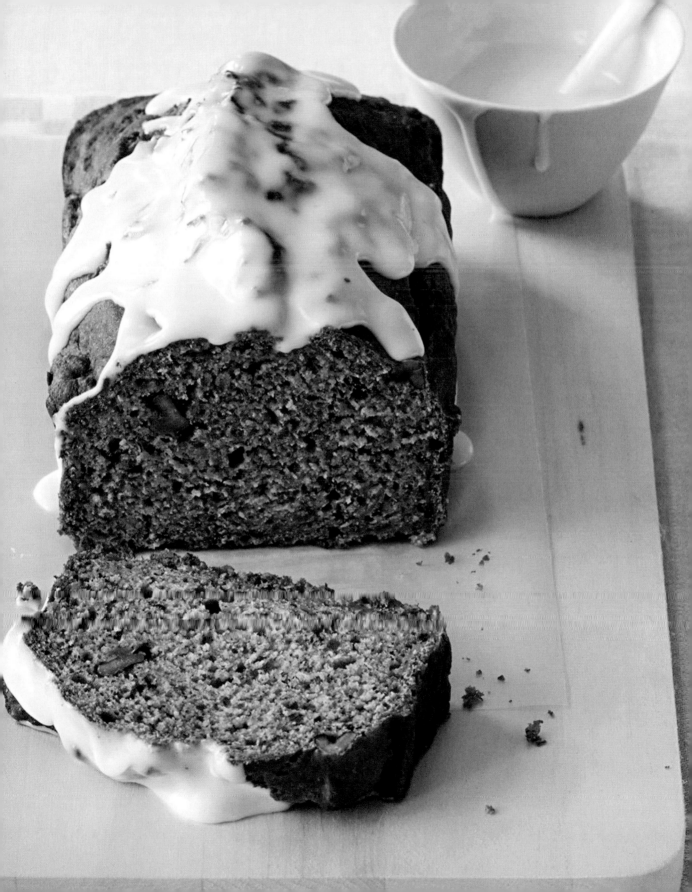

White Chocolate Banana Cream Pie

Prep: 15 minutes | *Cook:* 20 minutes | *Total time:* 35 minutes + 30 minutes cooling | *Makes:* 10 servings

We made this luscious dessert even more divine by adding a layer of white chocolate on top of the base. Make it for your next dinner party – it's a showstopper!

23cm (9 inch) shop-bought biscuit crumb pie
50g (2 oz) white chocolate, melted and cooled
2 bananas, sliced
125g (4oz) granulated sugar
50g (2oz) light brown sugar
40g (1½oz) plus 2 teaspoons cornflour
¼ teaspoon salt
750ml (1¼ pints) 2% fat milk
1 teaspoon pure vanilla extract
15g (½oz) butter
2 large egg whites, at room temperature
100g (3½oz) icing sugar

1. Brush bottom and sides of pie shell with white chocolate. Place bananas in shell and transfer to refrigerator.

2. Combine sugars, 40g (1½ oz) cornflour, and salt in a medium saucepan. Gradually whisk in milk; bring to the boil over medium heat, whisking constantly, then boil, whisking, 2 minutes. Whisk in vanilla and butter. Transfer pudding to a bowl. Cover with clingfilm, directly touching surface of pudding, and cool until just warm, about 30 minutes. Pour cooled pudding into shell.

3. Preheat grill, with rack in middle position. Beat egg whites and remaining 2 teaspoons cornflour in the bowl of an electric mixer until soft peaks form. Gradually add icing sugar until stiff peaks form, about 5–8 minutes. Spoon meringue over pudding to meet edge of pie shell and swirl with a spoon. Grill pie until browned in spots, rotating pie occasionally, about 2–3 minutes.

Serving size: 1 slice pie Calories 288; Fat 7.3g (sat 3.2g, mono 1.2g, poly 0.2g); Cholesterol 10mg; Protein 5g; Carbohydrate 53g; Sugars 39g; Fibre 1g; RS 0.9g; Sodium 191mg

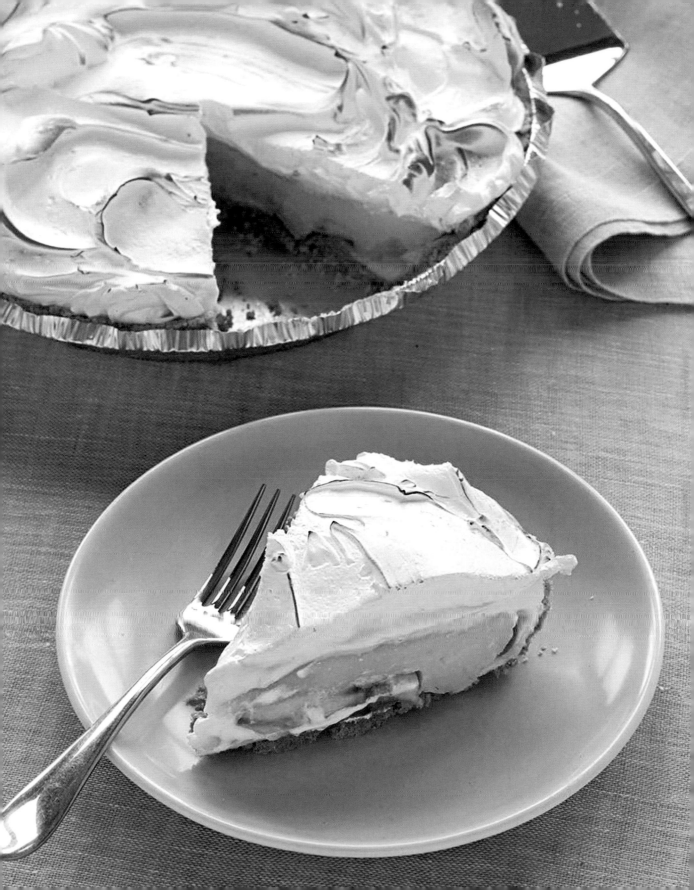

Bananas Foster

Prep: *5 minutes* | **Cook:** *10 minutes* | **Total time:** *15 minutes* | **Makes:** *4 servings*

RS 4.7g

Created in New Orleans in the 1950s, this easy – yet impressive – dessert is legendary. Not only is it delicious, a single serving also has nearly 5 grams of Resistant Starch.

40g (1½oz) tablespoons butter
75g (3oz) light brown sugar
½ teaspoon pure vanilla extract
¼ teaspoon cinnamon
⅛ teaspoon salt
4 ripe bananas, halved lengthwise
4 tablespoons dark rum
475ml (16fl oz) low-fat vanilla frozen
   yogurt (optional)

1. Melt butter in a large frying pan over medium-low heat. Add brown sugar, vanilla, cinnamon and salt; cook, stirring, until brown sugar melts, 2–3 minutes.

2. Raise heat to medium, add bananas, and cook, stirring, until caramelized on all sides, 3–4 minutes. Remove pan from flame, add rum and very carefully light with a match to ignite the alcohol. Shake carefully until flame dies (if you like a thicker sauce you can return the pan to the hob for an additional 1–2 minutes).

2. Divide bananas between 4 bowls and top with 125ml (4 fl oz) frozen yogurt, if liked. Serve immediately.

Serving size: 1 banana, 2 tablespoons butter-rum sauce
Calories 285; Fat 9g (sat 5.6g, mono 2.3g, poly 0.4g); Cholesterol 23mg; Protein 1g; Carbohydrate 45g; Sugars 32g; Fibre 3g; RS 4.7g; Sodium 80mg

TIP:
Caramelized bananas make an amazing topping for waffles and French toast. Just slice the bananas instead of halving lengthways.

Holiday Chocolate Bark

Prep: 5 minutes | **Cook:** 10 minutes | **Total time:** 15 minutes + 30 minutes chilling | **Makes:** 15 servings

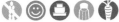

Great to give as a gift to friends and family during the holidays, this chocolate bark is bursting with winter's richest flavours.

175g (6 oz) plain chocolate
175g (6 oz) dark chocolate
 (70% cocoa solids)
¼ teaspoon salt
⅛ teaspoon ground cinnamon
15g (½ oz) puffed brown-rice cereal
75g (3 oz) pistachios, chopped
125g (4oz) dried cherries, chopped
50g (2 oz) white chocolate, melted

1. Line a rimmed 37 by 25cm (15 by 10 inch) baking sheet with foil; refrigerate.

2. Melt chocolates with salt and cinnamon in a large heatproof bowl set over simmering water, stirring often. Stir in cereal and half of pistachios and cherries. Immediately pour onto prepared baking sheet and spread with a spatula into a large rectangle, about 5mm (¼-inch) thick. Sprinkle with remaining pistachios and cherries; drizzle with white chocolate.

2. Refrigerate until firm, about 30 minutes. To serve, break into pieces. To store, transfer to an airtight container and refrigerate up to 3 days.

Serving size: About 25g (1 oz) Calories 198; Fat 12.7g (sat 6.2g, mono 1.7g, poly 0.8g); Cholesterol 1mg; Protein 3g; Carbohydrate 21g; Sugars 14g; Fibre 2g; RS 0g; Sodium 47mg

Mini Chocolate-Cinnamon Molten Cakes

Prep: 15 minutes | **Cook:** 12 minutes | **Total time:** 27 minutes | **Makes:** 8 servings

Warm and rich, this little pot of goodness is a chocolate lover's dream. If you've never made molten cakes before, go ahead and give them a try—they're easier than you think!

Cooking spray
100g (3½oz) wholemeal flour
50g (2 oz) unsweetened natural cocoa
  powder
1½ teaspoons baking powder
⅛ teaspoon salt
65g (2½oz) butter, room temperature
125g (4oz) sugar
2 eggs and 2 egg whites
2 teaspoons pure vanilla extract
50g (2oz) high-quality dark chocolate,
  melted
1 tablespoon coffee granules,
  dissolved in 1 teaspoon hot water
2 tablespoons icing sugar
Mixed berries and whipped cream,
  for serving (optional)

1. Preheat oven to 180°C/350°F/gas mark 4. Coat eight 125ml (4fl oz) ramekins with cooking spray and place on a baking sheet; set aside.

2. Sift flour, cocoa, baking powder and salt into a bowl.

3. In the bowl of an electric mixer, using the paddle attachment, cream butter and sugar until light and fluffy. Add eggs, egg whites and vanilla and beat until incorporated, 1 minute. Add flour mixture to butter-sugar mixture, and gently mix to combine. Add melted chocolate and dissolved coffee granules and gently fold in. Divide the mixture into the prepared ramekins.

4. Bake until cakes are puffy and cracked on top but still gooey in the middle, 12–13 minutes. Remove from oven and sift icing sugar over the top. Serve warm, with berries or cream, if liked.

Serving size: 1 cake Calories 232; Fat 11.4g (sat 6.6g, mono 2.3g, poly 0.5g); Cholesterol 66mg; Protein 5g; Carbohydrate 29g; Sugars 17g; Fibre 2g; RS 0g; Sodium 172mg

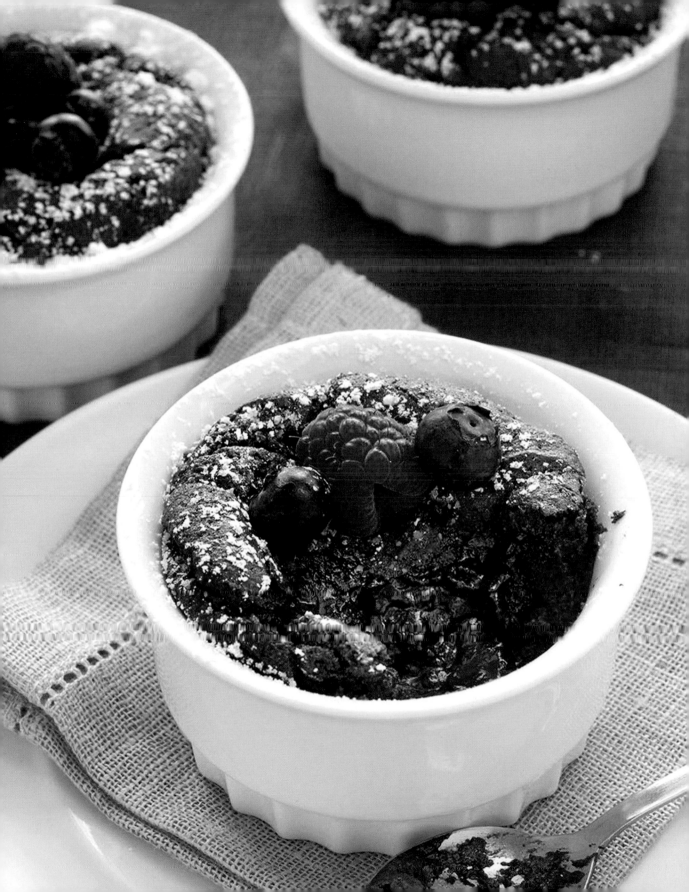

Coconut Cake with 7-Minute Frosting

Prep: *20 minutes* | **Cook:** *30–33 minutes + time for frosting* |
Total time: *55 minutes + 1 hour cooling* | **Makes:** *14 servings*

This gorgeous celebration cake deserves to be centre stage at your next gathering. We used tofu to help lower the fat, but we won't tell if you don't!

Cooking spray
375g (12oz) sugar
40g (1½oz) unsweetened desiccated
  coconut, plus more for serving
300g (10oz) plain flour, plus more
  for dusting
2½ teaspoons baking powder
½ teaspoon table salt
75g (3 oz) extra-firm tofu
175g (6fl oz) light coconut milk
1 teaspoon pure vanilla extract
125g (12 oz) vegetable oil

FOR FROSTING:

3 large egg whites
375g (12 oz) sugar
¼ teaspoon cream of tartar
Dash of salt
1 teaspoon vanilla extract

1. Preheat oven to 180°C/350°F/gas mark 4. Coat two 20cm (8 inch) round baking tins with cooking spray and line with baking paper. Coat with spray; dust with flour.

2. Combine 125g (4oz) sugar, 125g (4fl oz) water and coconut in a saucepan. Simmer until sugar dissolves, 2–3 minutes; cover and set aside. Strain and reserve coconut and syrup separately.

3. Combine flour, baking powder and salt in a large bowl. In a blender, combine tofu, coconut milk, vanilla, oil, reserved coconut and remaining sugar; blend until smooth. Add wet ingredients to dry ingredients and stir. Divide mixture between baking tins and spread evenly; bake until edges begin to pull away from sides of tin, 25–30 minutes.

4. Cool 5 minutes in tins; invert onto a wire rack to cool completely. As cake cools, brush with reserved coconut syrup.

5. Make frosting: Place first 4 ingredients (through to salt) in a large deep heatproof bowl set over about 3.5cm (1½ inches) of simmering water; beat with a handheld electric beater at low speed. Increase to medium-high, beating until peaks form when beaters are lifted (about 7 minutes). Remove bowl from saucepan; continue beating until frosting is cool (about 3 minutes). Beat in vanilla. Ice cakes; sprinkle with coconut.

Serving size: 1 slice cake Calories 370; Fat 12.1g (sat 3.8g, mono 2g, poly 5.4g); Cholesterol 0mg; Protein 4g; Carbohydrate 62g; Sugars 44g; Fibre 1g; RS 0g; Sodium 202mg

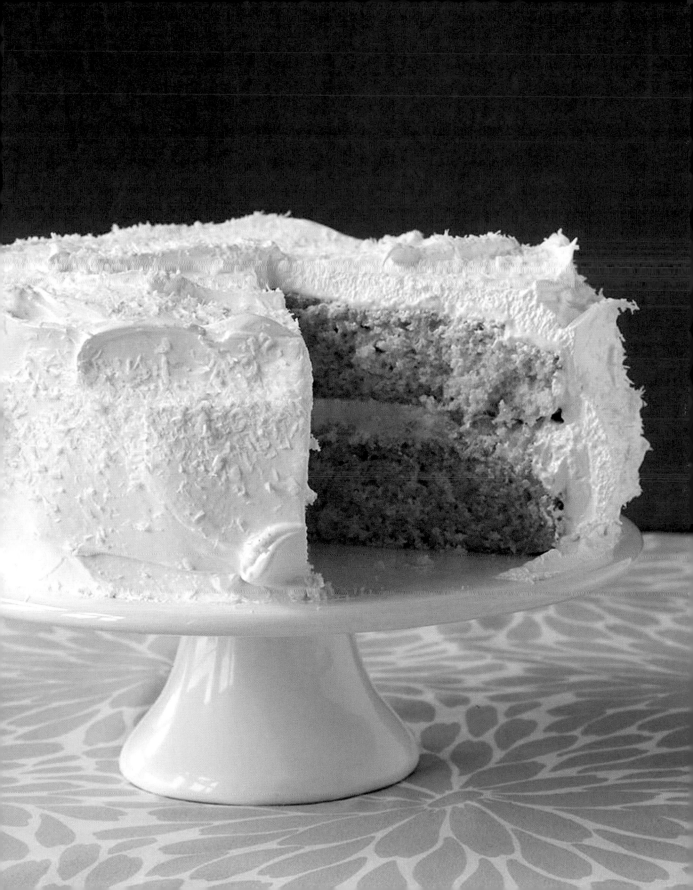

Oatmeal-Date-Chocolate Cookies

Prep: *10 minutes* | **Cook:** *12 minutes* | **Total time:** *22 minutes* | **Makes:** *32 cookies*

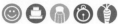

Chocolate chip cookies are the ultimate feel-good treat. And you'll feel even better about these because they're made with high-fiber dates and oats and chocolate chunks.

75g (3oz) unsalted butter
175g (6oz) light brown sugar
40g (1½oz) plain flour
40g (1½oz) wholemeal flour
¾ teaspoon bicarbonate of soda
150g (5oz) oats
½ teaspoon salt
1 egg, lightly beaten
1 teaspoon pure vanilla extract
175g (6oz) pitted dates, chopped
75g (3oz) coarsely chopped dark
   chocolate

1. Preheat oven to 180°C/350°F/gas mark 4.

2. Melt butter in a small saucepan over low heat. Remove from heat and stir in brown sugar until smooth. Combine flours, bicarbonate of soda, oats and salt in a medium bowl. Combine the butter mixture with the dry ingredients, and add egg, vanilla and dates. Fold in chocolate.

3. Mix well and spoon mixture by tablespoonfuls onto lightly greased (or baking paper–lined) baking sheets. Bake for 12 minutes, until tops are dry to the touch. Cool completely on wire rack.

Serving size: 1 cookie Calories 93; Fat 3.8g (sat 2.2g, mono 0.7g, poly 0.2g); Cholesterol 12mg; Protein 1g;Carbohydrate 14g; Sugars 9g; Fibre 1g, RS 1.1g; Sodium 70mg

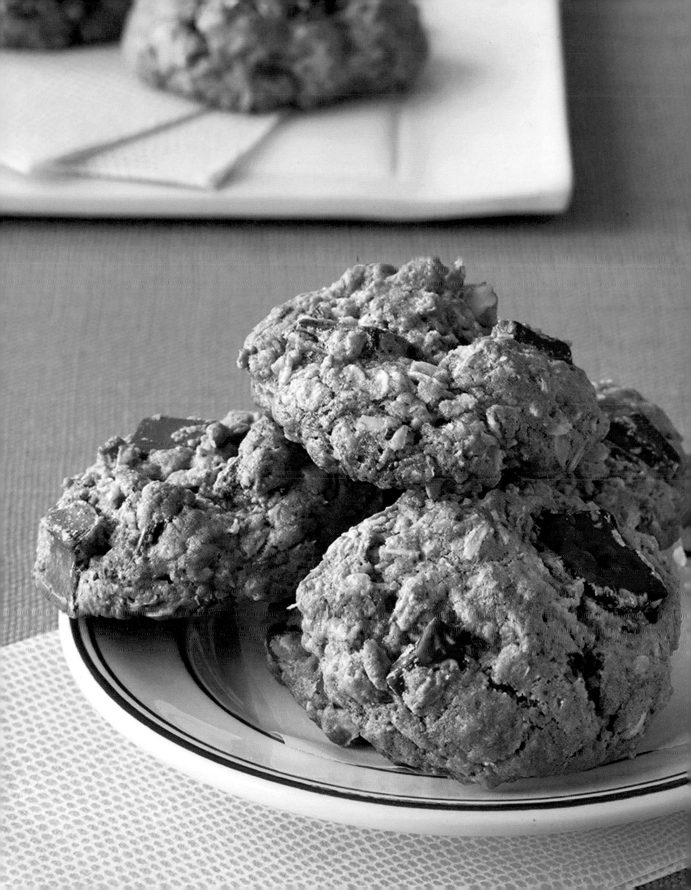

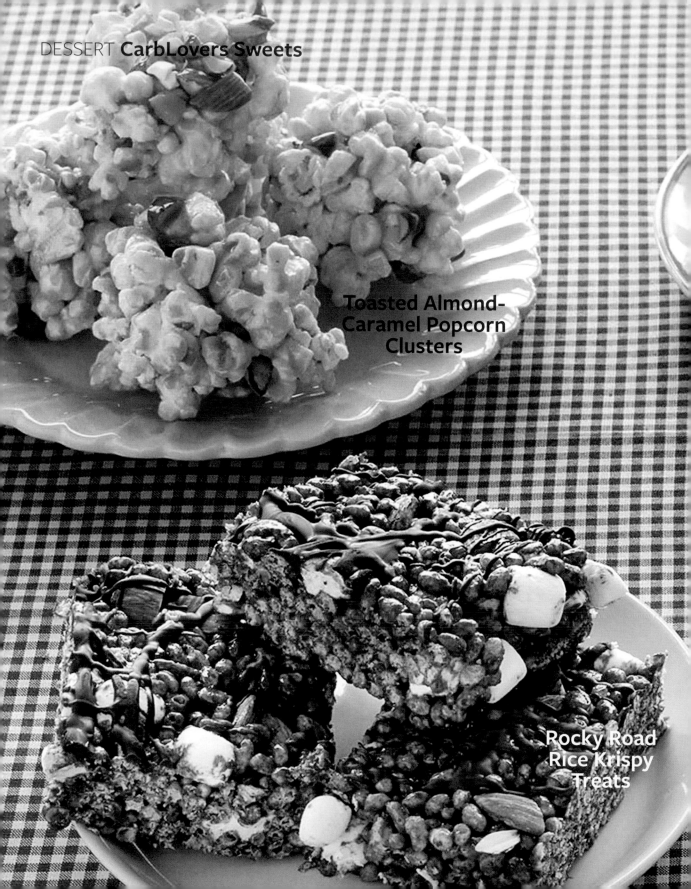

**Toasted Almond-
Caramel Popcorn
Clusters**

**Rocky Road
Rice Krispy
Treats**

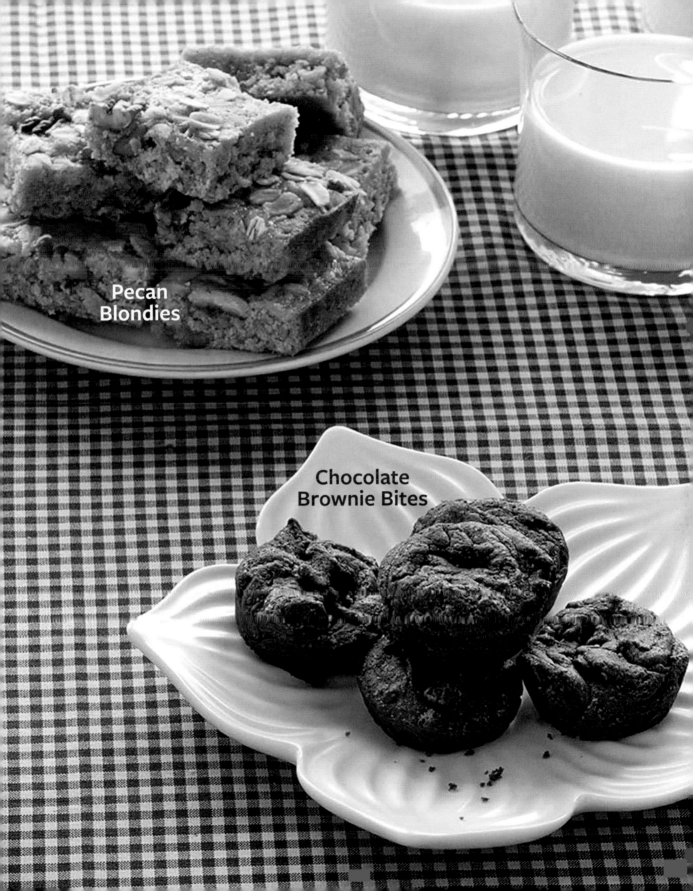

Pecan
Blondies

Chocolate
Brownie Bites

CarbLovers Sweets

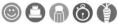

Have you ever seen a diet cookbook that featured so many delicous baked treats? Make a batch to share at your next book club meeting or girls' night in.

Toasted Almond-Caramel Popcorn Clusters

Prep: 5 minutes
Cook: 12 minutes
Total time: 17 minutes
Makes: 8 servings

Cooking spray
8 individually wrapped caramel sweets, unwrapped
⅛ teaspoon salt
25g (1oz) air-popped popcorn
2 tablespoons toasted unsalted chopped almonds

1. Coat foil-lined baking sheet with cooking spray; set aside.

2. Place caramels in double boiler and stir over medium heat until melted. Add salt and almonds and stir to combine. Add popcorn. Working quickly, stir to incorporate popcorn into caramel mixture.

3. Coat a measuring spoon with cooking spray. Drop popcorn mixture, 4 tablespoons for each cluster, onto prepared sheet; let cool until easy to handle, about 20 seconds. Roll into balls and let cool.

Serving size: 1 cluster Calories 58; Fat 2g (sat 0.3g, mono 0.7g, poly 0.6g); Cholesterol 1mg; Protein 1g; Carbohydrate 10g; Sugars 7g; Fibre 1g; RS 0g: Sodium 61mg

Rocky Road Rice Krispy Treats

Prep: 10 minutes
Cook: 10 minutes
Total time: 20 minutes + 30 minutes cooling
Makes: 15 bars

Cooking spray
300g (10½oz) miniature marshmallows
4 tablespoons unsalted butter
4 tablespoons cocoa powder
175g (6oz) crispy brown rice cereal
75g (3oz) almonds, chopped
50g (2oz) plain chocolate, chopped and melted

1. Coat a 23 by 33 cm (9 by 13 inch) tin with cooking spray; set aside. Reserve 50g (2oz) marshmallows.

2. Combine butter, cocoa and remaining marshmallows in a large saucepan; cook over medium-low heat until marshmallows are melted, 3–5 minutes. Add rice cereal, almonds and reserved marshmallows to mixture; stir until combined and sticky.

3. Press into prepared tin and drizzle with melted chocolate. Chill in refrigerator 30 minutes. Cut into 15 bars; serve.

Serving size: 1 rectangle Calories 176; Fat 6.8g (sat 3g, mono 2g, poly 0.6g); Cholesterol 8mg; Protein 2g; Carbohydrate 27g; Sugars 14g; Fibre 1g; RS 0.2g; Sodium 67mg

Chocolate Brownie Bites

Prep: 10 minutes
Cook: 10 minutes
Total time: 20 minutes
Makes: 12 servings

Cooking spray
75g (3oz) plain chocolate, finely chopped
40g (1½oz) butter
2 teaspoons coffee granules, dissolved in 1 tablespoon warm water
1 teaspoon pure vanilla extract
4 tablespoons plain flour
1 large egg, lightly beaten
3 tablespoons sugar
3 tablespoons light brown sugar

1. Preheat oven to 180°C/350°F/gas mark 4. Coat a mini muffin tin with cooking spray and set aside. Melt chocolate and butter in a small saucepan over low heat, stirring until smooth. Remove from heat, transfer to a medium bowl and add dissolved coffee granules and vanilla.

2. Add flour to chocolate mixture and stir well. Add egg and stir to incorporate. Add sugars and stir until smooth. Spoon mixture evenly into prepared tin. Bake until just cooked through and tops are smooth and slightly puffy, 10–12 minutes.

3. Cool completely (as bites cool, they will collapse and tops will invert) and enjoy.

Serving size: 1 brownie bite Calories 111; Fat 6.1g (sat 3.7g, mono 1.1g, poly 0.2g); Cholesterol 22mg; Protein 1g; Carbohydrate 13g; Sugars 9g; Fibre 0g; RS 0g; Sodium 8mg

Pecan Blondies

Prep: 10 minutes
Cook: 30 minutes
Total time: 40 minutes + cooling
Makes: 16 squares
Cooking spray
65g (2½oz) plain flour

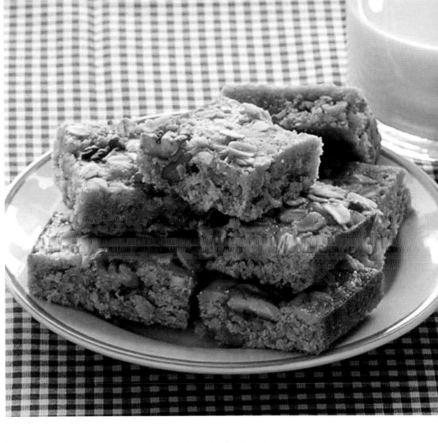

75g (3oz) old-fashioned rolled oats
150g (5oz) light brown sugar
½ teaspoon salt
50g (2oz) butter, melted
2 tablespoons vegetable oil
4 tablespoons apple juice
1 large egg
2 teaspoons pure vanilla extract
4 tablespoons pecans, roughly chopped

1. Preheat oven to 180°C/350°F/gas mark 4. Coat a 20cm (8 inch) square baking tin with cooking spray; line with baking paper (to overhang on two sides) and lightly coat paper.

2. Combine flour, 50g (2oz) oats, sugar and salt in the bowl of a food processor; pulse until oats are finely ground. Add butter, oil, juice, egg and vanilla; pulse until combined.

2. Transfer mixture to prepared tin; sprinkle with pecans and remaining oats. Bake until edges pull away from sides of tin, 25 to 30 minutes. Transfer to a wire rack to cool completely; cut into 16 squares.

Serving size: One square Calories 124; Fat 6.5g (sat 2.2g, mono 2.1g, poly 1.8g); Cholesterol 19mg; Protein 1g; Carbohydrate 15g; Sugars 10g; Fibre 1g; RS 1.1g; Sodium 81mg

Pavlova with Fresh Strawberries

Prep: *20 minutes* | **Cook:** *1 hour 30 minutes* | **Total time:** *1 hour 50 minutes + standing time* | **Makes:** *4 servings*

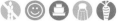

This popular meringue dessert was created in the 1920s for the Russian ballet dancer Anna Pavlova, and is just as light and airy as a grand jeté.

100g (3½oz) icing sugar
1 tablespoon cornflower
4 egg whites, at room temperature
¼ teaspoon cream of tartar
Pinch of salt
¼ teaspoon pure vanilla extract
4 tablespoons double cream
2 tablespoons agave nectar
1 tablespoon fresh lemon juice, plus
  ½ teaspoon finely grated zest
300g (10oz) strawberries, hulled and
  halved

1. Preheat oven to 110°C/225°F/gas mark ¼. Whisk together sugar and cornflower; set aside. Beat egg whites at medium-high speed with an electric mixer for 1 minute; add cream of tartar and salt, beating until blended. Gradually add sugar mixture 1 tablespoon at a time, beating at medium-high speed until mixture is glossy, stiff peaks form and sugar dissolves. (Do not overbeat.) Beat in vanilla. Gently spread mixture into an 18cm (7 inch) round on a baking paper-lined baking sheet, making an indentation in centre of meringue to hold filling.

2. Bake for 1 hour 30 minutes or until pale golden and the outside has formed a crust. Turn oven off; let meringue stand in oven, with door closed, 12 hours.

3. Before serving, whip cream until stiff peaks form; whisk in 1 tablespoon agave. In a separate bowl, whisk together remaining agave and lemon juice; toss with zest and strawberries.

4. Spoon whipped cream on top of meringue, and top with berries. (Centre of meringue may fall once the lemon mixture and strawberries have been added.)

Serving size: ¼ of meringue, 75g (3 oz) berries, 2 tablespoons whipped cream Calories 219; Fat 5.8g (sat 3.5g, mono 1.6g, poly 0.3g); Cholesterol 21mg; Protein 4g; Carbohydrate 39g; Sugars 34g; Fibre 2g; RS 0g; Sodium 97mg

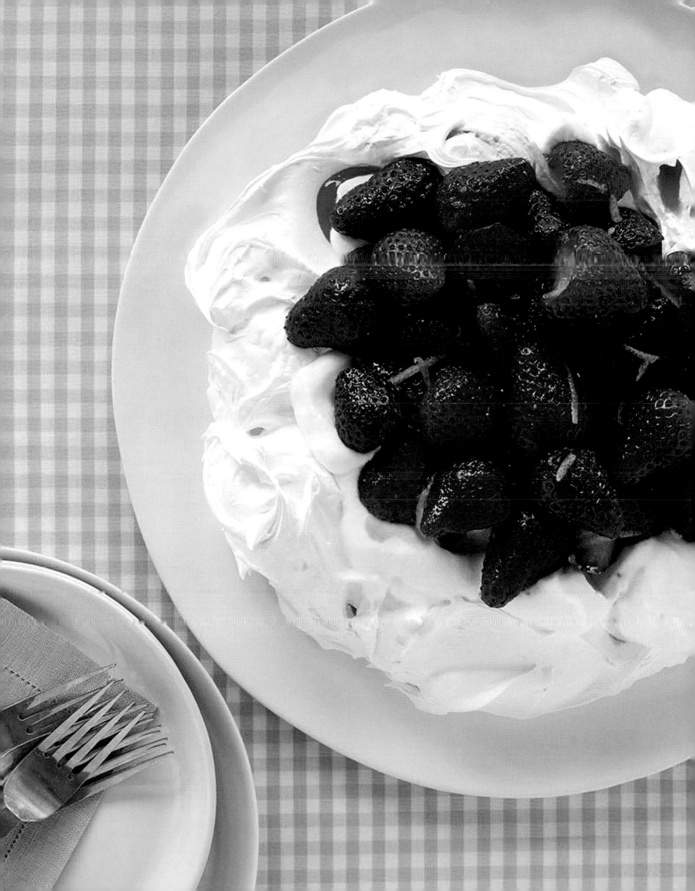

**RS
1.2g**

Brown Rice Pudding

Prep: *2 minutes* | **Cook:** *20 minutes (plus 10–15 minutes cooling)* | **Total time:** *32 minutes* | **Makes:** *4 servings*

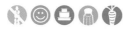

"I eat brown rice and veggies often for dinner. One night I had a sweet craving, so I turned my leftover brown rice into a quick and not too unhealthy dessert. The nutty rice goes well with the juicy ripe fruit." Emily Luchetti

475g (16fl oz) 1% fat milk
3 tablespoons brown sugar
275g (9 oz) cooked brown rice
2 tablespoons double cream
⅛ teaspoon salt
375g (12oz) fresh plums when in season (or 150g/5oz sultanas, dried apricots and/or sour cherries)

1. Combine milk and brown sugar in a medium saucepan. Briefly bring to the boil, whisking; reduce to a simmer. Cook, stirring occasionally, until liquid has reduced to 350ml (12fl oz), about 10 minutes.

2. Stir in rice and cook for 5–10 minutes, until some of the liquid has been absorbed. (There should still be some liquid in the pan; it will get firmer as it cools.)

3. Remove from heat and cool to room temperature. Stir in cream and salt.

4. Serve in bowls with fruit on top. (You can refrigerate the rice pudding overnight. If it is too thick for your liking the next day, whisk in a little milk.)

Serving size: 125g (4fl oz) rice pudding and 75g (3oz) fresh fruit or 40g (1½oz) dried fruit Calories 223; Fat 3.3g (sat 1.8g, mono 1g, poly 0.3g); Cholesterol 11mg; Protein 5g; Carbohydrate 44g; Sugars 23g; Fibre 4g; Iron 1mg; RS 1.2g; Sodium 93mg

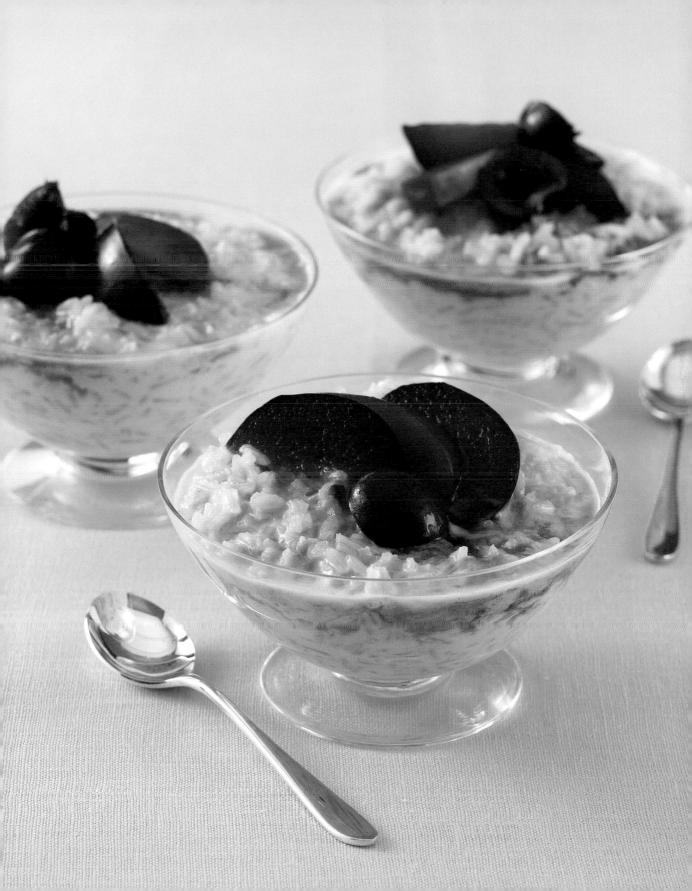

Date-Walnut Mini Cupcakes with Orange Cream Cheese Frosting

Prep: *20 minutes* | ***Cook:*** *15 minutes + cooling* | ***Total Time:*** *1 hour 20 minutes* | ***Makes:*** *48 servings*

"The inspiration for this recipe came from my memories of sitting round the kitchen table with my mom as a child and eating date-nut bread with cream cheese. My kids absolutely love these!" Allysa Torey

FOR CUPCAKES:

Cooking spray
250g (8oz) coarsely chopped pitted dates
150g (5oz) light brown sugar
5 tablespoons black treacle
50g (2oz) unsalted butter
125g (4oz) unbleached plain flour
5 tablespoons wholemeal flour
1 teaspoon bicarbonate of soda
½ teaspoon salt
1 large egg, lightly beaten, at room temperature
1 teaspoon pure vanilla extract
150g (5oz) walnuts, chopped

FOR FROSTING:

250g (8oz) cream cheese, softened
25g (1oz) unsalted butter, softened
125g (4oz) icing sugar, sifted
1 teaspoon freshly squeezed orange juice
½ teaspoon grated orange zest
½ teaspoon pure vanilla extract

GARNISH:

75g (3oz) walnuts, chopped

MAKE CUPCAKES:

1. Preheat oven to 180°C/350°F/gas mark 4 and coat four 12-hole mini muffin tins with cooking spray.

2. Combine dates, brown sugar, treacle, butter and 250ml (8fl oz) water in a medium saucepan over medium-high heat. Cover and bring to the boil. When mixture comes to the boil, remove from heat, transfer to a heatproof bowl, and allow to come to room temperature, about 45 minutes.

3. Combine flours, bicarbinate of soda and salt in a small bowl. Set aside.

4. When date mixture has cooled, place in a blender or food processor; process until smooth.

5. Transfer mixture to a large bowl. Add egg and vanilla; beat well. Add the dry ingredients in two parts; stir until incorporated, but do not overmix. Stir in the walnuts.

6. Carefully spoon mixture into prepared tins, filling each hole about ¾ full. Bake for 10–12 minutes, or until a skewer or knife inserted into centre of cupcake comes out clean.

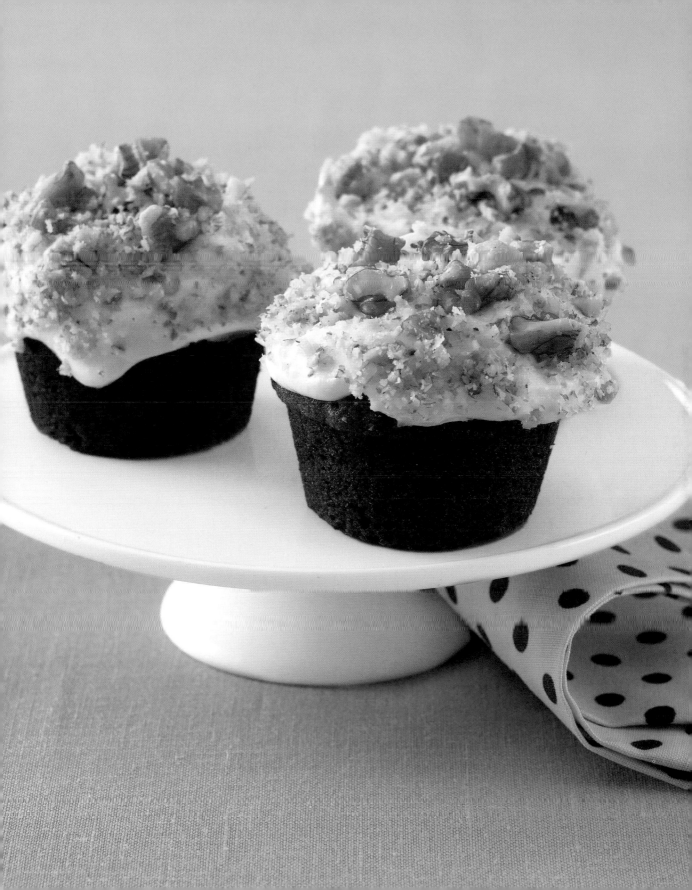

Date-Walnut Mini Cupcakes with Orange Cream Cheese Frosting

7. Cool cupcakes in the tins for 15 minutes. Remove from the tins and cool completely on a wire rack.

MAKE FROSTING:

1. Beat cream cheese and butter with an electric beater on medium speed in a large bowl until smooth, about 3 minutes.

2. Add sugar, orange juice, orange zest and vanilla; beat until creamy.

3. When cupcakes have cooled, decorate with frosting and sprinkle tops generously with walnuts. (Use frosting immediately, or cover and refrigerate for up to 2 hours, but no longer, before using.)

Serving size: 1 cupcake Calories 110; Fat 5.6g (sat 2.1g, mono 1.2g, poly 1.9g); Cholesterol 13mg; Protein 1g; Carbohydrate 14g; Sugars 10g; Fibre 1g; Iron 1mg; RS 0g; Sodium 69mg; Calcium 19mg

TIP:
If you're pressed for time, go ahead and use a lemon- or orange-flavoured shop-bought frosting on these yummy cupcakes.

Holiday Sugar Cookies

Prep: 20 minutes | **Cook:** 12 minutes | **Chill:** 4 hours | **Makes:** 24 (7cm/3 inch) cookies

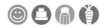

"For us, it is essential that sugar cookies taste as good as they look. Our wholemeal-sugar cookies hold their shape well, and they have a wonderful nutty note via the wholemeal flour" Matt Lewis and Renato Poliafito

FOR COOKIES:

150g (5 oz) plain flour, plus more
  for rolling
4 tablespoons wholemeal flour
¼ teaspoon salt
½ teaspoon bicarbonate of soda
125g (4oz) unsalted butter, softened
75g (3oz) granulated sugar
75g (3oz) light brown sugar
1 egg white
1¼ teaspoon pure vanilla extract
¼ teaspoon pure almond extract

FOR ICING:

250g (8oz) icing sugar, sifted
4 tablespoons pasteurized egg whites
2 teaspoons fresh lemon juice

MAKE COOKIES:

1. Preheat oven to 160°C/325°F/gas mark 3. Line 2 baking sheets with baking paper and set aside.

2. Whisk together flours, salt and bicarbonate of soda in a medium bowl.

3. Beat butter and sugars together in a separate medium bowl with an electric beater until light and fluffy. Scrape down sides and bottom of bowl. Add egg white and extracts; beat until just combined. Add flour mixture; stir until incorporated. Cover bowl with clingfilm, and chill for at least 4 hours.

4. Dust a work surface with flour. Turn out chilled dough directly onto work surface. Roll dough out to a 5mm (¼ inch) thickness. Use biscuit cutters to cut shapes in dough, and gently transfer them to baking sheets. (You can reroll the scraps, just be sure to chill in between.)

5. Bake cookies for 12 minutes or until set but not browned. Remove cookies from oven and cool for 5 minutes. Transfer cookies to a wire rack to cool completely.

Holiday Sugar Cookies

MAKE ICING:

1. Whisk together sugar, egg whites and lemon juice in a large bowl until completely smooth. (If the icing is too thin, add a bit more sugar. If it's too thick, add a few more drops of lemon juice.)

2. Transfer icing to a piping bag (or a resealable plastic bag with a small hole cut into one of the bottom corners). First, outline the cookie with icing, then fill it in, if liked. Let icing harden before serving. Cookies can be kept in an airtight container for up to 3 days.

Serving size: 1 cookie Calories 126; Fat 3.9g (sat 2.4g, mono 1g, poly 0.2g); Cholesterol 10mg; Protein 1g; Carbohydrate 22g; Sugars 16g; Fibre 0g; Iron 0mg; RS 0g; Sodium 59mg

TIP:
Don't stack your iced and decorated cookies until they are completely dry, preferably overnight.

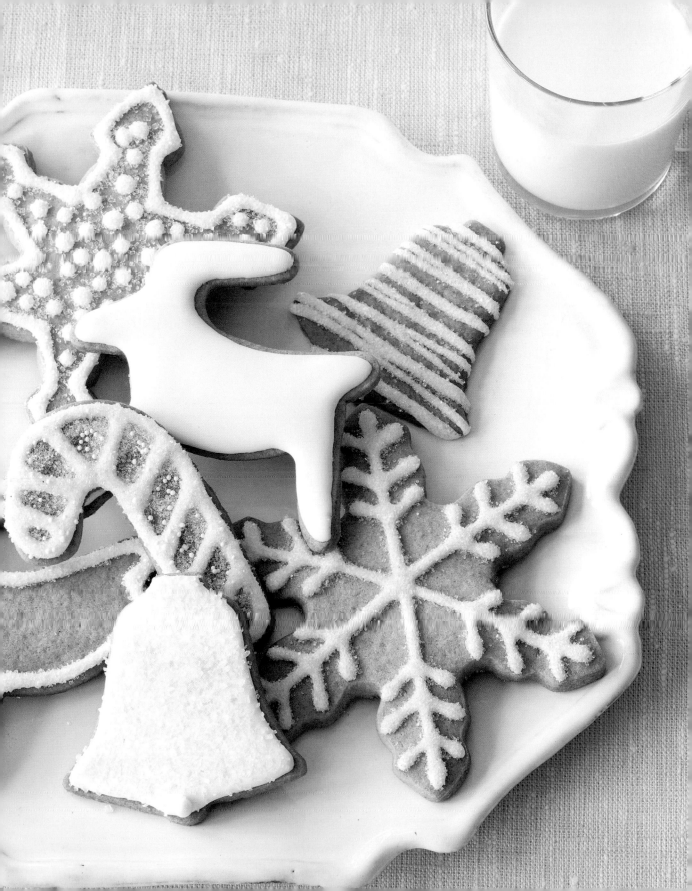

RS
1g

Bourbon Apple Crumble with Oats and Pecans

Prep: *15 minutes* | **Cook:** *45 minutes* | **Total time:** *1 hour* | **Makes:** *6 servings*

Sweet and fragrant with the luscious scent of spiced apples, this no-fail crumble makes a welcoming autumn or winter dessert.

Cooking spray
1kg (2lb) dessert apples, peeled and
  cut into 2.5cm (1 inch) pieces
1 tablespoon bourbon
5 tablespoons plain flour
4 tablespoons regular oats, uncooked
4 tablespoons light brown sugar
½ teaspoon mixed spice
⅛ teaspoon salt
40g (1½oz) chilled butter
4 tablespoons chopped pecans

1. Preheat oven to 190°C/375°F/gas mark 5.

2. Coat a 20cm (8 inch) square baking dish with cooking spray. Combine apples, bourbon and 1 tablespoon flour; arrange in prepared dish, pressing down lightly to compact.

3. Combine remaining flour, oats, sugar, spice and salt in a medium bowl; cut in butter using a pastry blender or 2 knives until mixture resembles coarse breadcrumbs. Stir in pecans. Sprinkle mixture over apples.

4. Bake for 45 minutes or until bubbly and golden brown. Serve warm.

Serving size: 10 tablespoons crumble Calories 245; Fat 10.2g (sat 4.1g, mono 3.9g, poly 1.5g); Cholesterol 15mg; Protein 2g; Carbohydrate 38g; Sugars 25g; Fibre 5g; RS 1g; Sodium 54mg

TIP:
Make this dessert special for company: Spoon low-fat vanilla yogurt into parfait glasses, alternating crumble layers with yogurt, ending with the crumble. Dig in!

Chocolate Drizzled Crepes with Fresh Banana Jam

Prep: *5 minutes* | **Cook:** *5 minutes* | **Total time:** *10 minutes* | **Makes:** *4 servings*

Say oui *to these delicious crepes! Not only can you make them in just 10 minutes, they're packed with more than 2 grams of Resistant Starch.*

2 bananas, peeled and coarsely
  chopped
350ml (12fl oz) skimmed milk
2 tablespoons sugar
4 x 30cm (12 inch) ready-made crepes
50g (2oz) dark chocolate, melted

1. Mash bananas, milk and sugar with a potato masher in a medium frying pan to combine. Cook over medium heat, stirring, until thick and almost smooth, about 5 minutes.

2. Fill each crepe with 4 tablespoons of the banana mixture; fold into a triangle. Drizzle with chocolate and serve.

Serving size: 1 crepe with 4 tablespoons banana mixture
Calories 277; Fat 9.1g (sat 5.8g, mono 2.6g, poly 0.3g); Cholesterol 27mg; Protein 7g; Carbohydrate 46g; Sugars 28g; Fibre 3g; RS 2.4g; Sodium 236mg

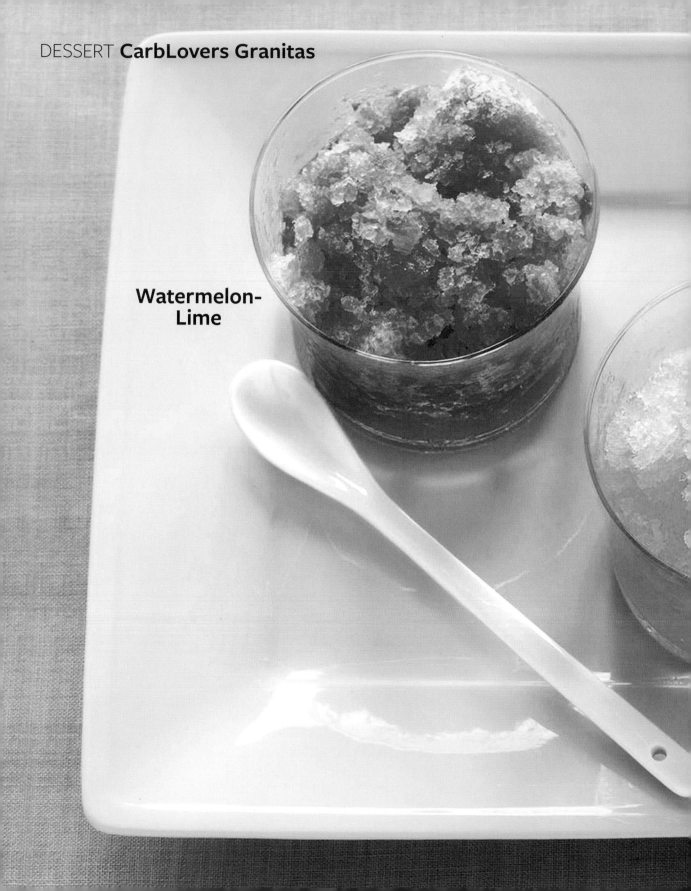

**Watermelon-
Lime**

Pineapple-Mint

Grapefruit-Prosecco

Icy, Refreshing Granitas

Prep: *5 minutes* | **Total time:** *2 hours 30 minutes* | **Makes:** *6 servings*

We love granitas because they're so light, refreshing, and incredibly low-cal. Experiment with your own flavour combinations!

Grapefruit-Prosecco

475g (16fl oz) grapefruit juice
250ml (8 fl oz) Prosecco or sparkling
  white grape juice
3 tablespoons agave nectar

Serving size: 250ml (8fl oz) Calories 95; Fat 0.1g (sat 0g, mono 0g, poly 0g); Cholesterol 0mg; Protein 0g; Carbohydrate 16g; Sugars 15g; Fibre 0g; RS 0g; Sodium 1mg

Pineapple-Mint

750ml (1¼ pints) pineapple juice
3 tablespoons finely chopped mint
2 tablespoons fresh lemon juice
2 tablespoons agave nectar

Serving size: 250ml (8fl oz) Calories 87; Fat 0g (sat 0g, mono 0g, poly 0g); Cholesterol 0mg; Protein 0g; Carbohydrate 21g; Sugars 17g; Fibre 0g; RS 0g; Sodium 6mg

Watermelon-Lime

1kg (2lb) seedless watermelon,
blended and sieved, solids discarded
(about 600ml/1 pint juice)
5 tablespoons fresh lime juice
3 tablespoons agave nectar

Serving size: 250ml (8fl oz) Calories 68; Fat 0g (sat 0g, mono 0g, poly 0g); Cholesterol 0mg; Protein 1g; Carbohydrate 19g; Sugars 16g; Fibre 1g; RS 0g; Sodium 3mg

1. Clear a large area in the freezer and place a 25 by 42cm (10 by 17 inch) rimmed baking sheet inside. Combine all ingredients in a jug and carefully pour onto baking sheet in freezer.

2. After 1 hour scrape a fork across the surface of the liquid (which will be partially frozen but still very slushy). Scrape surface every 30 minutes for the next 90 minutes until mixture has separated into icy crystals. Scoop into parfait glasses, martini glasses or glass dessert bowls.

TIP:
Make-ahead granitas? Sure. Just keep the mixture in an airtight container in your freezer for up to 2 weeks (mix with fork occasionally to keep icy consistency).

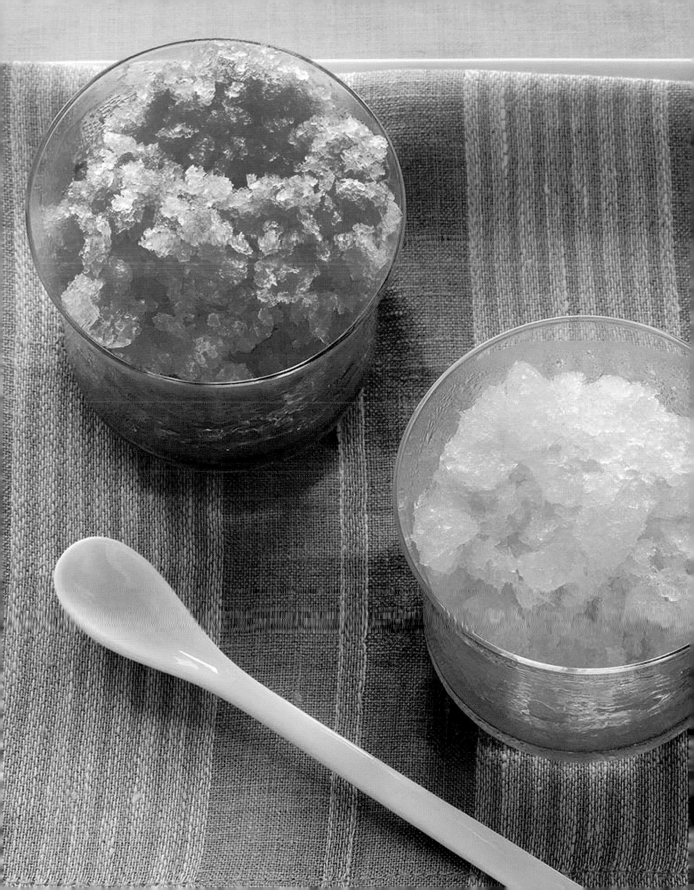

CarbLovers Party & Holiday Menus

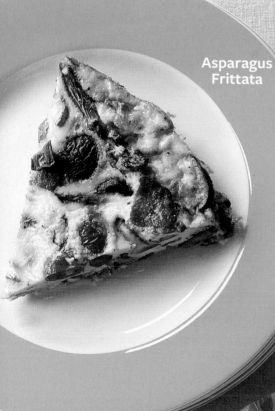

Asparagus Frittata

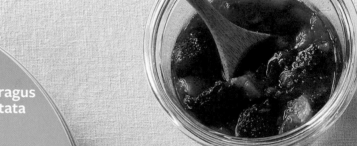

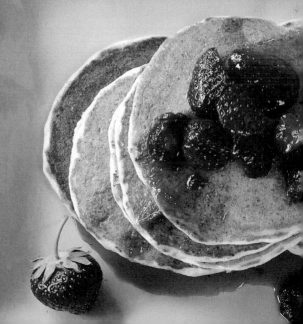

Oat and Honey Pancakes with Strawberry Syrup

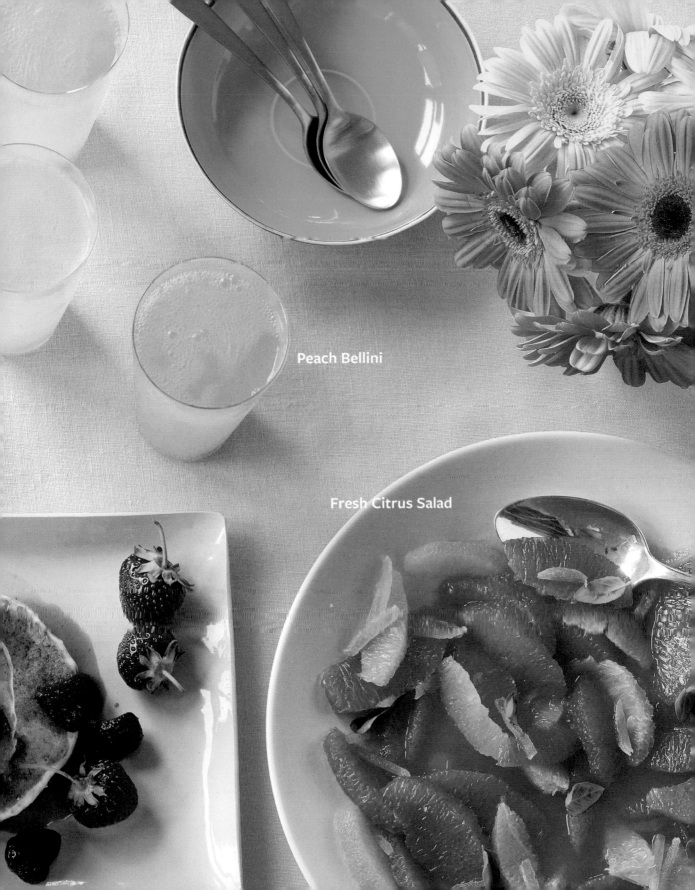

Peach Bellini

Fresh Citrus Salad

Think being on a diet and entertaining don't mix? We disagree! So we made sure the versatile and crowd-pleasing recipes in *The CarbLovers Diet Cookbook* were delicious enough to serve to guests. More important, we know from experience that it's a lot easier – and more fun – to lose weight while enjoying an active social life (saying no to party invitations and dinner with friends because you're afraid to overeat will just make you cranky . . . and even more vulnerable to bingeing). Our fun Match Day and Cocktail Party menus are the perfect blend of festive and filling, while our Spring Brunch, Romantic Dinner for Two and Instant Weeknight Get-Together menus are as easy as they are elegant. We even included a yummy Kids Menu with foods they'll love – no need to tell 'em they're healthy!

Family Night Menu

With today's overscheduled families, it's often tough to get everyone to sit down together for dinner. Try setting aside at least one night a week to really connect with your family over a menu like this one.

STARTERS: Chickpea and Artichoke Bruschetta (page 240)

MAIN: Fresh Mozzarella, Basil and Chicken-Sausage Pizza (page 136)

Green Salad with Vinaigrette

DESSERT: Toasted Almond-Caramel Popcorn Clusters (page 272)

1. Make popcorn clusters.

2. Preheat oven to 240°C/475°F/gas mark 9. Make bruschetta and place on a serving dish for everyone to eat. Assemble salad in a large bowl, but do not add dressing.

3. Assemble and bake pizza. Dress salad. Remove pizza from oven; cool, slice and serve.

4. Serve popcorn clusters for dessert.

Instant Weeknight Get-Together

Friends just told you they're in the neighbourhood? Your mother-in-law invited herself over? No worries – this menu comes together in just 15 minutes!

DRINK: Beer

STARTER: Guacamole and Tortilla Chips

MAIN: Prawn Tacos with Lime Crema (page 162)

DESSERT: Bananas Foster (page 262)

1. An hour or so before guests arrive, pick up fresh guacamole and prawns from the supermarket (or use frozen prawns that you have to hand). Buy beer if you'll be serving it.

2. Put beer in a large metal container with ice. When guests arrive, set out chips and guacamole, and let them serve themselves.

3. Make prawn tacos and serve while hot.

4. Make dessert and enjoy with your guests!

Spring Brunch Menu

Whether you're celebrating Easter, Mother's Day or a friend's new baby, spring always seems to bring lots of reasons to entertain. Our delicious menu has a little something for everyone and is gorgeous to boot.

COCKTAIL: Simple Peach Bellini (page 250)

STARTER: Fresh Citrus with Chopped Crystallized Ginger and Basil (page 40)

MAIN: Oat and Honey Pancakes with Strawberry Syrup (page 34)

Asparagus, Mushroom and Tomato Frittata (page 46)

DESSERT: White Chocolate Banana Cream Pie (page 260)

1. Make pie from start to finish up to 1 hour before the party and reserve at room temperature. Or, if making the morning of the party, make it through to step 2, cover surface of pudding with clingfilm, and refrigerate. Add meringue before serving.

2. Make frittata an hour before guests arrive (or up to 1 day before). Reheat before serving.

3. Make citrus salad. Cover and refrigerate. Uncover 10 minutes before guests arrive.

4. About 20 minutes before guests arrive, make strawberry syrup for pancakes, set aside. Cook pancakes and stack on a foil-lined baking sheet. Keep warm in a 110°C/225°F/gas mark ¼ oven until ready to serve.

5. Pour everyone a bellini. Sit down with your guests and enjoy.

Summer Grilling Menu

When the weather starts warming up, we can't wait to fire up the barbecue. It's such a simple and fun way to entertain friends and family. Clearing up is minimal, so it's easy on you.

STARTERS: German Potato Salad (page 211)

Creamy Spinach-Artichoke Dip (page 244)

MAIN: Burgers 4 Ways: Asian, Tuscan, Southwestern, Provençal (page 174)

DESSERT: Oatmeal-Date-Chocolate Cookies (page 268)

Fresh Watermelon Slices

1. Make potato salad and cookies the day before your party.

2. The morning of the party, slice watermelon, transfer to a serving dish, cover with clingfilm and refrigerate. Also, make the dip and cover the surface directly with clingfilm before refrigerating.

3. Decide which burgers you're going to make. Up to 3 hours before guests arrive, prep your burgers. Place burgers on a large plate, cover with foil and refrigerate. Prep any garnishes you'll be using for burgers.

4. About 30–40 minutes before guests arrive, preheat the barbecue. Remove potato salad and dip from fridge and bring to room temperature.

5. When guests arrive, start grilling!

Match Day Menu

Healthy food and sporting events don't usually go together, but our match-day eats are the exception. Of course, your guests don't need to know it's all good for them!

STARTERS: Layered Spicy Black Bean and Cheddar Dip (page 226)

Mexican Mole Chilli (page 84)

Mini Corn and Feta Muffins (page 234)

MAIN: Bison Sliders with Guacamole (page 166)

DESSERT: Pecan Blondies (page 272)

1. Make chilli and blondies the day before your party.

2. The morning of the party, bake muffins.

3. About an hour before company comes, make layered bean dip. Cover with clingfilm and refrigerate until guests arrive. Prepare the burgers for sliders, transfer to a large plate, cover with clingfilm and refrigerate.

4. Warm up chilli, covered, on the hob over low heat (or in a slow cooker) about 30 minutes before guests arrive.

5. Preheat oven to 200°C/400°F/gas mark 6. Wrap muffins in foil; heat for 10–15 minutes before guests arrive.

6. Uncover dip and set out with a bowl of tortilla chips. Welcome your guests! While they snack on dip and chilli, cook the sliders and make the guacamole. Serve hot.

Romantic Dinner for Two

Whether it's a first date or a night at home with your spouse, it's always fun to create a special meal for someone you love – and maybe stir up a little romance while you're at it! This menu is impressive *and* easy enough for you to focus on your company.

COCKTAIL: Simple Peach Bellini (page 250) or Champagne

STARTER: Edamame and Mushroom Potstickers (page 238)

MAIN: Spaghetti and Clams (page 116)

DESSERT: Mini Chocolate-Cinnamon Molten Cakes (page 264)

1. An hour or so before dinner, make the potstickers. Cover and refrigerate.

2. About 20 minutes before dinner, place a large saucepan of water on the hob to boil.

3. When your special guest arrives, pour him or her a bellini. Reheat potstickers in a frying pan over medium-high heat and place on a small serving plate, along with dipping sauce.

4. Assemble cakes in ramekins. Cover and refrigerate until ready to bake. Preheat oven to 180°C/350°F/gas mark 4.

5. Add pasta to boiling water and cook clams. Serve dinner.

6. Bring cakes to room temperature; bake.

Kids Menu

These recipes are a lot of fun and, most important, good for the kids – and you. Serve for a birthday party or sleepovers.

STARTER: Crispy Onion Rings (page 216)

MAIN: Individual Baked Macaroni Cheese (page 118)

Cornflake-Crusted Chicken Strips (page 182)

Steamed Broccoli with Parmesan

DESSERT: Rocky Road Rice Krispy Treats (page 272)

1. Make rice krispy treats a day in advance. Cover with clingfilm and store at room temperature.

2. Cook macaroni and assemble recipe in ramekins. Cover and refrigerate until ready to bake.

3. About 40 minutes before dinner, preheat oven to 200°C/400°F/gas mark 6. Bake ramekins.

3. Prepare and cook chicken strips and keep warm.

4. Place the contents of a 300g (10 oz) bag of frozen broccoli florets in a microwave-proof bowl. Microwave according to packet instructions, drain. Transfer to serving bowl and keep warm. Sprinkle with 2 tablespoons grated Parmesan before serving.

5. Make onion rings. Serve dinner.

Winter Holiday Meal

Holiday entertaining can be stressful because you already have a million things to do, right? We keep it simple by using recipes that can be made ahead and reheated – without losing their fresh taste. Make it even easier by serving this meal buffet-style.

COCKTAIL: Mulled Cranberry Cocktail (page 250)

STARTER: Butternut Squash Soup (page 80)

MAIN: Roast Beef Fillet with Rosemary Roasted Potatoes (page 176)

DESSERT: Holiday Sugar Cookies (page 281)

Holiday Chocolate Bark (page 263)

1. Make cookies and chocolate bark up to a day in advance. Transfer to separate airtight containers. Great gift idea: Package up a little of each for guests to take home.

2. Make squash soup. Cool, cover and refrigerate. An hour before the party, transfer soup to a slow cooker and heat to warm, or warm in a saucepan on the hob.

3. Up to 2 hours before guests arrive, make cranberry cocktail. Refrigerate or, if serving warm, keep on the hob over low heat.

4. About 1½ hours before guests arrive, make roast beef with potatoes. Slice beef and arrange on serving plate with poatoes and some fresh rosemary.

5. Serve guests. Or if serving buffet-style, place all items on a large table or sideboard, and have guests help themselves.

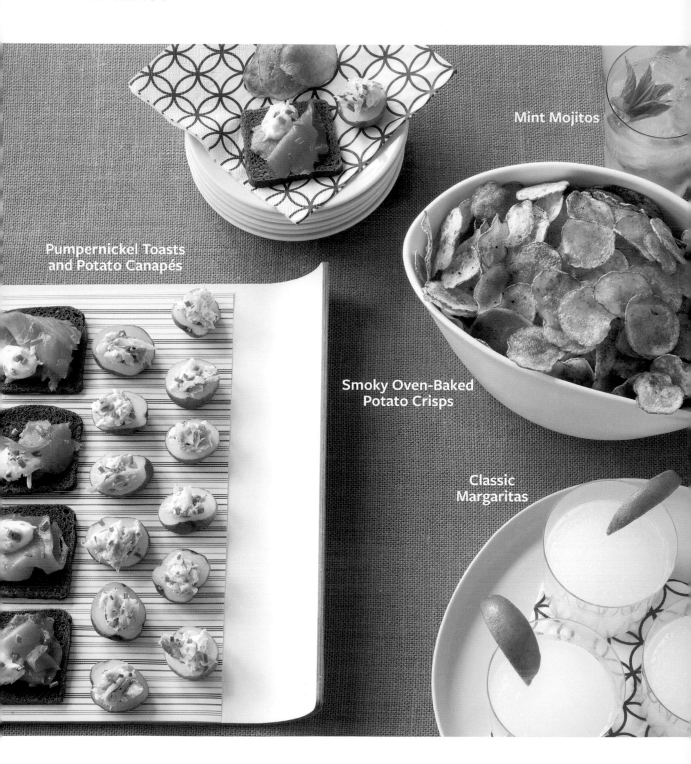

Mint Mojitos

Pumpernickel Toasts
and Potato Canapés

Smoky Oven-Baked
Potato Crisps

Classic
Margaritas

CarbLovers
Cocktail Party

Drinks and apps on a diet? Sure! Our light and delicious drinks and superslim bites will wow guests without weighing them down.

COCKTAILS: Mint Mojito,
Classic Frozen Margarita (page 250)

APPETIZERS: Pumpernickel Toasts
with Smoked Salmon and Lemon-Chive Cream (page 228)

Smoky Oven-Baked Potato Crisps (page 236)

Potato Canapés Stuffed with Soured Cream and Smoked Trout (page 246)

DESSERT: Chocolate Brownie Bites (page 272)

1. Make potato crisps the day before your party. Store in an airtight container. Bake brownie bites. Cover tightly with foil.

2. At least 3 hours before the party (or up to 2 days before), freeze the mixture for margaritas.

3. The day of the party, make canapés. Leave trout mixture (place, covered, in the refrigerator) off until ready to serve.

4. About 15 minutes before guests arrive, assemble pumpernickel toasts.

5. As guests arrive, blend margaritas and make mojitos. Have fun!

Book Club Menu

Don't get us wrong, we love our book club, but knowing that hosting duties are coming up always stresses us out. This menu – filled with totally doable recipes – will let you kick back and enjoy the conversation. And it's made up of recipes from Wolfgang Puck, Allysa Torey and other celeb chefs, so you'll have even more to talk about!

DRINK: Your favourite bottles of red and white, plus sparkling water

STARTER: Edamame and Pear
Crostini (page 230)

MAIN: Barbecue Chicken Pizza (page 144)

DESSERT: Date-Walnut Mini Cupcakes
with Orange Cream Cheese Frosting (page 278)

1. Make cupcakes and frosting up to 2 hours before party. Frost just before guests arrive.

2. Grill or bake bread for crostini. Make edamame mixture. Assemble crostini about 10 minutes before guests arrive.

3. About 20 minutes before guests arrive, preheat oven to 240°C/475°F/gas mark 9. Assemble pizza. Welcome guests, and once the discussion gets going, place pizza in oven.

4. Open wine and serve.

5. When pizza is done, slice into wedges or cut into bite-sized pieces, depending on number of guests.

6. As the book talk is wrapping up, serve cupcakes.

PART 3

The *CarbLovers* Cookbook Diet Plan

The 7-Day *CarbLovers* Kickstart Meal Plan

This week-long plan is the first phase of *The CarbLovers Diet*. It makes enjoying your favourite CarbLovers recipes – and losing up to 3kg (6lb) – so easy and satisfying you won't believe you're dieting. These meals were specially designed to satisfy your cravings for Resistant and body-nourishing nutrients that keep you feeling full, while clocking in at about 1,200 calories a day. Feel free to mix and match any of these meals, but please move on to Phase 2 of the diet after seven days (you can always come back to the Kickstart if you start gaining). Oh, and don't even think about skipping a meal! The 7-Day *CarbLovers* Kickstart Meal Plan purposely includes breakfast, lunch, dinner and one snack. You must stick to this pattern in order to maintain your energy and keep hunger at bay. Skipping just one meal might make you feel tired and stressed – and more likely to binge later. To keep it simple, every day we've included grab-and-go, and frozen options for dieters who are travelling or simply don't have time to cook. For even more no-cook options, go straight to page 316 for a list of *CarbLovers*-approved shop-bought foods.

Day 1 Monday

BREAKFAST: Grilled Banana on Toast (page 52)

LUNCH: Black Bean, Avocado, Brown Rice and Chicken Wrap (page 102)
OR
Levi Roots Reggae Reggae Chicken Curry

DINNER: Capellini with Bacon and Breadcrumbs (page 124)

SNACK: Rosemary and Garlic White Bean Dip (page 245) + 75g (3oz) raw vegetables

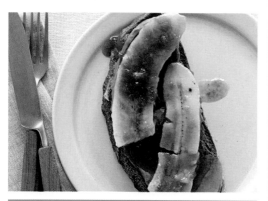

Day 2 Tuesday

BREAKFAST: Tropical Breeze Smoothie (page 66) + ½ medium slightly green banana

LUNCH: *CarbLovers* Club Sandwich (page 90)
OR
Innocent Mexican Veg Pot

DINNER: Prawn Tacos with Lime Crema (page 162)

SNACK: 2 Laughing Cow Mini Babybel Light cheese wheels + 4 Wheat Thins

Day 3 Wednesday

BREAKFAST: Spinach and Egg Breakfast Wrap with Avocado and Pepper Jack Cheese (page 60)

LUNCH: Broccoli and Cheese–Stuffed Baked Potato (page 206)

DINNER: Creamy Barley Risotto with Peas and Pesto (page 127)
OR
Amy's Kitchen Bean and Rice Burrito

SNACK: 10 baby carrots + 1 tablespoon low-fat ranch dressing

Day 4 Thursday

BREAKFAST: Banana Nut Porridge: Combine 50g (2oz) old-fashioned rolled oats and 250g (8fl oz) in a small bowl. Microwave on high for 3 minutes. Top with 1 sliced banana, 1 tablespoon walnuts, 1 teaspoon cinnamon.

LUNCH: Roast Beef Pumpernickel Sandwich with Roasted Red Pepper, Rocket and Goat's Cheese (page 98)

DINNER: Grilled Chicken Escalope with Summer Succotash (page 180) + side of whole-wheat vermicelli 50g (2oz) drizzled with 1 teaspoon extra virgin olive oil
OR
Weightwatchers' Vegetable Arrabiatta

SNACK: Toasted Almond-Caramel Popcorn Cluster (page 272)

Day 5 Friday

BREAKFAST: Tartine with Blackberry Thyme Salad (page 56) + 175ml (6fl oz) low-fat yogurt

LUNCH: Barley Salad with Corn, Feta, Basil and Charred Tomatoes (page 192) + 6 rye crackers
OR
Delphi Edamame Bean Salad

DINNER: Maple-Glazed Cod with Baby Pak Choi (page 150) + 65g (2½oz) cooked brown rice Edamame and Mushroom Potstickers (page 238)

SNACK: White Bean and Herb Hummus with crudités: Mash 50g (2oz) rinsed and drained cannellini beans, 1 tablespoon chopped chives, 1 tablespoon lemon juice and 2 teaspoons olive oil. Enjoy with 75g (3oz) fresh vegetables.

Day 6 Saturday

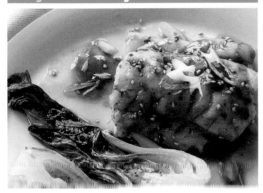

BREAKFAST: Oatmeal with Salted Caramel Topping (page 38)

LUNCH: Stacked Deli Sandwich with Homemade Coleslaw (page 92)
OR
Cauldron Vegetarian Lincolnshire Sausages + 150g (5oz) salad leaves and 125ml (4 fl oz) fat-free dressing

DINNER: Grilled Spice-Rubbed Pork Fillet (page 166)

SNACK: Medium (slightly green) banana

Day 7 Sunday

BREAKFAST: Oat and Honey Pancakes with Strawberry Syrup (page 34) + 250ml (8oz) 1% fat milk

LUNCH: Salmon Waldorf Salad (page 202) + 4 rye crispbread crackers

DINNER: Pasta Primavera (page 112)
OR
Innocent Thai Coconut Curry Veg Pot

SNACK: Trail Mix: Combine 15g (½oz) cornflakes, 2 tablespoons flaked almonds and 2 tablespoons dried cherries.

tip:
Love porridge? This is the plan for you! Our Banana Nut Porridge is the perfect go-to breakfast every day.

The 21-Day *CarbLovers* Immersion Meal Plan

By now you're probably eating and cooking more healthily and have lost about 3kg (6lb). You're slimmer, happier and ready for the next phase of *CarbLovers*. Boy, are you in for a treat! The 21-Day *CarbLovers* Immersion Meal Plan features bigger portions, more snacks (including cocktails!), more grab-and-go options, and even more delicious, indulgent recipes you can make yourself (think Buckwheat Crepes with Orange-Ricotta Filling for breakfast and Mini Chocolate-Cinnamon Molten Cakes for dessert!), as you eat about 1,600 calories a day. Just remember, you can mix and match any meal, even going back to the Phase 1 options if you like.

Your goal for the next three weeks is to lose about 1kg (2lb) a week. By the end of Phase 2, many dieters will have lost 6kg (12lb) or even more. If you still have more weight to lose, stick with the plan, returning to Phase 1 if you start to gain again. If you've met your weight-loss goal, congratulations! You can allow yourself a little more leeway when it comes to indulgences and eating out in restaurants. The dietitians who created *The CarbLovers Diet* have made sure that the newly slim you will stay that way as long as you stick to the *CarbLovers* way of eating.

The 21-DAY CARBLOVERS IMMERSION PLAN

WEEK1

Day 1 Monday

BREAKFAST: Grilled Banana on Toast (page 52)

LUNCH: CarbLovers Club Sandwich (page 90) + 25g (1oz) potato crisps
OR
Delphi Red Kidney Bean and Cracked Wheat Salad + Nakd Berry Delight Cereal Bar

DINNER: Penne with Sausage and Spinach (page 134)

SNACK 1: Coffee-Vanilla Smoothie (250ml/ 8fl oz serving; page 66)

SNACK 2: Toasted Almond-Caramel Popcorn Clusters (page 272)

Day 2 Tuesday

BREAKFAST: Cornflakes with milk and berries: 50g (2oz) cornflakes, 250ml (8fl oz) 1% fat milk + 125g (4oz) berries

LUNCH: Three Bean Soup with Bacon (page 72) + 1 wholemeal roll

DINNER: Grilled Chicken Escalope with Summer Succotash (page 180) + 150g (5oz) salad leaves and 2 tablespoons low-fat dressing
OR
Linda McCartney Deep Country Pie + 150g (5oz) salad leaves and 2 tablespoons low-fat dressing

SNACK 1: Rosemary and Garlic White Bean Dip (page 245) + 25g (1oz) pitta chips

SNACK 2: 2 Oatmeal-Date-Chocolate Cookies (page 246)

Day 3 Wednesday

BREAKFAST: Banana-Nut Porridge: Combine 50g (2oz) old-fashioned rolled oats + 250g (8fl oz) water; microwave on high 3 minutes. Top with 1 sliced banana + 1 tablespoon chopped walnuts + 1 tablespoon cinnamon. Serve with 250ml (8oz) glass of 1% fat milk.

LUNCH: Teriyaki Steak Sandwich (page 96) + medium apple
OR
Innocent Red Pepper Piri Piri Veg Pot + piece of fruit

DINNER: Sausage, Tomato, White Bean and Corkscrew Pasta Toss (page 120)

SNACK 1: 250ml (8fl oz) of fat-free or low-fat Greek yogurt, plain or with fruit

SNACK 2: 150ml (¼ pint) glass of wine

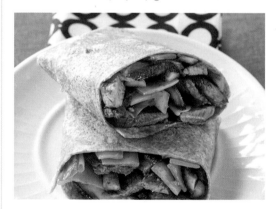

TIP:
Tell the world you're on a diet: OK, maybe not everyone, but letting a few close friends know will help keep you motivated.

Day 4 Thursday

BREAKFAST: Chocolate Antioxidant Boost Smoothie (page 66)

LUNCH: Grilled Cheese and Tomato on Rye (page 106) + Barley Salad with Corn, Feta, Basil and Charred Tomatoes (page 192)

DINNER: Penne with Grilled Chicken and Vodka Sauce (page 121)
OR
Garden Gourmet Vegetarian Burgers + 150g (5oz) salad leaves and 2 tablespoons low-fat dressing

SNACK 1: Trail mix: Combine 15g (½oz) cornflakes, 2 tablespoons flaked almonds and 2 tablespoons dried cherries.

SNACK 2: Roasted Red Pepper and Courgette Spread (page 242) + 3 baguette slices

Day 5 Friday

BREAKFAST: Grilled Banana on Toast (page 52)

LUNCH: Falafel Pitta with Tahini Sauce (page 94)

DINNER: Creamy Barley Risotto with Peas and Pesto (page 127) + 150g (5oz) mixed leaves + 2 tablespoons low-fat dressing
OR
Linda McCartney Lasagne + 150g (5oz) mixed leaves + 2 tablespoons low-fat dressing

SNACK 1: Smoky Oven-Baked Potato Crisps (11 chips; page 236)

SNACK 2: 150ml (¼ pint) glass of wine

Day 6 Saturday

BREAKFAST: Oat and Honey Pancakes with Strawberry Syrup (page 34) + 175ml (6fl oz) 1% fat milk

LUNCH: Creamy Cobb Salad (page 200) + Roasted Red Pepper and Courgette Spread (page 242) + 3 slices baguette
OR
Cauldron Moorish Felafels + 2 slices wholegrain bread

DINNER: Mexican Mole Chilli (page 84) with 2 Mini Corn and Feta Muffins (page 234)

SNACK 1: Chocolate Brownie Bite (page 272)

SNACK 2: 350ml (12fl oz) light beer

Day 7 Sunday

BREAKFAST: Oatmeal-Cranberry Muffin (page 63)

LUNCH: Pan Bagnat (page 109)

DINNER: Spaghetti and Turkey Meatballs with Tomato Sauce (page 130) + 150g (5oz) mixed leaves + 2 tablespoons low-fat dressing
OR
Higgidy Spinach, Feta and Roasted Red Pepper Quiche + 150g (5oz) mixed leaves + 2 tablespoons low-fat dressing

SNACK 1: Antipasto platter: 12 black olives + 50g (2oz) bottled marinated artichoke hearts, drained, + ½ roasted red pepper, sliced

SNACK 2: Banana "Ice Cream": Place 2 small frozen, sliced bananas + 6 tablespoons 1% fat milk in a blender or food processor and process until thick. Top with 2 tablespoons chopped walnuts.

The 21-DAY CARBLOVERS IMMERSION PLAN

WEEK 2

Day 8 Monday

BREAKFAST: Oatmeal-Cranberry Muffin (from batch that was made on Sunday) + Banana Shake: In a blender, combine 1 banana + 350ml (12fl oz) 1% fat milk + 125ml (4fl oz) ice and blend.

LUNCH: Grilled Chicken Caesar with Pumpernickel Croutons (page 201)

DINNER: Grilled Steak Fajitas (page 168)
OR
Amy's Kitchen Gluten-Free Bean and Cheese Burrito

SNACK 1: 8 baked tortilla chips + 125g (4oz) black beans mixed with 125ml (4fl oz) salsa

SNACK 2: Classic Frozen Margarita (page 250)

Day 9 Tuesday

BREAKFAST: Grilled Banana on Toast (page 52)

LUNCH: Hoppin' John (page 220) and 175g (6oz) cup cooked quinoa
OR
Linda McCartney Rosemary Vegetarian Sausages + 150g (5oz) mixed leaves + 2 tablespoons low-fat dressing

DINNER: Spaghetti and Clams (page 116) + 150g (5oz) mixed leaves + 2 tablespoons low-fat dressing

SNACK 1: 25g (1oz) Brie + 1 small apple

SNACK 2: 25g (1oz) plain chocolate

Day 10 Wednesday

BREAKFAST: Peanut Butter-Banana Blast Smoothie (page 66)

LUNCH: Curried Tuna Salad Sandwich (page 93)

DINNER: Tortilla Chicken Soup (page 82)
OR
Innocent Masala Veg Pot

SNACK 1: 2 tablespoons shop-bought hummus and 10 baby carrots

SNACK 2: 350ml (12fl oz) light beer

Day 11 Thursday

BREAKFAST: Oatmeal with Salted Caramel Topping (page 38) + green tea

LUNCH: Roasted Corn and Black Bean Burrito (page 104) + Heinz Classic Vegetable Soup (250ml/8fl oz)

DINNER: Fried Brown Rice with Edamame (page 218) + Edamame and Mushroom Potstickers (page 238)

SNACK 1: Granola with Pecans, Pumpkin Seeds and Dried Mango (page 44)

SNACK 2: 175g (6oz) low-fat vanilla yogurt

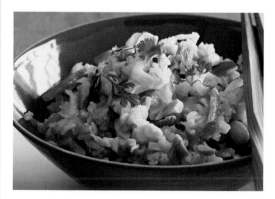

Day 12 **Friday**

BREAKFAST: Oat and Honey Pancakes with Strawberry Syrup (page 34)

LUNCH: Berry-Kale Smoothie (page 68) + 2 tablespoons shop-bought hummus + one 15cm (6 inch) pitta

DINNER: Polenta Crusted Tilapia with Sautéed Greens and Whipped Honey Yams (page 160)
OR
Levi Roots Hot Hot Chilli Beef

SNACK 1: 350ml (12fl oz) low-fat latte

SNACK 2: Chocolate Brownie Bite (page 272)

Day 13 **Saturday**

BREAKFAST: Eggs Benedict Florentine (page 36)

LUNCH: Roast Beef Pumpernickel Sandwich with Roasted Red Pepper, Rocket and Goats' Cheese (page 98)
OR
Baxter's Chunky Smoked Bacon and Three Bean Soup + 1 Laughing Cow Mini Babybel Original cheese + 3 rye crackers

DINNER: Fresh Mozzarella, Basil and Chicken Sausage Pizza (page 136)

SNACK 1: Granola with Pecans, Pumpkin Seeds and Dried Mango (page 44) + 350ml (12oz) skimmed latte

SNACK 2: 150ml (¼ pint) glass of wine

Day 14 **Sunday**

BREAKFAST: Asparagus, Mushroom and Tomato Frittata (page 46) + 250ml (8fl oz) orange juice

LUNCH: Barley Salad with Corn, Feta, Basil and Charred Tomatoes (page 192) + 6 rye crackers

DINNER: Orange Chicken Stir-Fry (page 186)
OR
Linda McCartney Deep Country Pie

SNACK 1: 1 medium banana + 2 tablespoons almond butter

SNACK 2: Rosemary and Garlic White Bean Dip with 25g (1oz) pitta chips (page 245)

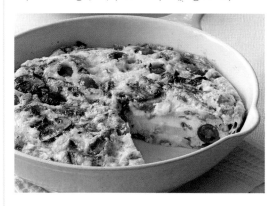

TIP:
Sip smarter with the delicious, super-slimming *CarbLovers* Fat-Flushing Cocktail (page 28).

The 21–DAY CARBLOVERS IMMERSION PLAN

Day 15 **Monday**

BREAKFAST: 50g (2oz) cornflakes + 250ml (8 fl oz) 1% fat milk + 125g (4oz) berries

LUNCH: Tuna and White Bean Crostino (page 100) + 250ml (8fl oz) New Covent Garden Heart-Warming Soup
OR
Delphi Felafel + Penn State Original Pretzels

DINNER: Capellini with Bacon and Breadcrumbs (page 124)

SNACK 1: Fat-free or low-fat Greek yogurt, plain or with fruit

SNACK 2: 25g (1oz) air-popped popcorn

Day 16 **Tuesday**

BREAKFAST: Double Berry Smoothie (page 66)

LUNCH: Stacked Deli Sandwich with Homemade Coleslaw (page 92)

DINNER: Penne with Sausage and Spinach (page 134)
OR
Sharwood's Sag Aloo + 150g (5oz) mixed leaves + 2 tablespoons low-fat dressing

SNACK 1: Trail mix: Combine 15g (½oz) cornflakes + 2 tablespoons flaked almonds + 2 tablespoons dried cherries

SNACK 2: 25g (1oz) plain chocolate

Day 17 **Wednesday**

BREAKFAST: Tartine with Blackberry Thyme Salad (page 56) +175ml (6fl oz) grapefruit or orange juice

LUNCH: Niçoise Salad (page 203) + 4 rye crispbreads or melba toast

DINNER: Mini Mediterranean Pizza (page 140)
OR
Quorn Burgers, Southern Style + 150ml (5oz) mixed leaves + 2 tablespoons low-fat dressing

SNACK 1: Medium banana + 2 tablespoons almond butter

SNACK 2: 2 Toasted Almond-Caramel Popcorn Clusters (page 272)

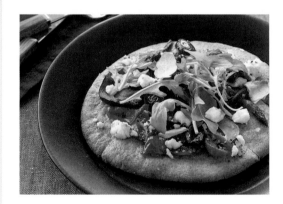

> **TIP:**
> Use fresh, in-season produce whenever possible. You'll get the most nutrients for your buck.

Day 18 Thursday

BREAKFAST: Banana-Nut Porridge: Combine 50g (2oz) old–fashioned rolled oats + 250ml (8fl oz) water; microwave on high 3 minutes. Top with 1 sliced banana + 1 tablespoon chopped walnuts + 1 teaspoon cinnamon.

LUNCH: Chunky Tomato-Basil Soup with Pasta (page 76) + Grilled Cheese and Tomato on Rye (page 106)
OR
Amy's Kitchen Gluten-Free Bean and Cheese Burrito

DINNER: Gnocchi with Walnut-Rocket Pesto (page 128) + 150g salad leaves + 2 tablespoons low-fat dressing

SNACK 1: Chickpea and Artichoke Bruschetta (4 pieces; page 240)

SNACK 2: 2 Oatmeal-Date-Chocolate Cookies (page 268)

Day 19 Friday

BREAKFAST: Banana-Nut Elvis Wrap (page 108) + 250g (8oz) 1% fat milk

LUNCH: Broccoli and Cheese–Stuffed Baked Potato (page 206)
OR
Hungry Joe's Jalapeno Chilli con Carne + Tyrells Habas Fritas

DINNER: Creamy Barley Risotto with Peas and Pesto (page 127) + 150g (5oz) mixed leaves + 2 tablespoons low-fat dressing

SNACK 1: Medium apple, pear or 125g (4oz) grapes + 8 crackers

SNACK 2: 150ml (¼ pint) glass of wine

Day 20 Saturday

BREAKFAST: Huevos Rancheros (page 42)

LUNCH: Chicken Noodle Soup with Autumn Vegetables (page 86)
OR
New Covent Garden Minestrone

DINNER: Provençal Burger (page 174) + Sweet Potato Chips with Curried Ketchup (page 208)

SNACK 1: Medium slightly green banana

SNACK 2: Watermelon-Lime Granita (page 288)

Day 21 Sunday

BREAKFAST: Banana-Pecan Breakfast Bread (page 59) + ½ slightly green banana + Coffee-Vanilla Smoothie (250ml/8fl oz portion; page 66)
OR
Kellogg's Fruit'n'Fibre + 125ml (4fl oz) 1% fat milk + 2 slices of wholemeal toast

LUNCH: Black Bean, Avocado, Brown Rice and Chicken Wrap (page 102)

DINNER: Ultimate Spinach and Turkey Lasagne (page 114) + 150g (5oz) mixed leaves + 2 tablespoons low-fat salad dressing

SNACK 1: Rosemary and Garlic White Bean Dip (page 245) with 25g (1 oz) pitta chips

SNACK 2: 150ml (¼ pint) glass of wine

Grab and Go

We're all for you preparing your own delicious *CarbLovers* recipes from scratch, and even serving them on your best china by candlelight when the mood strikes. But we also know that's not always realistic. Sometimes you're just too busy, or too far from home, to even *think* about cooking. That's why we created this carefully curated list of *CarbLovers*-approved foods, which you can find at most major supermarkets or gourmet delicatessens. (For more, check out *The CarbLovers Diet Pocket Guide* or carblovers.com.) Our expert RDs screened each food to make sure it has the right components to be part of a *CarbLovers* weight-loss plan. Oh, and they taste good too (real dieters tried 'em all). So go ahead: Stock your freezer with frozen meals and your office drawers with cereal bars and snacks. As long as you stick to the recommended portion sizes, you can slim down without ever slowing down.

For the healthiest, tastiest ingredients, packaged meals,

	CALORIES	FAT	FIBRE	CARBS	SODIUM
BAKERY					
Allinson Wholemeal Bread	233	37	3	7	0.4
Biona Organic Gluten-Free, Yeast-Free Millet Bread	214	38	4	6	0.39
Biona Organic Rye Bread, plain	164	35	0.5	10	0.45
Biona Organic Rye Bread, with golden linseed	197	33	5.5	7	0.46
Burgen Buckwheat and Poppyseed Loaf	248	38.5	5	5	0.31
Burgen Soya and Linseed Loaf	282	27	10	9	0.3
Genius Wheat-Free, Gluten-Free Bread, brown	314	44	14	8.5	0.64
Genius Wheat-Free, Gluten-Free Bread, white	311	42	14	7	0.58
Healthguard Sunflower Bread	256	43	8.5	6	0.43
Hovis Granary Loaf	256	46	2	4	0.41
Hovis Hearty Oats Loaf	248	37	4	6	0.42
Hovis Wheatgerm Loaf	225	39	2	5	0.39
Hovis Wholemeal Seeded Granary Loaf	237	40	2	7	0.39
Kelderman German-Style Rye Bread	190	37	2	8	0.5
Rankin Selection Brown Soda Bread	204	40	3	6	0.43
Vogel Sunflower and Barley Bread	239	40	4.5	7	0.5
Vogel Wholemeal Oat and Barley Rolls - per roll (72g)	166	25	3	5	0.86
Warburton's Wholemeal Soft Rolls - per roll (79g)	179	28	4	5	0.33
Warburton's Wholemeal Bread with Rye	246	41	2.5	7.5	0.4
BAKERY - WRAPS, BAGELS, PITTAS AND MUFFINS					
Food Doctor Multiseed and Cereal Pittas	224	40	3	10	0.43
Eghoyan Wholemeal Pitta Breads	260	51	2	6	0.7
Hollyland Bakery Wholemeal Pittas	242	44	2	6	0.4

Nutritional information is per individual portion. Check labels for portion size.

and treats, look for these *CarbLovers*-approved brands!

	CALORIES	FAT	FIBRE	CARBS	SODIUM
Kingsmill 50/50 Wraps - per wrap (75g)	208	41	3	3	0.11
Mission Deli Tortilla Wrap, herb - per wrap (61g)	200	31.5	6	2	0.34
Mission Deli Wraps, mulitgrain - per wrap (61g)	202	31	6	2	0.33
Mission Deli Wraps, plain - per wrap (61g)	207	31	7	2	0.35
New York Bagel Co, multiseed - per bagel (90g)	244	37	4	5	0.36
New York Bagel Co, wholemeal - per bagel (90g)	223	37	2	7	0.36
Old El Paso Tortilla Wraps - per wrap (60g)	200	28.5	7	1	0.3
Old El Paso Wholewheat Tortillas - per tortilla (60g)	205	29	7.5	4.5	0.32
Starbucks Skinny Blueberry Muffin, per muffin	370	72	5.5	2	0.2
Starbucks Rise and Shine Muffin, per muffin	428	56	19	4	0.2
Warburton's Toasting Muffins, per muffin	138	26.5	1	2	0.22
CEREALS - COLD					
Alpen Original Swiss Recipe Muesli	357	67	5	7	trace
Bird's Grape Nuts	345	71	2	11.5	0.5
Dorset Cereals Simply Fruity Muesli	301	64	2.5	8	trace
Dorset Cereals Super High Fibre Muesli	357	60	9	8	trace
Jordan's Country Crisp (Oat, Barley, Strawberries)	440	67.5	15.5	6	trace
Jordan's Truly Fruity Muesli	335	72	2	6.5	trace
Kallo WholeEarth Classic Cornflakes	359	80	1	5	0.6
Kallo WholeEarth Swiss-Style Muesli	340	59	7	10	0.06
Kellogg's All Bran	334	48	3.5	27	0.45
Kellogg's Bran Flakes	356	67	2	15	0.4
Kellogg's Cornflakes	372	84	1	3	0.5
Kellogg's Fruit'n'Fibre	380	69	6	9	0.45

	CALORIES	FAT	FIBRE	CARBS	SODIUM
Nestle Shredded Wheat	340	68.5	2	12	trace
Nestle Shreddies	371	74	2	10	0.3
Quaker Oat Crisp	364	61	7	13	0.3
Quaker Oat Granola	411	73	8.8	5.2	trace
Rude Health Apple and Cinnamon 7-Grain Granola	437	64	13	7	trace
Rude Health Ultimate Muesli	326	50.5	9	12	trace
Weetabic Minis, wholegrain	343	73	2	10	0.08
Weetabix Organic	338	68	2	10	0.26
Weetabix' Oatibix Flakes	381	73	6	6	trace
Weetabix' Oatibix Flakes with Fruit	381	74	5	6	0.1
CEREALS - HOT					
Jordan's Organic Porridge Oats	364	58.5	9	9	trace
Moonflake Medium Oatmeal	356	60	8	9	trace
One Organic Oaty Goodness Porridge Oats	370	56	8	11	trace
Quaker Oats So Simple, original	364	60	8.5	9	trace
Ready Brek Oat Cereal	373	58	9	8	trace
Rude Health Organic Fruity Date Porridge	333	69	5	8	trace
Rude Health Top Banana Porridge	361	65	7	6	trace
CRACKERS AND CRISPBREADS					
Amisa Organic Crispbread, spelt and muesli	348	53	9	17	0.5
Amisa Organic Crispbread, wholegrain buckwheat	340	68	3	8	0.5
Clearspring Oatcakes, sea vegetable and black pepper	452	59.5	11	7	0.9
Clearspring Oatcakes, sundried tomato and herb	389	62	10	7	0.1
Dr Karg Organic Emmenthal Crispbreads	408	51	15	10	0.8
Finn Crisp Five Wholegrains Crispbread	350	50	6	21	0.5
Finn Crisp Multigrain Crispbread	340	61	6	15	0.8
Finn Crisp Original Rye Crispbread	350	58	3	18	0.6

	CALORIES	FAT	FIBRE	CARBS	SODIUM
Food Doctor Fennel and Carraway Crackers - per cracker (8g)	42	8.5	0.2	1	trace
Fox's Wholemeal Crackers - per cracker (8g)	57	7.5	3	1	trace
Hovis Crackers - per cracker (6g)	27	4	1	0.3	trace
Nairns Organic Oatcakes	418	58	16	7	0.6
Nairns Rough Oatcakes	421	53	19	10	0.7
No-No Low-Fat Mixed Seed-Topped Flatbreads	412	69	10	4	0.7
Paterson's Oatcakes with Olive Oil	429	58	17	9	0.7
Paterson's Rough Oatcakes	431	58	17	8	0.8
Real Foods Multigrain Corn Thins	388	71	4	10	0.24
Ryvita Crispbread, dark rye - per crispbread (10g)	34	7	0.1	1.5	trace
Ryvita Crispbread, multigrain - per crispbread (11g)	41	6	1	2	trace
Ryvita Crispbread, original - per crispbread (10g)	35	7	0.2	2	trace
Ryvita Crispbread, pumpkin and oat - per crispbread (12g)	44	7	1	2	trace
Ryvita Crispbread, sunflower and oat - per crispbread (12g)	46	7	1	2	trace
Ryvita Wholegrain Crackerbread, per cracker (6g)	20	4	0.2	0.6	trace
Stockan's Thin Oatcakes	453	50	23	6	0.77

CRISPS

	CALORIES	FAT	FIBRE	CARBS	SODIUM
Amazin' Bio Corn Chips, Natural	493	67	22	n/a	n/a
Garcia Organic Veggie Tortilla Chips	485	66	21	8	0.2
Garden of Eatin' Sesame Blue Corn Chips	500	50	29	4	0.3
Kettle No Added Salt Crisps	517	52	30	6.5	0.08
Kettle Vegetable Chips	487	39	34	13	0.38
Tyrell's Naked Crisps	464	51	28	5	trace
Tyrell's Parsnip Crisps	504	57	33.5	10.5	0.2
Tyrell's Vegetable Crips	492	37	35	14	0.6
Walker's Sunbites Crisps, lightly salted	481	61	22	7	0.38
Walker's Sunbites Crisps, sweet chilli	479	61	21.5	7	0.26

	CALORIES	FAT	FIBRE	CARBS	SODIUM
FLOUR					
Dove's Farm Gram (chickpea) Flour	336	60	5	10	trace
Doves' Farm Organic Plain Wholemeal Flour	319	64	2	11	trace
Doves' Farm Organic Wholegrain Spelt Flour	330	64	2.5	8.5	trace
Marriage's Organic Strong Wholemeal Flour	322	70	2	8.5	trace
Shipton Mill Three Malts and Sunflower Flour	351	62	3	6	4
PASTA, RICE, NOODLES AND GRAINS					
Ainsley Harriot Roasted Vegetable Cous Cous	144	27	1	1.5	0.2
Amoy Udon Noodles	134	27	2	2	0.1
Blue Dragon Wholemeal Noodle Nests	351	76	trace	6	0.7
Biona Organic Spelt Pasta	362	71	2	4	trace
Biona Organic Wholewheat Fusilli	326	65	2	9	n/a
Biona Organic Wild Rice Mix	332	74	2	2.5	trace
Clearspring Organic Soba Noodles (buckwheat)	342	71	2	2	0.9
Del Ugo Organic Gluten-Free Spaghetti	271	44	4	6	trace
Del Ugo Pea and Pancetta Ravioli	235	30	7.5	2	0.33
Dove's Farm Organic Gluten-Free Pasta	347	76	1	2.5	trace
Garofolo Organic Wholewheat Spaghetti	350	65	2	8	trace
Merchant Gourmet Ready-to-Eat Red and White Quinoa	202	31	6	4	0.3
Merchant Gourmet Ready-to-Eat Wholesome Mixed Grains	204	25	7	3	0.25
Napolina Wholewheat Penne	335	63	3	9	trace
Seeds of Change Organic Semi-Wholewheat Tortiglioni	348	72	1.5	3	trace
Seeds of Change Organic Spinach Trotolle	348	72	1.5	3	0
Sun Grown Mediterranean Cous Cous	145	26	1.5	2	0.3
Tilda Brown Wholegrain Basmati Rice	351	72	3	3	trace
Tilda Pure Basmati Rice	355	76	1.5	1	trace
Tilda Steamed Brown Basmati Rice	136	26	2	2	0.1
Tilda Steamed Basmati - coconut, chilli and lemongrass	145	22.5	5	2	0.2

	CALORIES	FAT	FIBRE	CARBS	SODIUM
Tilda Steamed Basmati - Mexican chilli and bean	117	21.5	2	3	0.3
Tilda Steamed Basmati - pilau rice	120	22	2	2	0.3
Uncle Ben's Boil in the Bag Wholegrain Rice	344	73	2	3	trace
Veetee Dine In Pilau Rice	140	26	3	2	0.24
Veetee Dine In Vegetable Pilau Rice	140	26	3	1	0.3

PREPARED MEALS, CHILLED AND FROZEN (including vegetarian meat substitutes)

	CALORIES	FAT	FIBRE	CARBS	SODIUM
Amy's Kitchen All-American Veggie Burger	172	16	5	6	1.3
Amy's Kitchen Bean and Rice Burrito	165	28	3.5	3	0.3
Amy's Kitchen Gluten-Free Bean and Cheese Burrito	167	24	5	3	0.7
Amy's Kitchen Gluten-Free Country Vegetable and Pasta	162	16	8	2	0.2
Amy's Kitchen Gluten-Free Lasagne	122	14	5	1	0.3
Aunt Bessie's Vegetarian Toad in the Hole	264	27.5	10	3	0.9
Biona Mexican Refried Beans	121	12	4	10	0.41
Biona Organic Energy Vegetarian Mini Burgers	112	26	14	n/a	n/a
Cauldron Moorish Felafels	257	30	11	6.5	0.2
Cauldron Mushroom Burgers	171	16	8	1.5	0.5
Cauldron Vegetarian Lincolnshire Sausages	159	4	9	3	0.7
Delphi Edamame Bean Salad	138	9	8	4	1
Delphi Felafel	355	36	22.5	8	0.6
Delphi Lentil Salad	142	18	9	9	0.4
Delphi Red Kidney Bean and Cracked Wheat Salad	112	13	6	3	0.9
Garden Gourmet Vegetarian Burgers	168	9	6	2	0.6
Goodlife Nut Cutlets	279	22	17	6	n/a
Goodlife Root Vegetable Roasts	166	22.5	7	2.5	0.4
Goodlife Spicy Bean Quarter Pounders	221	24	11	8	n/a
Goodlife Vegetarian Glamorgan Sausages	234	23	12	5	n/a
Higgidy Spinach, Feta and Roasted Red Pepper Quiche	222	20	13	2	0.17

	CALORIES	FAT	FIBRE	CARBS	SODIUM
Hungry Joe's Jalapeno Chilli con Carne	78	9	2	2	0.12
Innocent Indian Dhal Curry Veg Pot	350	10	3	5	0.19
Innocent Masala Veg Pot	367	12	2.5	4	0.23
Innocent Mexican Veg Pot	83	11	2	5.5	0.17
Innocent Red Pepper Piri Piri Veg Pot	79	11	2	4	0.17
Innocent Thai Coconut Curry Veg Pot	337	10	2.5	3	0.16
Levi Roots Coconut Chicken Curry	155	19	5	2	0.17
Levi Roots Hot Hot Chilli Beef	180	21	7	3	0.24
Levi Roots Pepper Pot Chicken	130	16	3	2	0.3
Levi Roots Reggae Reggae Chicken Curry	139	18	4	3	0.2
Linda McCartney Cheese, Leek and Red Onion Plaits	278	26	16.5	2	0.3
Linda McCartney Cranberry and Camembert Burgers	220	10	12.5	4	0.5
Linda McCartney Deep Country Pie	248	25	14	3	0.3
Linda McCartney Lasagne	125	12	6	1	0.5
Linda McCartney Original Vegetarian Sausages	202	8	9	2	1.8
Linda McCartney Rosemary Vegetarian Sausages	128	10	4	6	0.5
Merchant Gourmet Ready-to-Eat Beluga Lentils	148	20.5	1	5	0.34
Quorn Burgers	160	8	7	2	0.4
Quorn Burgers, Southern Style	195	14.5	10	3	0.8
Quorn Cheese and Broccoli Escalope	209	16.5	11	3	0.5
Sharwood's Sag Aloo	92	10	5	1.5	0.3
Tivall Vegetarian Burgers	141	6	5	4	0.6
Weightwatchers' Moroccan Vegetable Tagine Pot	91	15	1.5	2.5	trace
Weightwatchers' Vegetable Arrabiatta	68	11	0.4	3	trace
SNACKS					
Alpen Fruit and Nut Bar - per bar (28g)	109	20.5	2	1	trace
Babybel Mini, per cheese (20g)	63	0	5	0	n/a
Babybel Mini Cheddar, per cheese (20g)	75	trace	6	0	0.14

	CALORIES	FAT	FIBRE	CARBS	SODIUM
Babybel Mini Gouda, per cheese (20g)	68	0	6	0	0.14
Babybel Mini Light, per cheese (20g)	42	trace	0.4	0	n/a
Be Fruity Apricot Bar - per bar (25g)	80	16	1	2.5	0
Be Fruity Strawberry Bar - per bar (25g)	80	16	1.5	2.5	0
Delphi Chunky Roasted Vegetable Houmous	190	16	12.5	5	1.2
Delphi Chargrilled Red Pepper Houmous Dip	178	20	10	6	1.2
Food Doctor Roasted Bean Mix	393	23.5	13	21	0.1
Fruitus Apricot Oat Bars - per bar (35g)	129	19	5	2	trace
Geobar, apricot and raisin - per bar (32g)	126	26	2	2	trace
Geobar, chocolate - per bar (32g)	130	25	3	1	trace
Jordan's Breakfast in a Bar - per bar (40g)	157	25	5	2	trace
Jordan's Cereal Bars, Apple and Sultana - per bar (30g)	111	21	2	1	trace
Jordan's Frusli Bars, Blackberry Burst - per bar (30g)	113	21	2	1	trace
Jordan's Frusli Bars, Cranberry and Apple - per bar (30g)	114	22	2.5	1	trace
Kelloggs Nutri-Grain Blackberry and Apple Bar - per bar (37g)	133	26	3	1.5	0.15
Kelloggs Nutri-Grain Elevenses Raisin Bakes - per bar (45g)	164	30	4	1	0.1
Kelloggs Nutri-Grain Golden Oat Bakes - per bake (50g)	204	32	8	1.5	0.1
Kelloggs Special K Bars, plain - per bar (23g)	90	17	2	0.5	0.25
Kelloggs Special K Bars, peach and apricots - per bar (23g)	88	17	1	0.5	0.1
Marmite Rice Cakes	391	77	2	3.5	2
Nakd Berry Delight Cereal Bar - per bar (35g)	135	18	5	2	trace
Nakd Cocia Delight Wholefood Cereal Bar - per bar (134	135	17	5	2	trace
Nature Valley Blackcurrant, Cherry and Raspberry Bar - per bar (30g)	112	24	1	1	trace
Nature Valley Trail Mix Bar, fruit and nut - per bar (30g)	118	19	3	2	trace
Nature Valley Trail Mix Bar, mixed berry - per bar (30g)	118	20	3	2	trace
Organix Multigrain Rice Cakes	388	80	3	4	trace
Penn State Original Pretzels	376	19	1	1	0.3

	CALORIES	FAT	FIBRE	CARBS	SODIUM
Penn State Sour Cream and Chive Pretzels	410	73	9	4	0.76
Twiglets, original	386	57.5	12	12	0.7
Tyrells Habas Fritas	526	52	29	13	0.1
Urban Fresh Foods Dried Black Cherry	287	76	0.2	8	trace
Weetabix Oaty Milk Chocolate Cereal Bar - per bar (23g)	79	12	1	6	trace
Weetabix Oaty Strawberry Cereal Bar - per bar (23g)	79	13	1.5	5	trace
Whitworth's Snacking Apricots	210	47	0.3	7	0.1
SOUPS					
Amy's Kitchen Low-Fat Lentil Soup	62	8	2	2.5	0.2
Amy's Kitchen Low-Fat Vegetable Barley Soup	27	5	0.4	1	0.3
Amy's Kitchen Split Pea Soup	44	8	0.1	1	0.3
Baxter's Chunky Carrot, Bean and Coriander Soup	53	10	0.6	2	0.24
Baxter's Chunky Smoked Bacon and Three Bean Soup	58	9	1	2	0.21
Baxter's Italian Bean and Pasta Soup	51	10	0.2	2	0.22
Baxter's Lentil and Bacon Soup	55	8	1	1	0.25
Baxter's Pea and Ham Soup	60	8	1	1	0.23
Geo Organics Chickpea and Lentil Soup	97	14	2	n/a	n/a
Heinz Big Soup Tomato and Butterbean	45	8	1	1	0.25
Heinz Classic Lentil Soup	46	8.5	0.2	1	0.5
Heinz Classic Vegetable Soup	45	8	1	1	0.3
Heinz Farmer's Market Three Bean and Red Pepper Soup	62	9	1.5	2	0.2
New Covent Garden Heart-Warming (tomato, vegetable and lentil) Soup	46	6	1	2	0.3
New Covent Garden Lentil and Bacon Soup	77	10	2	2.5	0.3
New Covent Garden Minestrone	34	5	1	1	0.4
New Covent Garden Moroccan Tagine Soup (with chickpeas and lentils)	53	8	1	2	0.4
New Covent Garden Souper Greens	39	3	2	1	0.3

	CALORIES	FAT	FIBRE	CARBS	SODIUM
Rakusen's Carrot and Lentil Soup	59	9	1	n/a	n/a
Suma Spicy Organic Lentil Soup	58	9	1	2	trace
Suma Tuscan Bean Soup	43	6	1	2	0.2

Index

Conversion Tables

The recipes that appear in this cookery book use metric measurements with imperial equivalents. All spoon measurements are level unless specified otherwise. The information in the following charts is provided to help cooks who prefer to measure both liquid and dry or solid ingredients by volume in cups. All equivalents are approximate.

Cup Equivalents for Different Types of Ingredients

A standard cup measure of a dry or solid ingredient will vary in weight depending on the type of ingredient. A standard cup of liquid is the same volume for any type of liquid. Use the following chart when converting grams (weight) or millilitres (volume) to standard cup measures.

Standard Cup	Fine Powder (e.g., flour)	Grain (e.g., rice)	Granular (e.g., sugar)	Liquid Solids (e.g., butter)	Liquid (e.g., milk)
1	125g	200g	225g	250g	240 ml
¾	90g	150g	175g	180g	240 ml
⅔	80g	125g	150g	160g	160 ml
½	50g	100g	100g	125g	120 ml
⅓	40g	75g	75g	80g	80 ml
¼	25g	50g	50g	60g	60 ml
⅛	15g	25g	25g	35g	30 ml

Useful Equivalents for Liquid Ingredients by Volume

¼ tsp					=		1 ml
½ tsp					=		2 ml
1 tsp					=		5 ml
3 tsp	=	1 Tbsp			=	½ fl oz =	15 ml
		2 Tbsp	=	⅛ cup	=	1 fl oz =	30 ml
		4 Tbsp	=	¼ cup	=	2 fl oz =	60 ml
		5⅓ Tbsp	=	⅓ cup	=	3 fl oz =	80 ml
		8 Tbsp	=	½ cup	=	4 fl oz =	120 ml
		10⅔ Tbsp	=	⅔ cup	=	5 fl oz =	160 ml
		12 Tbsp	=	¾ cup	=	6 fl oz =	180 ml
		16 Tbsp	=	1 cup	=	8 fl oz =	240 ml
		1 pt	=	2½ cups	=	1 pint =	480 ml
		1 qt	=	4 cups	=	1 ¾ pints =	1 litre

Useful Equivalents for Dry Ingredients by Weight

(To convert grams to ounces, divide the number of grams by 30.)

1 oz	=	¹⁄₁₆ lb	=	25g
4 oz	=	¼ lb	=	125g
8 oz	=	½ lb	=	250g
12 oz	=	¾ lb	=	350g
16 oz	=	1 lb	=	500g

Useful Equivalents for Length

(To convert centimetres to inches, divide the number of centimetres by 2.5.)

1 in				=	2.5 cm		
6 in	=	½ ft		=	15 cm		
12 in	=	1 ft		=	30 cm		
36 in	=	3 ft	= 1 yd	=	90 cm		
40 in				=	100 cm	=	1 m

Useful Equivalents for Cooking/Oven Temperatures

	Fahrenheit	Celsius	Gas Mark
Freeze water	32° F	0° C	
Room temperature	68°F	20°C	
Boil water	212°F	100°C	
Bake	325°F	160°C	3
	350°F	180°C	4
	375°F	190°C	5
	400°F	200°C	6
	425°F	220°C	7
	450°F	230°C	8

Recipe Index

INDEX

INDEX

INDEX

INDEX

Finally, a diet that really works!

Look for more great CarbLover's products to help you shed pounds – while eating your favourite foods!

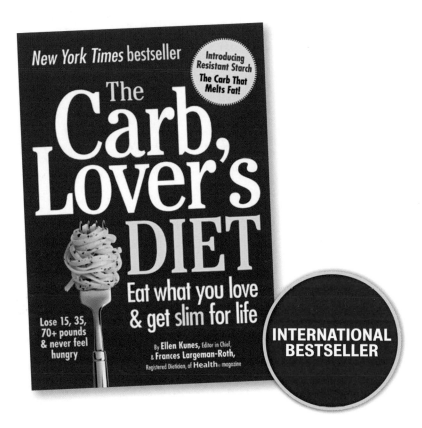

The CarbLover's Diet is the book that started a weight-loss revolution, inspiring thousands to drop all theweight they wanted without ever feeling hungry! Filled with hundreds of tips, expert advice, delicious recipes and real-life success stories, it's the diet book you'll turn to again and again.

Get Slim Now!
The CarbLover's Diet is available in all good bookshops.
Become a fan of CarbLovers on Facebook.
Follow @Carbloversdiet on Twitter.

Oxmoor House
VP, Publishing
Jim Childs

Editorial Director
Susan Payne Dobbs

Creative Director
Felicity Keane

Brand Manager
Vanessa Tiongson

Managing Editor
Laurie S. Herr

Project Editor
Holly D. Smith

Production Manager
Sue Chodakiewicz

Time Home Entertainment Inc.
Publisher
Richard Fraiman

VP, Strategy &
Business Development
Steven Sandonato

Executive Director,
Marketing Services
Carol Pittard

Executive Director,
Retail & Special Sales
Tom Mifsud

Executive Director,
New Product Development
Peter Harper

Director, Bookazine
Development & Marketing
Laura Adam

Publishing Director
Joy Butts

Finance Director
Glenn Buonocore

Assistant General Counsel
Helen Wan

Credits
Cover and main photography by **Andrew McCaul**
Food styling by **Stephana Bottom**
Prop styling by **Alistair Turnbull for Pat Bates**

p. 39, 45, 73, 75, 91, 99, 103, 107, 129, 133, 139, 153, 189, Melissa Punch

p. 143 Pasta shells, Con Poulos
p. 145 BBQ pizza, Kate Sears
p. 159 Sushi, Melissa Punch
p. 189 Chicken mole, Quentin Bacon
p. 147 Fusilli, Kate Sears
p. 231 Crostini, Joseph De Leo
p. 277 Rice pudding, Melissa Punch
p. 197 Barley, Quentin Bacon
p. 233 Polenta, Andrew McCaul
p. 148 Scoglio, Andrew McCaul
p. 153 Pizza, Andrew McCaul
p. 278 Cupcakes, Melissa Punch
p. 283 Cookies, Andrew McCaul

Cover: Pasta shells, page 143
Back Cover: (left to right), Oat and Honey Pancakes
with Strawberry Syrup, page 34; Bison Sliders, page 166;
Fresh Mozzarella, Basil and Chicken Sausage Pizza, page 137;
Mini Chocolate Cinnamon Molten Cakes, page 264